ROYAL HISTORICAL SOCIETY

STUDIES IN HISTORY

New Series

CHARITY AND THE LONDON HOSPITALS
1850–1898

T0355528

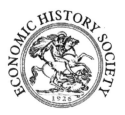

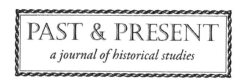

CHARITY AND THE LONDON
HOSPITALS
1850–1898

Keir Waddington

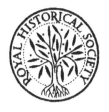

THE ROYAL HISTORICAL SOCIETY
THE BOYDELL PRESS

First published 2000
Paperback edition 2015

A Royal Historical Society publication
Published by The Boydell Press
an imprint of Boydell & Brewer Ltd
PO Box 9, Woodbridge, Suffolk IP12 3DF, UK
and of Boydell & Brewer Inc.
668 Mt Hope Avenue, Rochester, NY 14620–2731, USA
website: www.boydellandbrewer.com

ISBN 978 0 86193 246 7 hardback
ISBN 978 0 86193 331 0 paperback

ISSN 0269–2244

A CIP catalogue record for this book is available
from the British Library

This publication is printed on acid-free paper

Contents

List of Figures

List of Tables

TO BARRY, GILL AND GEMMA

Publication of this volume was aided by a generous grant
from the Scouloudi Foundation, in association with the
Institute of Historical Research.

Acknowledgements

This book started as an MA dissertation on charity in Victorian London and developed from there into the thesis on nineteenth-century metropolitan hospitals upon which this book is based. Much of the original work was inspired by debates in the early 1990s about the structure of healthcare in London, and in particular by the King's Fund Report and the Tomlinson Report on hospital provision. Along the way more and more medical history has crept in.

Throughout the process of researching and writing both thesis and book I have had the support of many to whom it is hard to express enough acknowledgement and gratitude. I have been left with a large debt to all those who have freely given their help and encouragement along the way. My main debt is to Martin Daunton who saved me from working on social control and introduced me to the social history of medicine. His unerring questioning, patience, guidance and support helped guide my research and his faith in my work encouraged me to publish. The same needs to be said of Anne Hardy who provided a critical eye on the medical side and has faithfully read and commented on everything that I have produced. Colin Jones, as advisory editor for the Royal Historical Society, has provided too many useful comments to mention and has proved patient throughout especially when the manuscript did not arrive when it was supposed to. Special thanks is also due to Abigail Beach, Bill Bynum, Roy Church, Joanne Edwards, Caroline Overy, Elsbeth Heaman, Negley Harte, Michelle Morgan, Frank Prochaska, Roy Porter, Harish Rao and Richard Weight and those at the Centre for Medical and Dental Education, St Bartholomew's, for all their suggestions and support, for their time and help. Much appreciation also goes to John Beckerson, Amanda Berry, Steven Cherry, Anne Crowther, Bronwyn Croxson, Anne Digby, Patricia Garside, Martin Gorsky, Paul Johnson, Graham Mooney, Patrick O'Brien, Sally Sheard and Jeremy Taylor for their advice. A special debt is owed to Mark Allinson and Michelle Elvin whose invaluable comments were so important to me while I was writing my thesis. In the writing of the final drafts of the book the support offered by Jennifer Haynes and her unqualified encouragement has been invaluable.

This book would not have been possible without the willing help, assistance and kindness shown to me by the archivists and librarians who have helped me along the way. In particular I wish to thank the archivists at the many institutions at which I have studied: Gillian Furlong at University College; Andrew Griffen, Caroline Jones, Marion Rae and Sally Thompson at St Bartholomew's; Nicholas Baldwin at Great Ormond Street; Jonathan Evans at the Royal London. I am also grateful to the staff of the London Metropolitan Archive for their support during the many months I spent in their reading room, and to those at the British Library, the Public Record Office, the Bodleian Library, University College Library and the Guildhall Library for their valuable help. A debt is owed to Sue Gold and Kaye Bagshaw and the staff of the library at the Wellcome Institute for the History of Medicine for their encouragement, support, enthusiasm and help. Without them I am sure I would not have found half the information I have.

Finally I wish to acknowledge the support of the British Academy, the Institute of Historical Research and the Royal Historical Society, whose funding made my research possible. Any mistakes are of course my own.

Keir Waddington
May 1999

Abbreviations

BHM	*Bulletin of the History of Medicine*
BMA	British Medical Association
BMJ	*British Medical Journal*
COS	Charitable Organisation Society
EcHR	*Economic History Review*
FWA	Family Welfare Association
GOSH	Great Ormond Street Hospital Archive
LCC	London County Council
LGB	Local Government Board
LH	Royal London Hospital Archive and Museum
LMA	London Metropolitan Archive
MAB	Metropolitan Asylums Board
NHS	National Health Service
PP	Parliamentary papers
RCH	Royal Hospital for Diseases of the Chest
SBH	St Bartholomew's Hospital Archive
SC	Select Committee
SHM	*Social History of Medicine*
SSA	Social Science Association
UCH	University College Hospital
UCL	University College London Archive

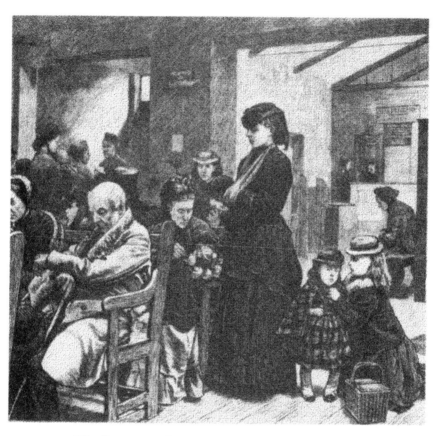

The Outpatients Room in University College Hospital

1

Introduction:
Philanthropy and the London Hospitals

The publication of the Turnberg Report in 1998, the twenty-first inquiry into London's health services during the twentieth century, ended the period of uncertainty following the 1992 Tomlinson Report.[1] The report's proposals partly reversed the recommendations made by Tomlinson and followed a promise of £140m. extra for the National Health Service. After five years of reform, Turnberg called for 'a more coherent approach to London's health needs than the mere arbitrary cost-cutting' of previous governments.[2] The report was not universally welcomed, but it was greeted with more enthusiasm than its predecessor, which had sent a wave of panic through London's hospitals already anxious about the future after NHS reforms had introduced the internal market.[3] In questioning the pattern of development, organisation of finance and nature of healthcare in London, Tomlinson had renewed public interest in the funding of London's hospitals. In such a climate, finance and the role of the state became central to any discussion of the NHS.

One hundred years before the Tomlinson Report had shaken hospital administrators similar concerns were being expressed when the Select Committee of the House of Lords on Metropolitan Hospitals delivered its final report. To what extent London's hospitals were adequately financed had long interested Victorian hospital reformers, medical profession and public, who were under constant pressure to contribute. By the 1890s many felt that the situation had become intolerable. An apparent endemic financial crisis, which had been building up since the 1860s, was seen to be facing London's voluntary hospitals and the need for investigation both as a palliative and as a solution was believed necessary. Unlike its twentieth-century counterparts, the select committee defended the existing system and concluded that state interference was incompatible with the principles of voluntarism that under-

---

1 *Evening Standard*, 3 Feb. 1998, 7; Bernard Tomlinson, *Report of the inquiry into London's health service, medical education and research*, London 1992.
2 *Evening Standard*, 3 Feb. 1998, 11.
3 For NHS reforms and the development of the internal market see Julian Le Grand, David Winter and Francis Woolley, 'The National Health Service: safe in whose hands?', in John Hills (ed.), *The state of welfare: the welfare state in Britain since 1974*, Oxford 1990, 88–134.

pinned London's hospital.[4] Only those on the margins of reform suggested that the state should intervene. With the foundation of the Prince of Wales Hospital Fund for London in 1897 and the surge of philanthropy that surrounded Queen Victoria's diamond jubilee, contemporaries felt that London's hospitals had once more been saved by charity. It was not until the 1920s that the state was finally forced to intervene.

Whereas the 1890–2 select committee vacillated, weakly recommending a modicum of central supervision and relocation, its twentieth-century counterparts questioned a pattern of development that had its origins in the Victorian London hospital system. The ethos that hospitals functioned to assist 'suitable cases for charity' had already been undermined before 1948, but the institutional legacy of the nineteenth century continued to confront health reformers. Resemblances to the Victorian medical market did not stop there. Thatcherite economics encouraged the renewed growth of private healthcare, if not a return to the principle of less eligibility enshrined in the 1834 Poor Law. In the mid-1990s the state started to devolve its statutory obligations and hospitals were encouraged to opt out of regional control to establish self-governing trusts. If this was not the 'subscriber democracy' of the nineteenth century, the trusts did make claims to an independent management of resources. When searching in 1975 for new sources of funding for the health service, the Resources Allocation Working Party turned to charity to 'bail out a debilitated health service'.[5] In 1987/8 charitable resources within the NHS produced an annual income of £130m. from rents and dividends. Non-NHS charities contributed a further £200m. and voluntary effort alone saved the NHS £24,000m. These contributions were not unusual. They can be seen as part of an on-going process within which the boundaries between voluntarism and the state have been constantly shifting.[6]

Parallels between debates on the structure and finance of healthcare in the nineteenth and twentieth centuries, and the on-going argument over the funding of London's hospitals underlie the writing of this book. This in not to claim that the concerns of the present have been projected back to explain the past. The need for late twentieth-century hospitals to appeal to charity is but a poor reflection of the central role philanthropy played in the construction of the Victorian hospital system. Contemporary debates do raise, however, important questions about how London's hospitals were funded and run in the nineteenth century, and about the discussions that surrounded their finance and organisation. It is these concerns that are the starting point for this book. As part of a growing interest in the economic history of medicine,

---

[4] *Select Committee of the House of Lords on Metropolitan Hospitals, Third Report*, PP 1892 xiii.

[5] Frank K. Prochaska, *Philanthropy and the hospitals of London: the King's Fund, 1897–1990*, Oxford 1992, 229.

[6] L. Fitzherbert, *Charity and the National Health Service*, London 1989, 11–17; Martin Daunton, 'Payment and participation: welfare and state formation in Britain, 1900–51', *Past and Present* cl (1996), 169–70.

it can be located within a new body of work by Steven Cherry and others that has started to see a more complex system of hospital finance and connections between patronage, management, patients and funding than earlier, less critical studies of hospitals have revealed.[7] It seeks to go beyond the study of great men and women, medical advances and medical education, that have characterised old-style hospital histories, where patients are often second to royal occasions or new buildings, to look at how London's hospitals were financed and administered in the nineteenth century.[8]

Hospitals and charity, 1850–98

In a society wedded to a voluntary ethic and where hospital administrators were constantly worried about fundraising, studying hospitals in London in the years between 1850 and 1898 reveals the inter-relationship between the metropolitan benevolent economy, hospital finance, hospital governors and medical authority in an institution that was undergoing a process of medicalisation and change. In doing so, it challenges the assumption that 'from the establishment of the great London hospitals in the eighteenth century charitable donations formed the economic base' of free medical care. Financial crisis was not simply a symptom of managerial inefficiency or a failure to attract philanthropy, but was rooted in the nature of what might loosely be called the 'benevolent economy' – those charitable resources available to voluntary institutions – and in the pressures exerted on London's hospitals.[9] The voluntary ethic that characterised hospital development was more than just a system of funding however. It effectively limited medical authority at a time when doctors were trying to extend their formal influence over the

7   See Anne Digby, *Making a medical living: doctors and patients in the English market for medicine, 1720–1911*, Cambridge 1994; Steven Cherry, 'Beyond national health insurance: the voluntary hospitals and the hospital contributory schemes', SHM v (1992), 455–82, and 'Before the National Health Service: financing the voluntary hospitals', EcHR c (1997), 305–26; Keir Waddington, ' "Bastard benevolence": centralisation, voluntarism and the Sunday Fund, 1873–1898', *London Journal* ix (1995), 151–67, and ' "Grasping gratitude": hospitals and charity in late Victorian London', in Martin Daunton (ed.), *Charity, self-interest and welfare in the English past*, London 1996, 181–202; Anne Borsay, 'Cash and conscience: financing the General Hospital at Bath, c. 1738–50', SHM iv (1991), 207–29; Amanda Berry, 'Charity, patronage and medical men: philanthropy and provincial hospitals', unpubl. DPhil diss. Oxford 1995; Martin Gorsky, 'Philanthropy in Bristol, 1800–50', unpubl. PhD diss. Bristol 1995.
8   For a discussion of hospital historiography see Lindsay Granshaw, 'Introduction', in Lindsay Granshaw and Roy Porter (eds), *The hospital in history*, London 1989, 1–17.
9   Jeanne L. Brand, *Doctors and the state: the British medical profession and government action in public health, 1870–1912*, Baltimore 1965, 192; N. Evans, ' "The first charity in Wales": Cardiff Infirmary and South Wales society, 1837–1914', *Welsh History Review* ix (1978/9), 332.

hospital's management. The result was conflict, rather than a harmonious assertion of doctors' authority, and this raises questions about how historians and sociologists have characterised the professionalisation of medicine during the nineteenth century.[10] London's hospitals, as I hope to show, are neither monolithic institutions, open to an easy analysis, nor simply the sites for medical advances or social control.

To look at one or two hospitals in London would not be enough. I have therefore examined seven – St Bartholomew's, Guy's, the London, University College Hospital, the German, the Royal Hospital for Diseases of the Chest and the Hospital for Sick Children. Each is indicative of the experiences of a particular type of Victorian hospital. St Bartholomew's and Guy's represent the varying fortunes of the endowed hospitals, while the London was an early eighteenth-century voluntary hospital. University College Hospital was the epitome of a nineteenth-century teaching hospital; the German was one of the few hospitals that sought to provide medical care for a particular immigrant group. The Royal Hospital for Diseases of the Chest and the Hospital for Sick Children represented the two types of specialist hospital, the former treating one category of disease, the latter a particular group of patients.[11] Additional material on other London and provincial hospitals has been drawn from contemporary and secondary sources to produce a comparative account of how hospitals were financed and administered between 1850 and 1898.

It was during this period that the Metropolitan Hospital Sunday Fund and Saturday Fund were founded and hospitals experienced a need to diversify their income in a situation where 'income barely keeps pace with the unavoidable expenditure'.[12] It witnessed not only the development of more scientific practices, forcing hospitals to conform to different standards, but also saw the expansion of the medical profession and a change in social attitudes towards medicine. Under these conditions hospitals were increasingly seen as a viable location for medical relief, even if there was not the sudden

---

[10] For the sociological discussion of the professionalisation see Eliot Freidson, *Professional powers: a study of the institutionalisation of formal knowledge*, London 1986, and T. J. Johnson, *Professions and power*, London 1972. These ideas have been used by historians such as M. Jeanne Peterson, *The medical profession in mid Victorian London*, Berkeley 1978; Irvine Loudon, *Medical care and the general practitioner, 1750–1850*, Oxford 1986; and Ivan Waddington, *The medical profession in the industrial revolution*, Dublin 1984, to help interpret the changes in the medical profession during the late eighteenth and early nineteenth century.

[11] For histories of these institutions see Victor C. Medvei and John L. Thornton, *The royal hospital of Saint Bartholomew's, 1123–1973*, London 1974; H. C. Cameron, *Mr Guy's Hospital, 1726–1948*, London 1954; A. E. Clark-Kennedy, *The London: a study in the voluntary hospital system*, ii, London 1963; W. R. Merrington, *University College Hospital and its medical school*, London 1976; C. McKellar, *The German Hospital, Hackney: a social and architectural history*, London 1991, and Jules Kosky, *Mutual friends: Charles Dickens and Great Ormond Street Children's Hospital*, London 1989.

[12] RCH, annual report 1850, LMA.

influx of middle-class patients that contemporaries feared.[13] With the foundation of the Prince of Wales Hospital Fund in 1897 a new era in active philanthropic control was ushered in, partly in response to fears over state intervention. It used grants to influence policy and organisation in order to provide the element of co-ordination that the select committee had recommended.[14] At the same time, London's hospitals were moving towards closer co-operation with the creation of the Central Hospital Council in which the major hospitals joined to discuss matters of mutual interest.

Voluntarism and the rise of the modern hospital

To understand how Victorian London hospitals worked it is necessary to look at their development and the voluntary system that underpinned them. Health took many forms in the nineteenth century. In its name 'Victorians flocked to the seaside, tramped about the Alps or Cotswolds, dieted, took pills, sweated themselves in Turkish baths, adopted this "system of medicine" or that' and attended hospitals in ever increasing numbers. The public health movement was a further manifestation of this anxiety that became a crusade for some, while for others it raised questions about the role of the state.[15] Concerns about sickness, healthcare, sanitation and preventive medicine were not merely an irrational or hypochondriac preoccupation in an age when few people could enjoy good health and no family, no matter what their social status, seemed safe from illness.

This consumer, cultural and political preoccupation with health helps explain why, during the nineteenth century, medical charity was able to thrive in a highly stratified market for medicine. The fact that a large proportion of healthcare for the sick and ill-defined 'deserving' poor took on a philanthropic dimension was a reflection of how Victorians defined their approach to social problems. The late eighteenth century, according to the historian Donna Andrew, had seen a change in the nature of benevolence with a shift away from posthumous bequests to a more active form of charity through voluntary organisations as an agent of 'national regeneration'.[16] In a society weaned on a voluntary ethos, philanthropy was seen as the main vehicle through which the problems generated by industrialisation and rapid

---

13 See Keir Waddington, ' "Unsuitable cases": the debate over out-patient admissions, the medical profession and late Victorian London hospitals', *Medical History* xlii (1998), 26–46.
14 Prochaska, *Philanthropy and the hospitals of London*.
15 Bruce Haley, *The healthy body and the Victorian culture*, Cambridge, Mass. 1978, 3. See also Christopher Hamlin, 'State medicine in Great Britain', in Dorothy Porter (ed.), *The history of public health and the modern state*, Amsterdam 1994, 132–64; Anne Hardy, *Epidemic streets: infectious disease and the rise of preventive medicine, 1856–1900*, Oxford 1993; Anthony S. Wohl, *Endangered lives: public health in Victorian Britain*, London 1983.
16 Donna T. Andrew, *Philanthropy and police: London charity in the eighteenth century*, Princeton 1989.

urbanisation could be relieved. Structural faults in society and the economy were rarely acknowledged and faith was placed in the curative value of self-help and charity, even after Charles Booth's social surveys of London in the 1890s hinted at philanthropy's inadequacies. At the same time as providing relief, such associational charity assisted and encouraged bourgeois integration. It offered a means towards establishing a consensus within the middle classes and between classes against the 'undeserving' poor.[17] Though this had started to weaken by the end of the nineteenth century, the proliferation of voluntary agencies it produced allied itself with the assumption that the state should play a minimal role, leaving philanthropy in co-operation with local government to 'superintend most moral, charitable, education and welfare services'.[18] If the reality of government action did not match this ideal, charity was a central element in what might be termed the Victorian 'welfare' state. There was scarcely 'a form of human want or wretchedness for which a special and appropriate provision [had] not been made'.[19] Charity was a source of national pride and new ways were devised to encourage the largely middle-class benevolent public to give. In financial terms the amount contributed by 1885 was greater than the budgets of many European states; by 1910 £2m. was being given in London alone.[20]

Medical charity was an important element in this multi-million benevolent economy and London's voluntary hospitals were the most dynamic part.[21] Integral to civil society, hospitals provided an institutional intermediary between the charitable and the recipients of relief. Though the nineteenth century saw a dramatic change in the nature of hospitals, they had a long and varied history that confirmed their philanthropic credentials. The first authentic hospital in Britain was established at York in 947, but it was not until Rahere's foundation of St Bartholomew's Hospital and Priory in 1123 that an institution was created specifically as a hospital and not as a hostel for travellers and pilgrims.[22] The number of hospitals increased in the

---

[17] Robert J. Morris, *Class, sect and party: the making of the British middle class, Leeds 1820–50*, Manchester 1990; Brian Harrison, *Peaceable kingdom: stability and change in modern Britain*, Oxford 1982; Frank K. Prochaska, *The voluntary impulse: philanthropy in modern Britain*, London 1988.

[18] Pat Thane, 'Government and society in England and Wales 1750–1914', in F. M. L. Thompson (ed.), *The Cambridge social history of Britain, 1750–1950*, III: *Social agencies and institutions*, Cambridge 1990, 33.

[19] Charles S. Loch, 'Charity: noxious and beneficent', *Westminster Review and Foreign Quarterly Review* iii (1853), 65.

[20] Cited in David E. Owen, *English philanthropy, 1660–1960*, Cambridge, Mass. 1964, 469; Charles S. Loch, *Charity and social life: a study of religious and social thought in relation to charitable methods and institutions*, London 1910, 487–8.

[21] For a discussion of medicine and charity see Jonathan Barry and Colin Jones (eds), *Medicine and charity before the welfare state*, London 1994; W. F. Bynum, 'Medical philanthropy after 1850', in W. F. Bynum and Roy Porter (eds), *Companion encyclopedia of the history of medicine*, ii, London 1997, 1480–94.

[22] John Woodward, *To do the sick no harm: a study of the British voluntary hospital system to 1875*, London 1974, 1.

thirteenth and fourteenth centuries in parallel with the growth of towns and trade. Early institutions like St Bartholomew's and St Thomas's (founded between 1106 and 1212) were not simply monastic preserves or necessarily committed to the care of the sick. They served a significant social role for benefactors and urban society alike.[23] At first such hospitals offered little more than rest, good diet and spiritual comfort rather than medical care in an institution where medically-minded clerics and the pious outnumbered lay medical practitioners.[24] By the time of the Henrican Reformation cure had started to replace care, but traditions and the social importance of hospitals were maintained, encouraging the development of a voluntary ideology that continued to shape hospital development.[25]

It was in the eighteenth century, with the foundation of the Westminster Hospital in 1719, that a new phase of development extended the relief provided by the five surviving medieval hospitals. The Westminster set the pattern for others to follow, resulting in a hospital boom in London that was more than an attempt to absorb excess charity created by a growing metropolitan economy. General hospitals in London were the first to be established, followed by similar institutions in provincial cities, and then by specialist hospitals in London, such as the London Lock Hospital in 1746. Founded by small groups within the social elite or by doctors working with them (as in the case of the London Hospital in 1740), these new hospitals were expressions of Andrew's associational organisations of 'national regeneration' and acted to unify or represent political or religious groups. They built on philanthropic principles encouraged by Enlightenment ideas and were not just expressions of a conspicuous and self-congratulatory benevolence.[26] Not every institution was welcomed or proved uncontroversial. Thomas Guy's endowment of Guy's Hospital in 1724 using the gains he had made from his dealings in the South Sea Bubble was not well received. Drawing inspiration from St Thomas's, where Guy had been a governor, his bequest was made just when posthumous charity was moving out of fashion.[27] Though Guy's Hospital dovetailed neatly into the institutional expansion of

23 Lindsay Granshaw, 'The hospital', in Bynum and Porter, *Companion encyclopedia*, ii. 1182.
24 Carole Rawcliffe, 'Hospitals of later medieval London', *Medical History* xxviii (1984), 1–3; Martha Carlin, 'Medieval English hospitals', in Granshaw and Porter, *The hospital in history*, 21–39; Miri Rubin, 'Development and change in English hospitals, 1100–1500', ibid. 41–59.
25 Paul Slack, 'Social policy and the constraints of government, 1547–58', in Jennifer Loach and Robert Tittler (eds), *The mid-Tudor polity, c. 1540–60*, London 1980, 110–14.
26 Roy Porter, 'The gift relationship: philanthropy and provincial hospitals in eighteenth-century England', in Granshaw and Porter, *The hospital in history*, 49–78; Charles Webster, 'The crisis of the hospital during the industrial revolution', in E. G. Forbes (ed.), *Human implications of scientific advance*, Edinburgh 1978, 214–15.
27 *Thirty-Second Report of the Charity Commission*, PP 1840 xxxii. 711.

the period, the large endowment ensured that it had more in common with surviving medieval hospitals.

The Westminster, the London and the other new voluntary hospitals were characteristic of eighteenth-century benevolence at a time when debate started to focus on the proper mix between the role of the state and the duties of the benevolent. Collecting charities rather than endowed medieval institutions like St Bartholomew's, they set the pattern for other voluntary organisations. Designed solely for the 'deserving' poor they represented a 'medico-charitable space' in which doctors were able to exert more authority over their patients and all those who gave could nominate suitable objects for care and also participate in the hospital's management.[28] Access to facilities was not a right. Voluntary hospitals were a hybrid that not only borrowed their management style and restricted definition of the sick poor from the medieval endowed hospitals, but also had a marked influence on later foundations. At the centre of these new institutions was a hierarchy of subscribers who supervised the running of the hospital, appointed the staff, admitted the patients and shaped how the institution was financed. Doctors, whose training and practice had lost part of its guild status and were more under the influence of free market forces, had a marginal administrative role that reflected economic and social constraints on Enlightenment practitioners. The small size of these early hospitals, which were to grow into the large general hospitals of the nineteenth century, was initially an advantage. They required a few hundred supporters and limited management to a group of active but wealthy men, leading others to found similar institutions.[29]

In institutional terms there was no significant disjunction between the eighteenth and nineteenth century. Building on the Hanoverian voluntary hospital 'movement', similar institutions were founded, encouraged by a new anatomico-clinical approach to medicine and professional demands. Urbanisation and the consequent extent of disease and ill-health in the nineteenth century pressurised the Victorians into further institutionalising medical services. New hospitals were relatively easy to establish and reflected Britain's entrepreneurial nature, but evolution was haphazard and erratic, responding to concerns over the high mortality and low morality of the poor.[30] Humanity, self-interest, religion and the pursuit of social status made common cause to help those deemed unable to meet the cost of private medical care.

London was at the centre of these developments. The particular qualities of the Victorian metropolis captivated contemporaries. To Dickens, Disraeli

[28] Adrian Wilson, 'Politics of medical improvement in early Hanoverian London', in Andrew Cunningham and Roger French (eds), *The medical enlightenment of the eighteenth century*, Cambridge 1990, 15.
[29] Ibid. 12–13.
[30] Lindsay Granshaw, 'The rise of the modern hospital in Britain', in Andrew Wear (ed.), *Medicine in society: historical essays*, Cambridge 1994, 205–6.

and Tennyson it was a city like no other; Bagehot equated London with a newspaper: everything was there and nothing was connected to anything else.[31] The author of *Suffering London* felt that London was the 'pale spectre', an 'agglomeration of energy [that] should present a panorama of life and activity intense enough to strike the minds of strangers with awe and admiration'.[32] London defied precise definition and had a village-like character ensuring that the Victorian Londoner remained 'long diffident about his metropolitan identity'. With a high degree of localism it was a city of contradictions that was kept together by the 'irrigations of commercial capital'.[33] According to the historian Patricia Garside it was 'central yet peripheral, economically secondary yet socially dominant, culturally inspirational yet parasitic'.[34] No other city in Victorian Britain offered such a diversity of medical services in a single urban context. London's social, political and medical importance helped fuel the development of new hospitals and the growth of existing ones. They were underwritten by an expanding middle class that was a result of an economy biased towards consumer-oriented enterprises largely organised in small workshops, the service sector and specialist financial and banking activities centred on the City from which it led the domestic and international money markets. Just as London increased in size from a population of half a million in the early eighteenth century to five million in 1900, so too did the number and size of its hospitals. In 1809 London could boast seven general hospitals, four lying-in and two for infectious diseases.[35] By 1890 provision had expanded to include twenty-one general hospitals, eleven with medical schools, and sixty-seven specialist hospitals. Concentration was greater in north London, for ten of the fifteen largest hospitals, with three-quarters of the beds, were within one mile of the Charing Cross.[36]

For all this, and the public attention they attracted, hospitals were not the main providers of healthcare in London. In an effort to keep deaths in the hospital to a minimum, governors tried to avoid admitting the chronic sick or the incurable, leaving the state (through the poor law) to care for these patients.[37] The workhouse infirmaries existed side-by-side with hospitals and

---

31 Cited in Patrica Garside, 'London and the home counties', in F. M. L. Thompson (ed.), *The Cambridge social history of Britain 1750–1950*, I: *Regions and communities*, Cambridge 1990, 489.

32 A. E. Hake, *Suffering London*, London 1892, 3.

33 John Davis, *Reforming London: the London government problem, 1855–1900*, Oxford 1988, 5; H. J. Dyos and D. A. Reeder, 'Slums and suburbs', in H. J. Dyos and M. Wolff (eds), *The Victorian city*, i, London 1973, 359.

34 Garside, 'London and the home counties', 490.

35 Geoffrey Rivett, *The development of the London hospital system, 1832–1982*, Oxford 1986, 25.

36 *Select Committee of the House of Lords on Metropolitan Hospitals etc.*, First Report, PP 1890 xvi. 3–4.

37 For the restrictions placed on early nineteenth-century hospital admissions see Woodward, *To do the sick no harm*.

a myriad of provident and free dispensaries and the friendly societies; between them were the numerous private practices from the fashionable Harley Street to the warrens of St Giles. It was not until the establishment of the Metropolitan Asylums Board in 1867 that any systematic effort was made to provide public institutions for the sick.[38]

The nineteenth century not only saw an expansion in the number of hospitals but also in the number of hospital types. St Bartholomew's, St Thomas's and Guy's, as endowed hospitals, continued to flourish at least until the onset of the agricultural depression in the 1870s when the fact that land was the major source of income for Guy's and St Thomas's resulted in a sharp fall in funding. St Bartholomew's was more fortunate. With its income derived primarily from metropolitan property, which was immune from the effects of the agricultural depression, it was regarded as the premier endowed hospital, 'one of the richest, most reputed and oldest hospitals in England'.[39] Until the First World War it had no need to appeal to the benevolent public for support, but this did not place it in the vanguard of development. Like many other endowed institutions, its management was attacked as corrupt and inefficient.[40]

The type of care these medieval hospitals had offered was mirrored in the nineteenth century by those hospitals established for immigrant groups like the French and the Italian hospitals. Founded by wealthy or naturalised immigrants for the benefit of London's alien communities, these institutions offered relief and medical care within an environment where immigrants' religious, cultural and linguistic differences were catered for. Whereas the French and Italian hospitals were more like hospices than medical institutions, the German Hospital was not run as a mission but as a voluntary hospital. Founded in Dalston in 1845 with support from the king of Prussia and the British royal family, the German modelled itself on its English counterparts.[41] Charity was solicited from the German community in London and from the German states, but the governors also encouraged local contributions and admitted English patients as out-patients and, in exceptional case, as in-patients. From the start, the hospital's ethnic base was an asset.

A shift in emphasis to clinical study in medical education and pressure from the Royal College of Surgeons and 1815 Apothecaries Act undermined training in private medical schools, promoting a shift in education into hospitals. From the 1800s onwards hospital schools emerged, either attached to existing general hospitals like the London, or to the new teaching hospi-

[38] Ruth G. Hodgkinson, *The origins of the National Health Service: the medical services of the new poor law, 1834–71*, London 1967, 620–80.
[39] *SC on Metropolitan Hospitals, First Report*, 171.
[40] St Bartholomew's, general account books, SBH, Hb 23/3–4. In 1869 *The Lancet* launched an attack on the hospital which ran throughout the year that described St Bartholomew's as a 'closed corporation': *Lancet* ii (1869), 615.
[41] German Hospital, annual report 1850, SBH.

tals like King's College Hospital and Charing Cross Hospital that had been founded to provided charitable healthcare within an educational framework. Of these University College Hospital was archetype. Located in one of London's most fashionable and medically overcrowded districts, the hospital opened in 1834 to provide clinical experience and training as an ancillary to a university medical education. University College Hospital's educational role conflicted with available resources from the start, which is why it was all too often in debt and survived on erratic legacies and deficit financing. Although other teaching hospitals did not suffer to the same degree as University College, the same pressures worked against their financial stability.

The boundaries between endowed, ethnic, voluntary and teaching hospitals were often blurred but none proved as controversial as the specialist hospitals. These evolved in response to demands for care and medical specialisation, but unlike their eighteenth-century prototypes, they were also a result of professional monopoly in the large general hospitals. Enterprising medical men, excluded from profitable posts in existing institutions by the corrupt system of internal appointments, took the initiative and founded specialist hospitals with the help of London's philanthropic community. Modelled on the Royal Ophthalmic Hospital, Moorfields, founded in 1794, many of these new institutions were not established on a firm basis and often closed after their founder lost interest or moved on. Others quickly won a place in the hearts of the subscribing public. The Hospital for Sick Children combined specialism in patient type with general treatment. Inspired by Dr Charles West and Dr Henry Bence Jones, the hospital opened in Great Ormond Street in 1852 and quickly became popular with subscribers. The inspiration behind the hospital, which owed much to West, and its specialist nature, gave the medical staff a more influential position than their contemporaries in other hospitals, but internal conflict could not be avoided as governors' interests clashed with doctors keen to extend or defend their authority. Whereas the Hospital for Sick Children limited its care to one group of patients, the Royal Hospital for Diseases of the Chest, like many other specialist hospitals, treated one category of disease. Established as the Infirmary for Asthma, Consumption and Other Diseases of the Chest in 1814 by Dr Isaac Buxton, the hospital started admitting in-patients in 1850. Like doctors at the Hospital for Sick Children, the medical staff played a direct role in the hospital's management and likewise came into conflict with the governors. Contemporaries accused such doctors of Machiavellianism, but specialist hospitals allowed those on the edge of the medical world to advance their careers through an institutional appointment.[42] Popular with the

---

[42] Lindsay Granshaw, *St Mark's Hospital, London: a social history of a specialist hospital*, London 1985, and ' "Fame and fortune by means of bricks and mortar": the medical profession and specialist hospitals in Britain, 1800–1948', in Granshaw and Porter, *The hospital in history*, 199–220.

subscribing public, they gradually became an accepted part of London's hospital system and important for the medical elite. General hospitals leisurely established specialist departments and acquired their own specialist reputations. In this teaching hospitals, forced to adapt faster than other institutions because of their educational remit, often led the way. At Guy's an effort was made to treat more ophthalmic patients in an effort to lower the hospital's high mortality rates, while the Middlesex acquired a reputation for cancer treatment.

From the 1850s onwards, the hospitals' medical and administrative functions began to develop beyond the simple institutional arrangements needed to dispense relief to the sick poor. Gradually they moved away from their clerical and philanthropic roots into the mainstream of medicine. For the historian Charles Rosenberg this required a change in orientation as both governors and medical staff came to view themselves as providers of medical treatment, not as moral or social reformers.[43] The charitable relationship between the hospital, its governors, doctors and patients evolved into a complex set of service relationships that increasingly underwent managerial subdivision and bureaucratisation.[44] Subscriber recommendation of patients began to break down as doctors played a greater part in selecting patients for admission. In the process, hospitals were transformed from 'places which healthy people should avoid and the sick should shun' to expensive institutions for the treatment of illness that posed new financial problems which could not be met by traditional patterns of philanthropy alone. Anaesthetics, antiseptics, scientific medicine, X-rays, bacteriology and nursing all helped alter the public's low opinion of the hospital.[45]

The changes outlined above had an impact on the medical profession's relationship with the hospital. Increasingly it was incorporated in the professional career structure of London's medical elite. Hospitals became places where reputations were made and profitable practices were established; a necessary arena for practice, research and medical education. In a financially insecure and status-conscious profession, where fears of competition and overstocking were paramount, hospital posts came to represent status, security and, indirectly, income. At the same time as promoting professionalisation, they engendered new splits in the profession between general

---

[43] Charles E. Rosenberg, *The care of strangers*, New York 1987.

[44] B. Craig, 'A survey and study of hospital records and record keeping in London (England) and Ontario (Canada), c. 1850–1950', unpubl. PhD diss. London 1988.

[45] For a more extensive treatment of the advances in medical practice see chapter 6, though A. Youngson, *The scientific revolution in Victorian medicine*, London 1979, and Christopher Lawrence (ed.), *Medical theory, surgical practice*, London 1992, provide a conflict-based analysis of medical advance. Brian Abel-Smith, *A history of the nursing profession*, London 1960, and Monica E. Baly, *Nursing and social change*, London 1982, offer general surveys of nursing and Carole Helmstadter, 'Robert Bentley Todd, Saint John's House, and the origins of the modern trained nurse', *BHM* lxvii (1993), 282–319, studies the influence of the nursing sisterhoods on the development of nursing.

practitioners and the new group of elite hospital consultants, and became centres for conflict between doctors and lay governors.[46] Only gradually were doctors able to extend their medical authority over the running of London's hospitals. Control over how money was raised took longer to establish. During the nineteenth century, in a social climate in which voluntarism was revered, it was the governors who dominated.

Contemporary attitudes lagged behind institutional and medical development although, by the end of the nineteenth century, contemporaries no longer saw hospitals as 'gateways to death'.[47] Philanthropists, unlike patients, however, had always viewed hospitals with pride. One Edwardian commentator explained in 1908 that hospitals were 'still beyond a doubt the most popular of our private charities'.[48] For one hospital reformer it was London's hospitals 'not our bridges, or railways or telephones' that were 'the real glory and abiding distinction of our civilisation'.[49]

Slowly, hospitals overcame their institutional inertia and adjusted to changing demands to become the accepted work place for doctors and a solution to the demands for institutionalised care removed from treatment within the family. Change was not without a price. As hospitals became more complex, bureaucratic and medical after 1850, pressure was exerted on existing financial resources. Medicalisation and an increase in patient numbers had inevitable financial consequences, forcing expenditure to rise and straining hospitals' benevolent resources. At the Royal Hospital for Diseases of the Chest this led the governors to make strenuous efforts to restrict expenditure and pursue aggressive fundraising techniques. The London Hospital, the largest medical institution in the capital with 790 beds by 1877, faced particular problems. Its size and the predominance of accident cases after 1872, created administrative and financial difficulties that no other hospital in London experienced. Income lagged behind expenditure and in 1896 Sydney Holland, the hospital's chairman and the 'prince of beggars', described the London's financial position as 'depressing', though in the previous year it had an income of £61,916.[50] London's hospitals were forced to move away economically from their philanthropic base, develop new ways of raising money and diversify their income. It was this process, rather than charity, that dominated their finances during the nineteenth century.

46 Digby, *Making a medical living*; Peterson, *The medical profession in mid Victorian London*; Waddington, *The medical profession in the Industrial Revolution*.

47 Woodward, *To do the sick no harm*, 124–46.

48 B. Kirkman Gray, *Philanthropy and the state, or social politics*, London 1908, 222.

49 Henry Burdett, *Hospitals and charities annual: 1895*, London 1895, 3.

50 Clark-Kennedy, *The London*, ii. 129. For Holland see J. F. Gore, *Sydney Holland: Lord Knutsford, a memoir*, London 1936, while N. Barnes, 'The Docker's Hospital', unpubl. BSc. diss. London 1993, offers a more critical analysis of his work at the Poplar Hospital.

Finance, philanthropy and the London hospitals

How, when, and to what extent money was raised from the metropolitan benevolent economy were questions that had worried hospital administrators from the eighteenth century onwards. Whereas doctors were supposed to devote most of their time in the hospital to treating 'deserving' patients, hospital governors were preoccupied with managing their institution's resources. As the financial position of London's hospitals deteriorated they therefore spent 'a good deal of time, and not a little patience and ingenuity' raising money.[51] By the 1890s no pronouncement could be made on the London hospitals without some reference to their funding.

Given the historical belief that London's hospitals were supported by charity, it is essential to look at the nature of benevolence. Charity in London was influenced by a variety of factors to create an amorphous voluntarism. How and why people gave has troubled historians, giving rise to a series of interpretations that have seen benevolence as anything from an expression of altruism to a form of class hegemony.[52] Studying the motives of those who supported the Victorian London hospitals casts some light on this debate. Philanthropy in London was shaped by the nature of London society and economy and no single charitable object had a uniform appeal. It was motivated by a wide range of concerns from guilt to gratitude rather than any one set of values. The spectrum was broad: religious and humanitarian motives stirred by images of sickness existed side-by-side with local or personal sympathy for an institution, notions of guilt, paternalism, social control, fashion and the belief that hospitals benefited society. London's hospitals were adept at manipulating all these interests. If charity cannot be reduced to simple terms, neither can the means through which hospitals sought to pick the pockets of the benevolent public. Charitable giving was not simply a matter of subscriptions, donations and legacies as many historians have perceived and hospitals devised new and varied means to attract charity. The pressure to contribute was unrelenting. So many appeals were launched that by the 1890s the public had become wearied by them. Governors enthusiastically embraced the possibilities of the charity bazaar, along with the contributions from church sermons, charitable concerts and street collections. Institutions developed their own collection schemes, but the foundation of the Sunday Fund in 1873, followed by the Saturday Fund in 1874, signified a new departure in funding. These benevolent funds organised collections and removed the contributor from the choice of beneficiary, distributing the funds according to an assessment of the individual hospital's utility. The aim was to promote reform. Whereas the benevolent funds were unique to the hospital sector (but not to London) other charities adopted

---

[51] *Hospital*, 6 June 1891, 109.
[52] See Alan J. Kidd, 'Philanthropy and the "social history paradigm" ', *Social History* xxi (1996), 180–92, for a discussion of these views.

similar fundraising techniques. The means of giving were as varied as the reasons for philanthropy and the London hospitals in their anxious pursuit of funds left nothing to chance.

However, the *a priori* assumption that all hospitals were funded by charity alone is not borne out by a study of London's hospitals. Governors purpose-fully pursued money-saving initiatives, developed non-charitable sources of income and adopted active fundraising tactics. Benevolence remained important, with the Sunday and Saturday Funds helping to redirect philan-thropy into hospitals, but as the Royal Hospital for Diseases of the Chest admitted, hospital income came from 'great and widely spread source[s]'.[53] Standard interpretations exclude many basic aspects of hospital income where diversity was the rule rather than the exception, and not all hospitals relied on philanthropy as their main source of funding. Endowed hospitals like St Bartholomew's and St Thomas's drew a large portion of their funds from property and investments, while individual hospitals had different funding strategies. University College Hospital, for example, relied on loans and the London Hospital experimented with mortgages in the 1860s. How-ever, certain common forms of funding can be detected. Hospitals drew income from investments and property, from charges to their patients, from the sale of services particularly those connected with the training of nurses, turning the hospital's function to a financial benefit, and from borrowing and deficit financing. Only state funding was anathema; every other source was exploited. Hospital finance was multifaceted and erratic, conditioned by the resources available within the benevolent economy. At the same time, it was able to draw on a wider range of resources linked to the hospital's function and property.

Finance could not remain static as the hospital developed. Although the structure of income varied between institutions, each experienced a process of financial diversification. The development of hospital income can be located within Rosenberg's framework where both governors and doctors increasingly came to view themselves as providing medical treatment. Medical expansion, rebuilding and increased demand all influenced the hospital's financial structure, but at the same time it was shaped by volunta-rism and the nature of London's benevolent economy.[54] The need to develop new sources of funding was always present, especially as philanthropy proved to be unreliable. It was perhaps because London's hospitals did not rely on any one source but constantly diversified their financial base that they could expand in response to increased demand for institutional healthcare.

From these changes in the hospitals' structure of funding it might be assumed that finance had a considerable influence on an administration constructed around a source of funding that was declining in importance. However, whereas the hospitals' administration was undergoing a process of

---

53 RCH, annual report 1868, LMA.
54 Rosenberg, *Care of strangers.*

change it remained firmly committed to a voluntary ethos. Little historical attention has been paid to how hospitals were administered. Medicalisation, rebuilding and financial anxiety required bureaucratisation and administrative streamlining, but the gradual transformation of the hospital into a medical institution did not alter the voluntary rationale behind management. Hospitals varied, but a certain institutional managerial norm centred on a 'subscriber democracy' and a small active clique of governors persisted. With hospital administration in London dominated by a male social elite, this raises questions about the extent of women's influence in the hospital when in other areas their philanthropic role was expanding, and about the influence of the working classes when in the twentieth century their impact on the hospital was increasing through contribution schemes.[55] These men, however, were not arrogant, incompetent or ignorant but fearful of external pressure and working within an administration geared to financial concerns. They spent money when it was available and pursued economies when it was not. The prime concern was to keep the institution running. The governors' first reaction was invariably to defend the hospital rather than to change it, producing a re-active rather than a pro-active administrative structure.

Changing social *mores* and attitudes about the nature and extent of poverty, not an alteration in the structure of funding, produced a steady decline in philanthropy's domination, but in the London hospitals a contender for control emerged. An increasingly assertive medical profession used a rhetoric of science to extend its authority and attempted to realign the hospital to reflect medical (rather than moral) standards. Influence existed at an informal and formal level, but it was their formal authority that doctors wanted to expand. No one argued for complete medical control, only a sharing of managerial responsibility. This is not to suggest that by the turn of the century doctors were able to dominate; rather that the governors' authority was modified by the professionalisation of medicine and the medicalisation of the hospital. Not all institutions progressed at the same rate and, although the governors' hegemony was eroded, at best a dual administration was created. The extension of medical influence often involved a crisis as a result of which the doctors were defeated but from which a compromise emerged allowing them an increased role in management. Events at Guy's Hospital in 1879–80 surrounding the appointment of a new matron exemplify this process.[56] Conflict, tension and an alteration in the nature of the hospital conspired to increase the level of medical authority. Science and professionalisation were, however, ultimately too weak, even by 1900, to counter an authority based on charitable contributions and voluntarism.

By the 1880s an apparent financial crisis in London's hospitals encouraged

---

[55] See Frank K. Prochaska, *Woman and philanthropy in nineteenth-century England*, Oxford 1980; Cherry, 'Beyond national health insurance', 455–82.
[56] See Keir Waddington, 'The nursing dispute at Guy's Hospital, 1879–80', *SHM* viii (1995), 211–30.

fears about state intervention and debate about the boundaries between civil society and the state in healthcare. The Select Committee on Metropolitan Hospitals proposed a charitable solution to the problems facing London's hospitals and the Prince of Wales Hospital Fund for London and the Central Hospital Council were constructed as voluntary alternatives to state intervention. In the 1890s voluntarism was defended and a new means of collecting charity was developed through the Prince of Wales Hospital Fund to provide the funds deemed necessary. For a short time the position was stabilised, but by the early twentieth century hospitals' financial difficulties eventually forced them to turn to the state for aid.

The Tomlinson Report has shown that the structure of healthcare in the 1990s faced problems similar to those which confronted London's hospitals at the end of the nineteenth century. Historically, the metropolitan hospitals were an important part of a complicated benevolent economy in a period when the boundaries between civil society and the state were gradually being redefined and the roles of charity and taxation were beginning to be questioned. At the same time, professional values were starting to erode the *mores* of the established elite. A study of the financial and administrative development of the hospitals of Victorian London illustrates these themes and helps explain the pressures acting on charity and the growth of institutional charitable provision. Hospital finance therefore provides a starting point for a discussion of the wider issues affecting the development of the hospital, the nature of philanthropy and charitable contributions, and the process by which the medical profession attempted to gain control over their institutional working environment. In doing so, it locates the hospital within the broader context of voluntarism to explain the balance between charitable and non-charitable funding and authority in a charitable institution.

PART I

PHILANTHROPY AND FUNDING

2

The Philanthropic Imperative

Differing definitions

'The social fabric of Victorian England', according to Alan Kidd, 'was permeated by charity and the repercussions of the charitable relationship'. Benevolence extended through a wide range of social behaviour, 'from the informal
expression of kindness to a dependant at one end to legislative campaigning
for social justice'.[1] Whereas critics saw charity as thoughtless, self-satisfying,
unco-ordinated and pauperising, the product of a half-awakened conscience,
these challenges failed to undermine the Victorian confidence in the voluntary ethos. London's hospitals were built on this faith, which had maintained
them since the early eighteenth century. Philanthropists wanted to believe
that, like the Good Samaritan, 'an Englishman rarely stands aside from public
business' and was imbued with an 'obligation to contribute, in one way or
another to the common good'. It was a hope bolstered by the large sums
donated annually to benevolent societies and remained strong into the twentieth century.[2] With a self-conscious regard for public opinion, linked to an
anxious concern for finance, philanthropists sought to alleviate human mis-
ery and poverty. They revealed problems that could not be solved by the individual, prompting calls for legislative activity as they pioneered 'recognition
of new areas of concern but ultimately making it clear that voluntarism [was]
not enough'.[3] For all this, charity remained ubiquitous, both immune from
precise measurement and under constant scrutiny.

Charity, however, is a contested concept. The word 'philanthropy' first
appeared in 1625 in Misheu's *Guide to the tongue*. It was believed to be derived
from the Greek where it meant 'a loving of man' and was first used by Bacon
in 1625 in his essay on 'Goodness, and goodness of heart'.[4] He defined it as
'the affecting of the Weale of Men', but Victorian notions of benevolence
built on eighteenth-century traditions of commercial Christianity bolstered
by sermons and religious pamphlets, and continued to see philanthropy in
essentially Christian terms. Despite the growing debate over the desired function of charity and its nature, Victorians found little need to define philan-

---

[1] Kidd, 'Philanthropy and the "social history paradigm" ', 180; Harrison, *Peaceable kingdom*, 220.
[2] Owen, *English philanthropy*, 164; Geoffrey Finlayson, *Citizen, state, and social welfare in
Britain, 1830–1990*, Oxford 1994.
[3] Harrison, *Peaceable kingdom*, 234.
[4] Francis Bacon, *Goodness, and goodness of heart*, London 1625.

thropy. Where they presented a range of overlapping social, religious and philosophical rationales for benevolence contemporaries made no effort to clarify their reasons for giving. It was integral to their understanding of society and they remained confident that charity would continue to ameliorate the problems caused by industrialisation and urbanisation. Historians have subsequently puzzled over the exact meaning of philanthropy and offered their own rationales for giving. Some have gone so far as to assume that these motivations remain impossible to analyse, but this has not stopped their colleagues from constructing competing theories to explain the benevolent actions of the Victorians.

Traditional interpretations of philanthropy have been rooted in a liberal, essentially Whiggish, conception of history.[5] Concentration, especially in David Owen's work, focused on the endowed charities and the Charity Commission. Benevolence was shown to be progressive in an evolutionary model that culminated in the welfare state.[6] By the late 1970s a new critical approach had started to evolve, building on earlier moves to borrow from the social sciences. Marxist historians came to believe that industrialisation had imposed pressure on communal and deferential patterns of authority, creating anxiety within the ruling elite. In response philanthropy became an instrument of class domination, a means to assert Gramsci's idea of hegemony. According to this interpretation, endowed charities were marginalised and the new nineteenth-century voluntary associations came to the fore, imposing a middle-class ideology onto society. Gareth Stedman Jones in *Outcast London* wholeheartedly embraced this social control interpretation and applied anthropological ideas of the 'gift relationship' to notions of charity and power as part of a wider trend in historical inquiry.[7] Attention shifted to the activities of the Charitable Organisation Society (COS) and the modification of the 'gift relationship' as benevolence became more formalised. Philanthropy ceased to be progressive and became obligatory, motivated by more self-interested concerns. The idea that charity was a mechanism of power was not unique. It had been discussed by William Cobbet in 1816 and by Frederick Engels in his *The condition of the English working class in 1844*, but by the 1980s the construction of philanthropy as an instrument of social control had become a seductive view.[8] Marxist historians, however, were not the only

[5] For the historiography of charity see Kidd, 'Philanthropy and the "social history paradigm" ', 180–92, and Colin Jones, 'Some recent trends in the history of charity', in Daunton, *Charity, self-interest and welfare*, 51–63.
[6] See Owen, *English philanthropy*; Wilbur K. Jordan, *Philanthropy in England, 1460–1660: a study of the changing pattern of English social aspirations*, London 1959; Bernard Kirkman Gray, *A history of English philanthropy: from the dissolution of the monasteries to the taking of the first census*, London 1905.
[7] Gareth Stedman Jones, *Outcast London: a study of the relationship between classes in Victorian society*, London 1984; Kidd, 'Philanthropy and the "social history paradigm" ', 183.
[8] See Alan J. Kidd, 'Outcast Manchester: voluntary charity, poor relief and the casual poor, 1860–1905', in Alan J. Kidd and K. W. Roberts (eds), *City, class and culture: studies of*

ones to reinterpret the role of charity. Frank Prochaska equally redefined philanthropy, rejecting both earlier Whiggish models of the passage to modernity and the reductionist notion that charity was part of a middle-class conspiracy to inculcate its values into a susceptible working class. According to his interpretation benevolence was a positive concept inspired not by fear of social unrest but by kindness; it had an important function in society and helped to expand the social role of women.[9] Donna Andrew has adopted a similar framework. In *Philanthropy and police* she argues that eighteenth-century philanthropy was based on existing charitable traditions but was closely linked to a new understanding of commercial Christianity that took account of the process of industrialisation and the accumulation of wealth. Andrew, however, was not entirely convinced that benevolence was purely a product of a new sense of humanitarianism. For her those involved in voluntary organisations also used philanthropy as an agent of social regeneration.[10]

In recent years there has been a move against such interpretations as historians have returned to the pessimism of earlier Marxist assumptions. Once more they have come to doubt the altruistic dimension of charity. Robert Morris, in his study of middle-class and voluntary associations in early nineteenth-century Leeds, has become the main proponent of this view. He argues that voluntary societies were an important arena for middle-class activity, which provided common ground between religious sects and parties and a framework through which they established their class identity and negotiated urban social relations. Morris, like Yeo and Garrard before him, admits that voluntary societies were not perfect transmitters of class values, but he sees them as an established 'cultural norm'.[11] Richard Trainor in his analysis of the Black Country elites has extended Morris's argument. He notes that although charity was modified by new public initiatives, it remained crucial to the elite provision of medicine and recreation, reinforcing the 'benign use of middle class wealth'. For Trainor, voluntary societies 'reduced points of conflict between middle class and working class people', helping channel the latters' aspirations as subscribers and demonstrated 'the concerns of the upper orders for social problems'.[12] Others have followed his lead. Once more philanthropy has become a tool in class formation; an instrument of middle-class hegemony.

---

social policy and cultural production in Victorian Manchester, Manchester 1985, 48–73; Stephen Yeo, *Religion and voluntary organisation in crisis*, London 1979; John Garrard, *Leadership and power in Victorian industrial towns, 1830–80*, Manchester 1983.

9 See Prochaska, *Woman and philanthropy*, and *The voluntary impulse*, for an analysis of philanthropy's continued contribution to the welfare state, a view shared by Geoffrey Finlayson, 'A moving frontier: voluntarism and the state in British social welfare, 1911–49', *Twentieth Century British History* i (1990), 183–206.

10 Andrew, *Philanthropy and police*.

11 Morris, *Class, sect and party*.

12 Richard H. Trainor, *Black Country elites: the exercise of authority in an industrialised area, 1830–1900*, Oxford 1993, 351.

Where does this leave the historian? Was philanthropy such a muddled concept that Wilbur Jordan is correct in assuming that its inspiration is 'immune . . . from the fumbling probing of the historian'?[13] True, few Victorians have left detailed accounts of their motivations. Those who did talk publicly about charity either did so from the pulpit, stressing Christian virtues, or were critical of what they characterised as the unregulated and pauperising activities of benevolent societies. Victorian writers could be equally sceptical. In Victor Hugo's Les Misérables, Madeleine's endowment of the local hospital was attributed either to ambition or to a desire for recognition and social acceptance. The same motives were ascribed to Mr Bulstrode, the banker in George Eliot's Middlemarch.[14] More noble sentiments are often lacking. Whereas perceptive studies do exist for medical charity in sixteenth and seventeenth-century Turin, for eighteenth-century London dispensaries and provincial hospitals, and on medical charity in Huddersfield and Wakefield, there is less historical writing and contemporary information on why support was given to London's nineteenth-century hospitals. Reconstruction is, however, possible by synthesising the different historical approaches to charity. It is perhaps only by looking at how London's hospitals attempted to manipulate the hopes, fears and aspirations of the charitable, what Bronwyn Croxson has labelled the 'public face' of charity, that we might come closer to an understanding of why they were the most dynamic sector of the metropolitan benevolent economy.[15] An analysis of the fundraising vocabulary used by governors also helps to explain the wider impetus behind philanthropy when the subscriber's own voice was often absent. Continuities existed with eighteenth-century voluntary hospitals and dispensaries, and governors seemed to know instinctively what would motivate benevolence.

To give or not to give?: motivating the benevolent public

Metropolitan charity and support for London's hospitals was not the civic pride and social duty of the Manchester elite, the commercially-inspired benevolence of Wakefield and Huddersfield or the self-help of Oldham; it was something more imprecise.[16] London's size, economic concerns and

13 Jordan, Philanthropy, 144.
14 Cited in Robert H. Bremer, Giving: charity and philanthropy in history, New Brunswick 1996, 107.
15 Sandra Cavallo, 'Motivations of benefactors: an overview of approaches to the study of charity', in Barry and Jones, Medicine and charity, 46–62; Hilary Marland, 'Lay and medical conceptions of charity during the nineteenth century', ibid. 149–71; Porter, 'The gift relationship', 49–78; Bronwyn Croxson, 'Public and private faces of eighteenth-century London dispensary charity', Medical History xli (1997), 127–49; R. Kilpatrick, ' "Living in the light": dispensaries, philanthropy and medical reform in late eighteenth-century London', in Cunningham and French, Medical enlightenment, 254–80.
16 See John V. Pickstone, Medicine and industrial society: a history of hospital development in

society combined with the sheer number of charities (many of which had a national significance) to create an amorphous voluntarism. Influenced by a variety of factors and with a vast array of institutional and personal outlets, metropolitan charity had no uniform image. It was shaped by the resources and attitudes of the high concentration of middle-class and professional occupations that the growth of London's service sector encouraged, though it would be unwise to rule out the importance of working-class philanthropy.[17] The London middle classes were not, however, Stedman Jones's cynical supporters of the COS but a diverse class that shared a strong faith in voluntarism.[18] The same diversity can be seen in medical charity. In London's hospitals, philanthropy was built on a wide range of supporters, classes and ideas that embodied the spectrum Richard Titmus identified in his study of the blood donation service.[19] Hospital charity was a blend of 'altruistic' and 'egoistic' values; individuals were motivated by interests that extended from guilt to gratitude.

The Victorian 'religious boom' and the expansion of religious institutions played an important role in stimulating and justifying the charitable intentions of the benevolent. These sentiments appeared unaffected by the forces promoting secularisation that some historians have seen as characteristic of the late Victorian period.[20] A religious and moral imperative remained a recurrent theme in writing on charity after 1850: in the 750 works published on philanthropy between 1850 and 1898 Christian dogma remained prominent, reinvigorated after 1883 by the *Bitter cry of outcast London*. In its acceptance of the industrial city, Nonconformity embodied a social programme that embraced benevolence. In an attempt to reinforce the social role of the established Church and to make it appear more relevant to the problems facing urban society, ministers rushed to publish their sermons on Christian charity. They extolled readers to avoid posthumous benevolence and give

---

Manchester and its region, 1752–1946, Manchester 1985; Hilary Marland, *Medicine and society in Wakefield and Huddersfield, 1780–1879*, Cambridge 1987; John Foster, *Class structure and the industrial revolution: early industrial capitalism in three English towns*, London 1974.

17 Frank K. Prochaska, 'Philanthropy', in Thompson, *Cambridge social history of Britain*, iii. 357–94; Ellen Ross, 'Survival networks: women's neighbourhood sharing in London before World War One', *History Workshop* xv (1983), 4–27.

18 Stedman Jones, *Outcast London*, 241–315. For the COS see Charles L. Mowat, *The Charity Organisation Society, 1869–1913*, London 1961; Madeleine Rooff, *A hundred years of family welfare: a study of the Family Welfare Association (formerly the Charity Organisation Society)*, 1869–1969, London 1972. For a more critical interpretation see R. Humphreys, 'Poor law and charity: the Charity Organisation Society in the provinces 1870–1890', unpubl. PhD diss. London 1991, and Jane Lewis, *The voluntary sector, the state and social work in Britain*, Aldershot 1995.

19 Richard Titmus, *The gift relationship*, London 1950.

20 See Robert Currie, *Methodism divided: a study in the sociology of ecumenicalism*, London 1968; Alan D. Gilbert, *Religion and society in industrial England: Church, Chapel and social change, 1740–1914*, London 1976; Robert Currie, Alan D. Gilbert and Lee Horsley, *Churches and churchgoers*, London 1977.

during their lifetime; some went so far as to claim that philanthropy was the 'genius of Christianity', unquestionably belonging to the Church. With Victorian chapels and churches built on debt and not always able to fulfil their self-defined social role or combat the perceived growing social and geographical divide between rich (or middle class) and poor, it was important to encourage congregations to give generously.[21] Clerics found inspiration in the life of Christ and the gospel of St Paul, though the view that charity was a divinely ordained rent on property had already begun to fade by the start of the nineteenth century.[22] Victorian philanthropy continued to be idealised as a Christian virtue, epitomised by Christ and a Christ-like love of mankind. To be charitable was to serve God and, it was stressed, society by reducing the number of poor.[23] Here Christian ideas of benevolence merged with political debate. Even the hard-hearted COS, which sought to organise philanthropy and remove its pauperising and irrational sentimentalism, subscribed to this view.[24] In an environment that favoured an Evangelical approach to benevolence, action rested on a solid faith that philanthropy emanated from a sentiment of religious and personal sacrifice.

All religious denominations were actively involved in promoting charitable work, but it was the Evangelical revival at the end of the eighteenth century and a second Evangelical boom in London around 1859 that provided a powerful catalyst for Christian charity. Evangelism was 'a useful and timely ethic for the emerging middle class', rationalising worldly success as a product of providence and making it necessary to promote benevolence.[25] Conversion stood at the heart of Evangelism and good works, though not essential to salvation, were seen as evidence of true conversion.[26] Evangelists therefore craved philanthropic employment to answer the spiritual anxiety that a preoccupation with sin generated. Charity was used by some philanthropists to resolve tensions within their personality, but Evangelists felt that they could not ignore the suffering of their neighbour, especially when their neighbour was made in the image of God and had an immortal soul. This conferred a duty to raise individuals out of their suffering so that they might be prepared to meet their saviour.[27] Charity in this context became God's will and merged with the Evangelists' overwhelming desire to reform the morals of their fellow men. The impact these ideas had on Victorian society ensured that a political culture of Evangelicalism linked to social purity came to underlie

[21] John Horsford, *Philanthropy: the genius of Christianity*, London 1862, p. vii.
[22] Andrew, *Philanthropy and police*, 42.
[23] Frederick W. Farrar, *Social and present-day questions*, London 1891, 96.
[24] See Prochaska, *Women and philanthropy*.
[25] Ian Bradley, *The call to seriousness: the evangelical impact on the Victorians*, London 1976, 145, 157.
[26] Ibid. 21.
[27] Brian Harrison, 'Philanthropy and the Victorians', *Victorian Studies* ix (1966), 358. See Anon., *Charity: a tract for the times*, London 1874; S. Meacham, 'The evangelical inheritance', *Journal of British Studies* iii (1963/4), 92.

London society and for those who were not committed religionists, a secular form of Evangelicalism thrived.[28]

Evangelists were an important body of subscribers and philanthropic reformers, inspiring others to action. By 1850 an estimated three-quarters of the country's charities were under their control.[29] William Wilberforce, best known for his anti-slavery campaigns, was a tireless philanthropist whose name appeared on the subscription list of some seventy charities. At Guy's Hospital the administration was dominated by governors who came from an Evangelical background. The most prominent mirrored Wilberforce's enthusiasm for activity: Benjamin Harrison, the hospital's treasurer until 1876, gave to twenty-one societies; Charles and Robert Barclay, both prominent governors at Guy's, supported eighty-six voluntary organisations between them. Many, like the bankers Samuel Thornton and Charles Barclay, had known or worked with Wilberforce, while Harrison was familiar with the Clapham sect. Evangelists were not just involved in hospital administration: by means of their flower and letter missions they attempted to humanise the hospital and increase contact with the sick poor.[30] Evangelists seemed to be everywhere, not least on hospital subscription lists.

Charity in a Christian framework was regarded as its own reward, but the religious justification for benevolence was not completely disinterested. The Reverend Brook Lambert, writing in the *Contemporary Review* in 1873, saw the poor as a necessary evil designed by God to benefit the leisurely by giving them 'cases by which they might perfect themselves in spiritual medicine'.[31] Charity was projected as a means of buying admission to heaven, a form of fire insurance for the afterlife. From this perspective, Christian philanthropy could serve both the recipient and the giver, uniting humanitarian and selfish concerns under the general sanction of Christian theology. Hospital administrators recognised this and regularly appealed to religious sentiments. The relationship was not entirely one-sided: hospitals fulfilled a need for the religiously motivated. Their explicit humanitarian motive appeared to answer the spiritual and emotional poverty that had been generated by materialism.[32] It would be unwise, however, to see Victorian charity as entirely the consequence of an Evangelical revival and of religious sentimentality. Philanthropy was not simply, as the Evangelists would have it, the natural result of conversion or a product of a true acceptance of the Gospel. From the eight-

28 Susan D. Pennybacker, *A vision for London, 1889–1914: labour, everyday life and the LCC experiment*, London 1995, 3.

29 Kathleen Heasman, *Evangelicals in action: an appraisal of their social work in the Victorian era*, London 1962, 11.

30 Ford K. Brown, *Father to the Victorians: the age of Wilberforce*, Cambridge 1961, 71, 355–7; Heasman, *Evangelicals in action*, 225–31.

31 Brook Lambert, 'Charity: its aims and means', *Contemporary Review* xxiii (1873/4), 463.

32 Margaret B. Simey, *Charitable effort in Liverpool in the nineteenth century*, Liverpool 1951, 106.

eenth century charity had moved from a pure expression of Christian devotion to acquire temporal characteristics.[33]

One contemporary wrote that the English are 'most devoted to sympathy and commiseration, most tenderly alive to the softest impression of every affection', making benevolence a natural extension of this national characteristic.[34] The image of sickness was a compelling one that cut across social, political and religious boundaries. Governors carefully exploited such humanitarian sentiments and made 'piteous' appeals to public sympathy to alleviate the suffering of the sick.[35] A particularly emotive appeal was made by the governors of the Royal Hospital for Diseases of the Chest in 1857 when they claimed that in treating diseases of the chest the hospital was relieving a 'most fatal and distressing' form of illness.[36] The hospital was, however, regularly outdone by the Hospital for Sick Children. Tear-jerking appeals were launched and books published like James Greenwood's *Little Bob in hospital* in 1887, which explained the suffering of sick children and the hospital's good work in the most heart-rending terms. In 1858 the *London Journal* could write that 'there was no one with so many claims upon the sympathies of the benevolent' as the Hospital for Sick Children.[37] Only the most hard-hearted could ignore such appeals. That the hospital attracted an increasing amount of revenue from philanthropy where other hospitals experienced a decline is indicative of its success in encouraging contributions.

Sympathy did not have to be impersonal. Often it was generated by a familial or personal experience of sickness. For example, William Henry Lueade, long a sufferer from gout and rheumatism, left money to St Bartholomew's in 1868 to treat the 'necessitous poor' with these complaints.[38] Hospital appeals, local collections and sermons motivated in some subscribers a personal attachment to their local institution. The governors of the London Hospital played on this, asserting that it was 'the only hospital to the treacherous East End'.[39] The German immigrant community had a natural sympathy for the German Hospital, as did the local community in Dalston, which looked on the institution with pride. Personal association could work in a different way and familial or personal experience of a particular institution was a powerful generator of support. Elizabeth Baly, who left money to St Bartholomew's to found a scholarship, did so because her brother had been physician at the hospital.[40] The reason for her bequest was mirrored in other contributions. All hospital appeals built on an element of sympathy either for the sick,

---

[33] Andrew, *Philanthropy and police*, 14–15, 18–22.
[34] Cited in Woodward, *To do the sick no harm*, 21.
[35] Henry Davis, *Our hospitals: their difficulties and remedy*, London 1894.
[36] RCH, governors' minute book, 30 Oct. 1857, LMA, H33/RCH/A1/1.
[37] Hospital for Sick Children, press cuttings, GOSH, 8/153.
[38] St Bartholomew's, register of legacies, 1764–1917, SBH, Hb 5/3.
[39] *Truth*, 19 Apr. 1883.
[40] St Bartholomew's, register of legacies, 15 Feb. 1893, SBH, Hb 5/3.

for the hard work of the hospital staff, or for the financial plight of the institution.

Where religion created a theological impetus for benevolence, wealth created its own responsibility. 'Noblesse oblige', writes Finlayson, 'could merge into a way of quieting a conscience troubled by the possession of riches, or of justifying those riches by devoting a proportion of them to the benefits of others.'[41] Many 'a gambler and society miscreant found solace in channelling part of his ill-gotten gains to the cause of the sick poor'.[42] Guilt could be a powerful incentive to philanthropy, but hospitals preferred to dwell on 'a tremendous sense of social duty and responsibility'.[43] In Manchester Pickstone claims that this was paramount in motivating donations.[44] The traditional paternalistic ethos epitomised the social obligations of wealth. Paternalists were hostile to organised benevolence, but their emphasis on the duties, rather than the rights of property, and their stress on the role of the individual was a compelling argument in favour of charity. In espousing paternalism writers like Arthur Helps in his *Friends in council*, earnestly stressed the social duties of wealth.[45] Novelists like Elizabeth Gaskell in *Mary Barton* and Charles Dickens in *Hard times* both argued for greater social responsibility on the part of the industrial bourgeois. Similar ideas were developed by Walter Rathbone in the 1860s. His book, *Social duty*, expressed the widespread concern that the process of industrialisation and urbanisation had led to a breakdown in co-operation between classes.[46] Rathbone called for a renewed 'intercourse between rich and poor' where charity was no longer a sentimental response but the social duty of every man of wealth and leisure. It was only through voluntary organisations that personal efforts could be fully utilised; only through personal energy and devotion that organised associations could mitigate existing evils. Both, it was anticipated, would ultimately serve to promote social harmony and moral reform.[47] Charity as a social duty was widely confirmed by other authors. From the 1860s onwards recurrent social crises, a 'rediscovery of poverty' and the resurrection of the desire to bridge the gap between classes seen in the settlement movement renewed the emphasis on the idea of philanthropy as social duty.[48] It was widely acknowl-

41 Finlayson, *Citizen, state and welfare*, 49.
42 Woodward, *To do the sick no harm*, 19.
43 Brian Abel-Smith, *The hospitals, 1800–1948: a study in social administration in England and Wales*, London 1964, 5.
44 Pickstone, *Medicine and industrial society*, 138–47.
45 David Roberts, *Paternalism in early Victorian England*, London 1979, 4, 25.
46 Rathbone was a Unitarian and active in providing charitable nursing care in Liverpool: Heasman, *Evangelicals in action*, 285–6.
47 William Rathbone, *Social duties considered with reference to the organisation of efforts in works of benevolence and public utility*, London 1867, 30, 67–90, 109.
48 Kidd, 'Outcast Manchester', 49. See Asa Briggs and Anne Macartney, *Toynbee Hall: the first hundred years*, London 1984; Andrew Vincent and Raymond Plant, *Philosophy, politics and citizenship: the life and thought of the British idealists*, London 1984, 132–49.

edged that the community had a great responsibility to support the poor and the local hospitals. For Robert Fowler MP, this represented a 'debt' that could only be repaid through contribution.[49] Ideas of social duty were rejuvenated by T. H. Green's politics of conscience and the Idealist school of thought that incorporated philanthropy as one of the obligations of the 'active' citizen. Although Idealism reinvigorated existing rationales for giving and influenced debates on welfare into the late 1930s, hospital philanthropists made little reference to these ideas in their appeals and continued to talk about altruism, humanitarianism, religious sentiment and social duty.[50]

A feeling of altruism, a sense of humanitarian sympathy or religious senti-ment, were not charity's only sources of inspiration. Even Anglo-Jewry, which had its own philanthropic tradition and a strong sense of obligation to co-religionists, could not separate itself from secular concerns.[51] Less noble incentives were part of the morphological landscape of charity and hospital governors were adept at manipulating them. Foucault has argued that hospi-tals were part of an institutional effort to establish normative standards.[52] Other historians have developed this view, placing the hospital within a wider discussion of philanthropy as an instrument of social control.[53] How-ever, social control is a confused concept, supported more by hindsight than by evidence. It adopts a reductionist and mechanistic view of society, focus-ing on coercion and deviant behaviour, a conviction that takes Durkheim's notion of 'socialisation' to extremes. Social control is an idea that has been frequently misused; its proponents tend to generalise and place every action within some grand design. Even in sociology it has not had 'a very successful career'.[54] It is perhaps too much to argue that hospitals were part of a 'carca-rial archipelago' that strove to produce a docile deviant population.[55] For all this, there was an awareness that charity had a role to play in staving off social unrest by acting as 'a conspicuous symbol of the charitable impulses of the rich'.[56] Philanthropists like Shaftesbury and Barnardo shared this view, and the *Charity Record & Philanthropic News* commented that benevolence helped 'crush out that class feeling which at times threatens to turn this Eng-

---

[49] London Hospital, scrapbook, 11 Apr. 1888, LH, A/26/31.
[50] Melvin Richter, *The politics of conscience: T. H. Green and his age*, London 1964; Alan J. Milne, *The social philosophy of English idealism*, London 1962; Stefan Collini, 'Idealism and "Cambridge idealism" ', *Historical Journal* xviii (1975), 171–7; Vincent and Plant, *Philoso-phy, politics and citizenship*; José Harris, 'Political thought and the welfare state, 1870–1940: an intellectual framework for British social policy', *Past and Present* cxxxiv/v (1992), 116–41.
[51] See Eugene C. Black, *The social politics of Anglo-Jewry, 1880–1980*, Oxford 1988.
[52] Michel Foucault, *Discipline and punishment: the birth of the prison*, London 1979.
[53] See A. P. Donajgrodzki (ed.), *Social control in nineteenth-century Britain*, London 1977, for the use of the social control theory in a wider historical context.
[54] Cited in C. K. Watkins, *Social control*, London 1975, 2.
[55] C. Dandeker, *Surveillance, power and modernity: bureaucracy and discipline from 1700 to the present day*, Cambridge 1990, 27.
[56] Marland, *Medicine and society*, 140.

land of ours into two hostile camps'.[57] Charity was stimulated at times of stress. In 1885–6 a harsh winter and worker demonstrations in the West End in February 1886 saw a rush of charitable effort and the foundation of a special Mansion House Fund.[58] Hospital governors certainly expected gratitude and deference from their patients. The religious ministrations of a resident chaplain and the controlling rules on behaviour can be seen as a vehicle for instilling a bourgeois ethic. One writer felt that what was 'sown' in the hospital was liable to take root in society.[59] For the *Christian Times*, 'no child can have gone though [the Hospital for Sick Children] without having such a memory impressed upon its mind – a revelation of the great fact of charity, the great fact of devotion, the great fact that man lives not for self, but for God and his neighbours'.[60] In the northern industrial towns the hospital's practical benefits in the treatment of accident cases were made to serve an ideological purpose in the hospital's foundation and in their appeals for support. Local industrialists and factory owners used them to show that they cared for their workers as a balance to the exploitation of the factory system.[61] In London the situation was different, in part because of the diverse nature of the metropolitan economy. The governors of the London hospitals believed that they were answering a practical social need rather than acting as a bulwark against revolution. Some supporters may have been motivated by a desire to control patients, but this was not the view of the majority. Neither were London's hospitals an ideal vehicle for control and 'it seems that the intended recipients picked out what they wanted from the facilities on offer, and rejected the moral or authoritarian message'. Rules were more easily made than enforced and supplication was a ready façade to secure treatment. More patients discharged themselves than were removed by the governors and many of the rules reflected a shared system of social values.[62]

A different perspective does show that subscribers supported hospitals for more self-interested reasons that had less to do with the positive rhetoric hospitals constructed around their fundraising. Contemporaries warned against selfish philanthropy, but the repugnance ascribed to it was insufficient to have any major influence on subscribers.[63] Governors anxious for funds were prepared to utilise selfish concerns to elicit support. Hospitals, it was widely felt, offered 'the best guarantee that the money devoted to the purpose shall be judiciously expended'.[64] They were presented as an economical and effec-

---

57 *Charity Record & Philanthropic News*, 6 Jan. 1881, 2.

58 Stedman Jones, *Outcast London*, 290–8.

59 S. E., 'The poor and the hospital', *Fraser's Magazine* xiii (1876), 723.

60 Hospital for Sick Children, press cuttings, GOSH, 8/153.

61 See Pickstone, *Medicine and industrial society*; Marland, *Medicine and society*.

62 F. M. L. Thompson, 'Social control in Victorian England', *EcHR* xxxiv (1981), 206.

63 Francis Peck, *The uncharitableness of inadequate relief*, London 1879, on the hypocrisy of selfish charity.

64 S. E., 'The poor and the hospital', 715.

tive use of charity, in many cases giving superior returns to other forms of benevolence. It was a common claim put forward by voluntary organisations, and in particular by medical charities. In a society increasingly concerned about the problems of 'gratuitous' assistance, this was a powerful justification for support. The *Daily Telegraph* echoed these ideas in 1871, emphasising the benefits that hospitals presented to the subscribing public and to the nation:

> We know that they [hospitals] assist in the case of accidents that may happen to anybody in any class, we know that as schools of medical science they are equally useful to the rich and poor, and we know that they repay the cost to the community over and over again, in sending back to their work and homes, in health, men who if they had not been so attended to, would probably have left families destitute upon the world.[65]

Although contemporaries felt that it was impossible to 'accurately represent the service rendered to humanity' by hospitals, hospitals did try to quantify their contribution to the national good by parading patient statistics in front of the public.[66] They appealed to ideas of national efficiency and played on the long-standing view that sickness was a major cause of poverty that plunged families into crisis and hardship. Governors contended that hospitals removed a root cause of distress by rapid and effective treatment, while quick intervention prevented the spread of disease. This served a dual purpose. Industry and the economy benefited from a reduction in the time lost through sickness as patients were returned to work. Equally, charity and the poor law were spared the expense needed to support the families of the sick for prolonged periods. Hospitals were accordingly presented as 'an important agent against pauperism', reducing the general reliance on charitable relief.[67] In effect, support for the hospital was projected as a means of saving money, an idea that appealed to sentiments of local parsimony at a time when the poor rate was under pressure from an expanding metropolitan poor law. The governors of the Royal Hospital for Diseases of the Chest used these concerns when they claimed that many of their patients were able 'to resume their customary employ and support of themselves and their families'.[68] To the commercial classes the idea of utility and value for money in return for a modest subscription had a powerful appeal. Marland, in her study of Wakefield and Huddersfield, believes that it was such practical concerns that motivated many subscribers.[69]

The calculating extended this view of utility and argued that hospitals accorded a direct benefit to society through 'the experience which they afford

[65] *Daily Telegraph*, 20 Feb. 1871, 2.
[66] *Lancet* ii (1878), 23.
[67] Franz Oppert, *Hospitals, infirmaries and dispensaries: their construction, interior arrangements and management, etc.*, London 1867, 47.
[68] RCH, annual report 1850, LMA.
[69] Marland, *Medicine and society*, 130.

to the medical profession'.[70] In a society acutely worried about the extent of disease and fearful of contagion this is hardly surprising. Some writers stressed that hospitals benefited both the rich and the poor through their contribution to medical science. Others were more partisan: one anonymous writer in *Fraser's Magazine* claimed that the Hospital for Sick Children should be supported because it allowed doctors to gain 'that knowledge of special disease of infancy which might be applied to the benefit of the children of the rich'. For Lord Taunton this explained why the institution had so many supporters.[71] The governors of University College Hospital expressed similar sentiments in a more muted form. They asserted that the hospital was doing an 'incalculable good' which tended 'to the advancement of science and the relief of human suffering'.[72] Appeals on these grounds were widespread and formed part of the common vocabulary used in generating support.

In addition to these benefits, 'the majority of subscribers' still wanted 'a show for their money' and it was this 'show' that helped ease the flow of benevolence. Voluntary contributions to the hospital fitted within a hierarchy of giving. Each contribution attracted a certain number of privileges and hospitals matched these against a graduated scale based on the size, rather than the nature of the gift. At the top of the hierarchy were those entitled to become governors. Here the benefactor was given the right to take an active administrative role in return for their contribution, causing critics to fear that some only gave money to promote their candidates or to secure profitable contracts. However, the main physical return on a subscriber's contribution was the provision of a governor's 'letter'. The letter system had developed during the eighteenth and early nineteenth centuries with the growth of the London hospitals; such was its success that it was adopted throughout the country.[73] Procedures varied between institutions but the aim remained the same. Essentially it was a scheme of incentives designed to encourage or reward support, with each letter carrying the right to admit a patient. In theory this guaranteed treatment, or at least the attention of a doctor. Even within this system there were graduations: differences were made between the right to admit in-patients and the ability to recommend out-patients while the number of letters awarded was linked to the size of the contribution. Subscribers felt that they were a 'natural', a *quid pro quo* for their support, and patients made strenuous efforts to acquire them.

Although the number of patients admitted with governors' letters fell during the nineteenth century as doctors gained more control over the admis-

70 Richard Dawes, *The evils of indiscriminate charity and of careless administration of funds left of charitable purposes*, London 1856, 8.
71 Anon., 'A visit to the Hospital for Sick Children', *Fraser's Magazine of Town and Country* xlix (1854), 63; *Times*, 16 May 1861, 8.
72 UCH, annual report 1869, UCL.
73 H. Hart, 'Some notes on the sponsoring of patients for hospital treatment under the voluntary system', *Medical History* xxiv (1980), 447.

sions process, contemporaries continued to worry about how subscribers used their admission rights.[74] One speaker at a Social Science Association conference in Birmingham in 1868 feared that hospitals had become 'private institutions for the relief of subscribers' nominees'. Anxiety was expressed that many indiscriminately distributed their letters, 'often in favour of their own dependants, and to save their own pockets', and this matched wider concerns about the indiscriminate nature of giving and its pauperising effects on the recipient. Examples of abuse were paraded: one lady in Portland Place, who subscribed to a large number of hospitals, was accused of issuing 1,500 letters a year to her friends' servants.[75] Employers in particular were singled out for criticism. Many developed the exploitation of letters to a sophisticated level, contributing to the hospital instead of providing insurance for their employees. When the New River Company gave five guineas to the Royal Hospital for Diseases of the Chest in 1852 it stated that the donation was influenced by 'the liability of their outdoor servants to diseases of the chest'.[76] The COS claimed that such employers were invariably those who paid their workers low wages. It overlooked the fact that a small subscription rather than expensive insurance made good financial sense.[77] Hospital reformers campaigned noisily against the practice. In their calls for the abolition of the letter system they joined with doctors who argued that it was unethical to treat a patient simply because they had been recommended by a subscriber with no medical knowledge. Although admissions were increasingly being realigned on a medical footing, the letter system was too deeply entrenched for most hospitals to heed these calls and abandon letters altogether. Abuse was recognised, but governors did not protest too vehemently because money was at stake.

Contributions conferred other, more social benefits to subscribers. Those running London's hospitals were all too aware that charity was 'the most fashionable amusement of the present age'. It was a concern that had been repeated since the mid 1750s in tandem with the growing number of voluntary societies. Victorian critics of the 'telescopic philanthropy' and 'rapacious benevolence' epitomised by Mrs Jellyby and Mrs Partridge in *Bleak House*, realised that 'no small number of these benevolent persons are philanthropists because it is the fashion to be so'.[78] Charity offered 'a morally approved vehicle for self-aggrandisement' and played a status-giving and a status-

[74] Waterlow commented in 1890 that 'practically it makes no difference whether the person comes with a letter or not, excepting that the letter is accepted as some evidence that the patient is a person who ought to be treated; but really the eligibility to admission is the degree of suffering'. At the London subscribers' recommendations fell from 46% of cases treated in 1855 to 9% in 1898, a fall symptomatic of a general decline. By 1910 recommendations were rarely required: *Select Committee of the House of Lords on Metropolitan Hospitals, Second Report*, PP 1890/1 xiii. 164.

[75] *Lancet* i (1882), 407; *BMJ* ii (1868), 433; *Lancet* i (1868), 494.

[76] RCH, governors' minute book, 5 Feb. 1852, LMA, H33/RCH/A1/3.

[77] *Charity Organisation Reporter*, 4 Apr. 1878, 68.

[78] Cited in Simey, *Charitable effort*, 56.

maintaining role. Through the annual ceremonies of charitable organisation, which took place at the height of the season, a safe and ideal opportunity was provided to mix with the social elite. For the wealthy, it was a conspicuous act of benevolence that gave humanitarian satisfaction, neutralised some resentment at a local level and justified their wealth and position.[79] For the aspiring, subscription lists in the press and in the hospitals' annual reports allowed benevolent individuals to achieve public association with other members of civil society and helped them build a 'name' for themselves and their charitable intentions. It could also provide a means of furthering business and political careers.[80] According to one acidic critic in the *Westminster and Foreign Review Quarterly*, many subscriptions were largely dependent on the names attached. This was not limited to London. Evidence suggests that the names of prominent members of civil society helped stimulate local charity, and a number who gave money actively looked for their names on subscription lists and complained noisily when they were omitted.[81] Royal patronage had a particularly powerful appeal. Voluntary societies, realising the financial benefits that resulted, clamoured for royal support. In return the monarchy, according to Prochaska, benefited, winning loyalty and understanding at a time when their political influence was waning.[82]

Hospitals were adept at securing royal favour and support, but this aspect of philanthropy seldom entered their fundraising rhetoric. Governors offered no moral condemnation of those who wanted to use charity to improve or confirm their social position and indirectly advertised the social benefits associated with giving. Prominent and fashionable members of civil society were invited to fundraising events to lend hospitals social *cachet*. Their names were given all due prominence on subscription lists and acted as 'a kind of peg upon which to hang any number of appeals for support, and any number of schemes for bleeding the charitable public'. Patronage by the social elite, as David Cannadine argues, was widely seen as a necessary precondition for success in any charitable activity.[83] The governors of the London lamented the death of the duke of Cambridge in 1850 in these terms, noting that they had

79 Kidd, 'Philanthropy and the "social history paradigm" ', 189.
80 P. Shapley, 'Voluntary charities in nineteenth-century Manchester: organisational structure, social status and leadership', unpubl. PhD diss. Manchester Metropolitan University 1994, chap. vi.
81 Anon., 'Philanthropy of the age and its relation to social evils', *Westminster Review and Foreign Quarterly* xxxv (1869), 447; John Davies, 'Aristocratic town-makers and the coal metropolis', in David Cannadine (ed.), *Patricians, power and politics in nineteenth-century towns*, Leicester 1982, 196. For example, at the London in 1888 the East End Tradesmen's Association objected when their name was missed from the annual report: London Hospital, minutes of the court of governors, 6 June 1888, LH, A/2/14.
82 Frank K. Prochaska, *Royal bounty: the making of a welfare monarchy*, New Haven 1995.
83 *Charity Record* ii (1882), 70; David Cannadine, *Lords and landlords: the aristocracy and the towns, 1774–1967*, Leicester 1980, 221–2.

lost a 'generous contributor to its funds' and a powerful and unwavering friend, 'whose benevolent influence has been the means of permanently increasing the income of this important charity'.[84] The German Hospital equally felt the loss, especially as the duke had been instrumental in eliciting support from English subscribers.[85] Not all who were asked gave their support or time, but hospitals usually attracted enough prominent sponsors to confirm their social standing and to appeal to the snobbery of some of their contributors.

To these 'selfish' concerns must be added contributions that were given from a feeling of gratitude. Governors were occasionally rewarded with a donation from a patient. Invariably these contributions were small, but they served an important ideological function, highlighting the hospital's role in stimulating provident and deferential habits, and much was made of them. One patient at University College Hospital wrote that she 'desires to forward . . . a donation of £5 5s. as a small acknowledgement of the benefits she has received, and of her gratitude to all who have ministered to her'; another at the Royal Hospital for Diseases of the Chest offered to renovate the hospital's brass plate 'as a token of his gratitude for the benefit received'. Not all were in a position to give, but many expressed feelings of gratitude. One patient thanked the hospital for the treatment given to her daughter, but regretted 'that my position will not allow me a more substantial recognition than this'.[86] These were exactly the patients hospitals and philanthropists aspired to help.

Where does this leave us? Support for hospitals did not embody every concern that could motivate benevolence. Where they appealed to public and private sympathy, hospitals were not particularly seen as a bulwark against revolution. Contribution to medical charities might have highlighted a concern for the sick poor that ameliorated class tensions, but few hospitals in London directly played on these sentiments. They preferred instead to stress religious sentiments, humanitarianism and their social utility, appealing simultaneously to the selfish or altruistic concerns of their subscribers. All sections of society responded, but no individual did so from a single motive. Religion may have provided a strong context for inspiration, but the philanthropic psyche contained a conflicting mix of motivations that could be both altruistic and intrinsically selfish. Perhaps by playing on all these concerns hospitals ensured that their support was guaranteed, even if their demands eventually outstripped the charitable resources available.

---

[84] London Hospital, minutes of the court of governors, 23 July 1850, LH, A/2/10.
[85] German Hospital, annual report 1851, SBH.
[86] RCH, governors' minute book, 3 Nov. 1859, LMA, H33/RCH/A1/2; UCH, annual report 1884, UCL.

Ways of giving: philanthropy and hospital fundraising

Governors invested considerable time and effort in persuading potential contributors to give, using a common vocabulary of fundraising that was constantly refined and developed. A large part of the hospitals' administration was geared to finance and with doctors assuming a marginal role in the financial administration, sole responsibility rested with the governors. Income from charity dominated their concerns and it was to philanthropy that they turned first to solve their hospital's economic problems.

Benevolence took many forms, but donations, subscriptions and legacies in the form of a cash gift were the traditional ways to contribute.[87] Donations could fluctuate wildly from year to year while legacies were unpredictable, providing a form of 'windfall' philanthropy that could not be relied on. Although death could take a heavy toll, claiming an estimated 8–10 per cent of subscribers annually, subscriptions were without the same uncertainties.[88] Subscriptions were small annual contributions, usually one guinea, and though in theory any amount could be contributed few gave more than five guineas. Every effort was made to collect them, but as one philanthropist noted, 'the constant struggle of getting annual subscriptions is the one bit of weariness in hospital work'.[89] To ease this workload, charitable organisations employed paid collectors who took a commission on the total raised. After 1896 collectors could use a printed directory, *The charitable ten thousand*, to locate potential subscribers and they frequently crossed each other's paths in the pursuit of funds.[90] Cases of fraud were occasionally reported and Labouchère's *Truth* specialised in exposing charity swindles, but collectors had a monetary interest in ensuring that subscriptions were collected promptly and not allowed to lapse. Although Mr Ostermoor, the collector at the German Hospital, was required to visit the 'mercantile and manufacturing towns', few were expected to travel outside London and many carried out their work in the immediate locality of the hospitals.[91]

Governors were keen to build up a large body of subscribers and they attached considerable importance to them, but their fundraising efforts went far beyond this. Voluntary organisations, as Morris notes, rarely existed on subscriptions alone.[92] Hospitals perhaps more than any other type of benevolent society tried to attract philanthropy through a variety of channels.

The benevolent often found it easier to make a donation than the long-term commitment that subscribing entailed. To encourage donations hospital

---

87 The importance of these different charitable components are discussed in chapter 3 where they are put in the context of the hospitals' structure of income.
88 *Charity Record & Philanthropic News* iv (1884), 83.
89 Ibid. xvii (1897), 142.
90 Owen, *English philanthropy*, 480.
91 German Hospital, minutes of hospital committee, Oct. 1856, SBH, GHA 2/2.
92 Morris, *Class, sect and party*, 298.

governors awarded life or honorary governorships and subscribers' privileges. At the Hospital for Sick Children, for example, life governorships were given for any donation over £31 10s., and between 1850 and 1890 1,115 were granted.[93] No contribution was seen as too small and amounts varied considerably. Some like Baron de Hirsch, a Jewish financier and a member of the Marlborough House set, were major benefactors. In 1893 he gave the £28,000 he had won on the 'turf' to the London hospitals; the Hospital for Sick Children alone received £1,200.[94] Others gave what they could afford and, unlike subscriptions, there was no set amount. All donations were acknowledged with enthusiasm, from the £7 7s. received by the London from the workmen employed at Tebbutt and Company to the £10,000 given in 1896 to help rebuild University College Hospital by the furniture manufacturer Sir John Blundell Maple, whose premises adjoined the hospital's.[95] Major donations of this kind were invariably used to fund building and provided the financial foundation of several institutions, mostly outside London.[96] Large contributions of this kind were, however, rare and when they were received they were acknowledged with a greater show of publicity.

Donations were not limited to money. Land and stock, such as James Bentley's gift of £1,000 in 3 per cent consolidated stock to St Bartholomew's in 1857, were received, but contributions of this sort were infrequent. A gift of land created administrative problems and often entailed some degree of management and expense. They were therefore either invested, or more regularly sold in times of hardship.[97] Other types of non-monetary gifts were more common. The Hospital for Sick Children was particularly fortunate and received a large number of gifts, especially of toys and children's clothes. For example, in 1852 Charles West, the difficult founder of the hospital, donated both his library and a hot-air bath; the following year a Mr Jeggs gave a collection of toys and a Mrs Latham some flannel dressing gowns.[98] All hospitals were given flowers and paintings. Many were donated for reasons similar to those expressed by Lord Kirkaldie in his present of flowers to Guy's in 1875, 'for the decoration of the Hospital Wards'.[99] The royal household gave food,

---

[93] Hospital for Sick Children, register of life governors, GOSH, 6/1/1.

[94] *Hospital*, 21 Jan. 1893, 266.

[95] London Hospital, minutes of house committee, 23 Sept. 1856, LH, A/5/28; UCH, minutes of general committee, UCL, A1/2/8.

[96] Jeremy R. B. Taylor, *Hospital and asylum architecture in England, 1840–1914: buildings for health care*, London 1991, 34–5. At St Bartholomew's, the convalescent home at Swanley, Kent, was only made possible through the gift of £5,000 from Peter Reid (a friend of the hospital's secretary) and £16,000 from Kettlewell: Memoirs of William Henry Cross, 1866–1905, SBH, X 5/26.

[97] St Bartholomew's, register of legacies, 1764–1917, SBH, Hb 5/3.

[98] Hospital for Sick Children, minutes of the committee of management, 20 June 1852, GOSH, 1/2/3; 7 Apr. 1853, GOSH, 1/2/4.

[99] Guy's Hospital, minutes of the court of committees, 9 June 1875, LMA, H9/Gy/A3/10.

Figure 1: St Bartholomew's Hospital: legacies received, 1850–98

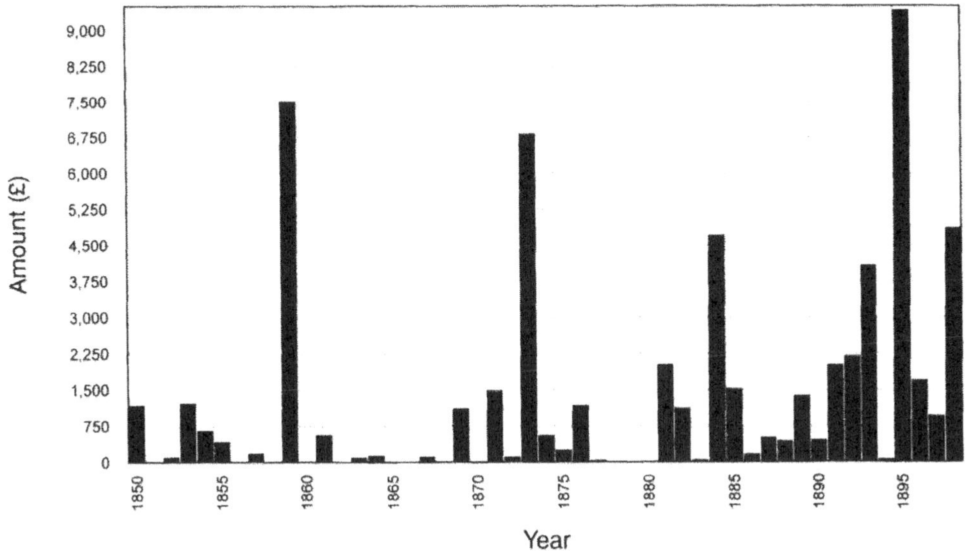

Source: General account books, SBH, H/b/5/3–4

especially pheasants, and old linen, presumably for bandages, and doctors donated books and medical equipment to the hospitals where they had trained or worked. Not all gifts were useful. The value to patients of a selection of tickets for the Princess, Globe and Shaftesbury theatres given to the Royal Hospital for Diseases of the Chest in 1896 must be doubted, though presumably the governors ensured that they were not wasted.[100] In 1892 one 'lady' gave 'several favoured institutions' a 'whole shopful of harmoniums' and the *Hospital* correctly realised that many hospitals 'prefer[red] the simplicity of cash gifts'.[101] Non-monetary donations were important in making hospitals a more pleasing environment, but governors attached greater significance to contributions of a more conventional nature.

Legacies were the most unpredictable source of charitable income, as shown by the amounts left to St Bartholomew's (see figure 1). Thomas Guy's endowment of Guy's Hospital in 1724 had encouraged a distrust of posthumous benevolence. Jealousy of Guy and rumours of his money-lending and miserly habits fuelled a concern about the 'dead hand' of charity that was never entirely shaken.[102] The 1736 Mortmain Act was the legal codification of this suspicion, strengthening testators' rights to overturn wills that left land to a charitable cause. Hardwicke, Lord Chief Justice in 1736, noted that the act was designed to prevent individuals from giving money in perpetuity

100 RCH, minutes of the house committee, 21 Sept. 1896, LMA, H33/RCH/A4/5.
101 *Hospital*, 6 Feb. 1892, 226.
102 Cameron, *Mr Guy's Hospital*, 13–34.

when they had not given during their lifetime, to ward against the 'locking-up' of land, and to prevent families from being disinherited. According to Andrew, this distrust of perpetual bequests had come to permeate the ethos of giving by the end of the eighteenth century. Those writing on philanthropy from the start of the nineteenth century certainly stressed that the charitable should give during their lifetime when they could control their benevolence, and a series of legal decisions under Lord Eldon's chancellorship strengthened the testators' position.[103] The Mortmain Act was modified in 1881 and 1891, but the desire to ensure that land was not 'locked-up' was maintained. Legislation and cultural trends in giving did have an effect. In 1890 the *Standard* noted that only one in seven testators left bequests, and most of those had no children.[104] A survey conducted by the *Daily Telegraph* in the following year found that only 13 per cent of all legacies went directly to charitable causes, though the proportion was higher among women.[105] Most large wills, however, did include some provision for philanthropy. Gifts in perpetuity were avoided; the aim was to assist the institution in the present by a cash gift that avoided all legal constraints.

The amounts left differed considerably. Between 1884 and 1898 the London received 660 legacies ranging from five guineas to an estate worth £119,423 from James Holden. Invariably bequests were given with no clear purpose in mind, but some had conditions attached. Lueade's legacy to St Bartholomew's mentioned above, or Jacob Gorfende's gift of £100 to the London in 1867 for the care of Jewish patients are just two examples.[106] However, where a clear purpose was stated it was usually in favour of the provision of aftercare through the hospital's convalescent home or Samaritan fund, which often depended on this source of funding. Governors did their best to attract legacies and frequently fought lengthy legal battles over contested wills: at Guy's the governors were even known to apply directly to the recently bereaved for funds. All bequests were dutifully acknowledged as governors sought to display the hospital's good fortune in the hope that other benefactors would follow their example. They were at pains, however, to avoid the impression that their hospital was a rich endowed institution for fear of discouraging charity. The poor wording of many bequests ensured that hospitals did not receive all the legacies they were entitled to, but in general the benevolent public favoured them.

The endowment of beds combined all these ways of giving. The arrangement was pioneered by the Hospital for Sick Children. In 1868 a collection of £1,000 raised by the *Aunt Judy Magazine* was awarded to the hospital. At the request of the editor, the money was 'invested' to support a bed and in

---

103 Andrew, *Philanthropy and police*, 46.
104 Ian Williams, *The alms trade: charities, past, present and future*, London 1989, 22–5; *Lancet* i (1890), 922.
105 Owen, *English philanthropy*, 470–1.
106 London Hospital, legacy book, LH, F/9/3.

recognition the governors named it the 'Aunt Judy Magazine cot'. Others quickly followed. The cost of endowing a bed was set at £1,000 and annual donations of £100 were accepted. In 1881 the first cot was funded by subscription, but most were created by bequest. In all between 1870 and 1900 seventy-four cots were endowed, the majority after 1890, while fourteen were funded by subscription.[107] With the addition of the 'Guildford Cot' in 1872 and the obvious success of the scheme, the British Medical Journal (BMJ) recommended that other hospitals should follow the Hospital for Sick Children's lead.[108] The practice was quickly adopted because it provided a guaranteed annual income and an attraction for large gifts. Guy's, because of its reliance on rental income, was one of the last major hospitals to adopt the practice and only in 1894 were two beds and one cot endowed.[109] The German Hospital, in contrast, refused to endow beds. When approached by the Woolwich German Club in 1867 the governors pointedly dismissed the suggestion, explaining that the hospital was a 'free' institution. A deterioration in the hospital's finances and pressure from benefactors eventually persuaded the governors to endow a bed in memory of Oscar van Ernsthausen in 1901.[110] Other hospitals, in urgent need of funds, could not afford to be so dogmatic and the endowment of beds became a common practice.

Subscriptions, donations and legacies were the traditional ways of collecting money from the benevolent public. However, to these must be added the 'endless variations and complications' of charitable funding.[111] Hospitals could not wait for philanthropists to favour them, so several active ways were employed to encourage benevolence. 'In order to stimulate the flow of funds', explained the Medical Times & Gazette in 1852, 'the charitable public is called upon to dine, to act, and to pray'.[112] One invention followed another and new devices were introduced mixing seriousness with entertainment. The Charity Record & Philanthropic News sardonically described charity's tactics as an 'amateur circus'. However, 'even the oldest and most meritorious of our philanthropic institutions would find itself completely neglected were it not continually to remind the public of its existence, either by festival, personal appeal, or effective advertisement'.[113] The Hospital disliked the fact that charitable organisations had to 'peg away' at benevolence, but many realised that despite the undignified nature of 'begging' it was often the only way to raise money.[114] Whereas specialist hospitals were singled out for their aggressive fundraising tactics, all hospitals survived by 'pleading in competi-

---

107 Hospital for Sick Children, register of special cots, GOSH, 6/1/25–7.
108 BMJ i (1872), 617.
109 Guy's Hospital, treasurer's report, LMA, H9/Gy/A94/1.
110 German Hospital, minutes of the board of household management, 19 Sept. 1867, SBH, GHA 8/5; papers concerning a bed endowment, GHB 10/21.
111 Quarterly Review clxxvii (1893), 466.
112 Medical Times & Gazette xxvi (1852), 39.
113 Charity Record & Philanthropic News ii (1882), 104.
114 Hospital, 6 Feb. 1892, 226.

tion'.[115] Although the rattling of boxes on street corners was viewed as undesirable and reminiscent of the worst excesses of street musicians, hospitals tried every money-raising tactic possible. The North West London Hospital, however, broke the law when it organised a 'Prize Distribution' in 1890. The initiative, though highly successful, collecting £1,500 in the first few weeks, was designated a lottery and declared technically illegal under the Lotteries Act. The governors, to avoid prosecution, were forced to return all the contributions.[116]

The pressure to contribute was unrelenting: 'it came from the pulpit and the platform, the reports and pamphlets of the charity societies, the numerous family and women's magazines' and especially from the press.[117] *The Times* devoted whole pages to advertisements from charitable societies and specialist journals were founded like the *Charity Record & Philanthropic Review* or *Charity*, which reflected charity's incessant advertising. Hospitals gradually developed more sophisticated methods. Both the London and the East London Hospital for Children incorporated the message 'Supported by Voluntary Contributions' into the facade to remind passers-by of the hospitals' charitable status.[118] The governors of the Royal Hospital for Diseases of the Chest were aware 'that publicity should be given to the charity': by the 1870s approximately 6 per cent of the hospital's expenditure was spent on advertising, and by the 1890s adverts were placed in fifteen different papers and journals.[119] The aim was to reach the largest possible audience. Not all campaigns met with approval, but the most common complaint was the frequency of adverts: 'day by day a column and a half of the most urgent advertisements assure the public that, unless immediate aid is given, half [the] wards must be shut up'.[120]

Hospitals extended their appeal beyond the press. Governors issued pamphlets with photographs showing pleasant wards, flowers and nurses to increase their hospital's public appeal. The effect was to multiply patient admissions and strain finances further. The Hospital for Sick Children was particularly good at this form of advertising. Dickens added his influential support shortly after the hospital opened in 1852 with his 'Darling Buds' in which he forcefully argued for the necessity of a children's hospital in London and recommended the Hospital for Sick Children to the public.[121] Others soon followed. Greenwood's *Little Bob in hospital* or Tom Hood's *Lilliput lodgers* explained the good work of the hospital in the most emotive terms.[122] The publication of *Suffering London* in 1892 took the same idea but extended the

[115] *BMJ* i (1892), 345.
[116] *Charity*, Jan. 1890, 205.
[117] Prochaska, *Women and philanthropy*, 39.
[118] Taylor, *Hospital and asylum architecture*, 34.
[119] RCH, minutes of the finance committee, LMA, H33/RCH/A5/2.
[120] *BMJ* (1860), 458.
[121] Kosky, *Mutual friends*, 4.
[122] Hospital for Sick Children, specimen appeals, GOSH, 14/18.

emotive appeal to cover every London hospital. In the wake of the Select Committee on Metropolitan Hospitals, it was a rare example of co-operation. The book was the idea of Henry Burdett, a leading expert on hospital charity and founder of the Hospitals Association.

From the 1870s onwards Burdett became synonymous with the voluntary hospital movement, playing a prominent role in the Sunday Fund, the Prince of Wales Hospital Fund and late nineteenth-century debates on the admission of paying patients and the relationship between hospitals and the state. In almost every issue affecting London's hospitals he was a prominent voice and an avid defender of the voluntary system. Burdett worked with the motto 'personal service to the sick in days of health' and became renowned for his business principles, financial acumen, expertise and bluntness. Bullying anyone who disagreed, he was often on better terms with the caged birds in his study than with his family or colleagues. As his influence grew in the 1880s he took to having a shorthand writer with him at meetings to prevent his blunt comments from being misquoted.[123] The son of a Leicestershire clergyman, Burdett had entered banking before being appointed superintendent of the Queen's Hospital, Birmingham. Within six years he had earned a considerable reputation having virtually doubled the hospital's income and as a result was made house governor of the ailing Seamen's Hospital, Greenwich. In a matter of years he had revitalised the hospital and trained several rising administrators. After a failed attempted to became a doctor, Burdett moved out of hospital administration to be secretary to the shares and loan department of the London stock exchange in 1881. Burdett, however, did not abandon his interest in hospital affairs. An avid sportsman and gambler, it was reputed that when he broke the bank of the casino in Monte Carlo he gave his winnings to the prince of Wales to be distributed to hospitals and other charitable causes.[124] Always willing to advise, he was regularly consulted but made enemies as quickly as he made friends, especially as he lacked patience with inefficient management. *Suffering London* was just one of his many projects. Burdett had persuaded a meeting of hospital secretaries in November 1891 that they should co-operate and produce a book to publicise the work and plight of the capital's hospitals. As a governor of a large number of London hospitals he had considerable leverage and it was probably this, rather than the possible benefits of the scheme, that made hospitals accept. Through Burdett's involvement a grant of £500 was secured from the Scientific Press. However, despite influential support, the venture had little impact on the financial problems facing the London hospitals and Burdett quickly

---

123 Prochaska, *Philanthropy and the hospitals of London*, 11; Rivett, *The London hospital system*, 373–4.
124 *Lancet* ii (1897), 1215–16; Christopher Maggs, *A century of change: story of the Royal National Pension Fund for Nurses*, London 1987, 13–22.

turned his attention to other projects to improve the metropolitan hospitals' income.[125]

The main purpose of publicity was to announce the hospital's financial needs and their public appeals. Appeals were launched at public meetings when the first collection was made and promises of support were received amid much publicity. They allowed hospitals to raise large amounts in a relatively short time. *The Times* was particularly impressed when the London collected £24,000 in a matter of months in 1860, but the hospital had a long history of using appeals to generate much-needed capital and was well suited to such efforts.[126] Appeals were often used to solve a particular financial problem or raise money for rebuilding. When Guy's faced a financial crisis in the early 1880s the governors launched a public appeal in 1886. Every effort was made to collect the largest amount possible and the governors exploited their connections to raise money. Messrs Louis Cohen and Messrs Bristowe Brothers purposefully went round the Stock Exchange collecting money and £256 4s. was collected from Lloyds. Within four months £56,000 had been raised.[127] At the Royal Hospital for Diseases of the Chest in 1891, after an uneasy start in October, an appeal brought in new subscribers 'almost daily' and by December £100 had been collected from this source.[128] Few hospitals, however, were as regular in their appeals as the London. The governors, worried that debt was becoming a constant feature of the hospital's finances, sought to circumvent the problem by founding a quinquennial appeal in 1878, legitimising a large funding drive every five years.[129] The move proved successful and each new appeal was widely supported.

Debt was recognised as an excellent opportunity for launching an appeal, a realisation shared by the NSPCC.[130] When Guy's launched its appeal in 1886 the governors stressed the hospital's financial plight. Responsibility was transferred from their financial management, which many critics considered responsible for the hospital's problems, to the effect the agricultural depression was having on the value of the hospital's landed estates and income.[131] More cynical observers felt that those running London's hospitals were deliberately irresponsible in their financial management in the hope that their financial problems would motivate more contributions. Patient numbers were paraded as each hospital attempted to display its public utility in quantitative terms. Often this led to the deliberate manipulation of statistics to produce the most favourable image. Frequently this backfired. Patients did die

---

[125] *Hospital*, 30 Apr. 1892, 70.
[126] *Times*, 7 May 1860, 9; London Hospital, annual report 1850, LH.
[127] Guy's Hospital, appeals cash book, LMA, H9/Gy/D45/1; *BMJ* i (1887), 739.
[128] *Charity Record* xi (1891), 393.
[129] London Hospital, minutes of the house committee, 29 Jan. 1878, LH, A/5/38.
[130] George K. Behlmer, *Child abuse and moral reform in England, 1870–1908*, Stanford, Ca. 1982, 142.
[131] Guy's Hospital, appeals cash book, LMA, H9/Gy/D45/1.

immediately after being discharged, resulting in scandals that greatly affected income.[132]

The regularity of appeals became a distressing feature of hospital finance in London, matching the incessant charitable activity in other cities and tiring the patience of the public.[133] Governors nevertheless continued to launch appeals because help was always forthcoming in response to their 'pathetic' pleas for support.[134] By the late 1860s only three of the twelve general hospitals in London did not have to make continuous calls on the public.[135] A further spate of appeals in the early 1880s created concern that the charitable nexus of hospital funding was beginning to break down. Under these conditions, philanthropists began to fear that the state might have to intervene to prevent the widespread closure of beds. Governors, as shown in chapter 7, willingly used this fear to encourage further contributions, drawing on the hostility civil society felt towards state intervention.

Appeals, however, were limited by their very nature. Governors could not constantly launch appeals for fear that they would antagonise the public and discourage contributions. To maintain an annual influx of charitable contributions hospitals organised an annual dinner or ball. Philanthropists, as Prochaska observes, tried to make the act of giving a pleasurable occupation and the annual dinner was a successful formula.[136] From the foundation of the voluntary hospitals in the eighteenth century, governors had held an annual dinner and they became the focus of the hospital's year, both socially and financially. Even St Bartholomew's, which as an old endowed hospital did not have to attract philanthropy until the start of the twentieth century, organised periodic dinners. Dinners at St Bartholomew's, like those at the voluntary hospitals, had an inherent fundraising aspect. They were seen as 'a well chosen opportunity' to enable 'many of the Tenants to learn the vast amount of good which the punctual payment of rents ensured to the Poor Patients'.[137] The Charity Record & Philanthropic Messenger understood that dinners were often the only way to persuade more reluctant supporters to contribute, but not all journals were entirely sympathetic. Charity carried a scurrilous attack on how these dinners often degenerated into an excuse for social snobbery, gluttony and false appeals.[138] Dinners were seen as a burden 'on the time and patience of public men', but their highly successful nature made them impossible to abandon.[139] The governors of the German Hospital

132 Abel-Smith, The hospitals, 39–40.
133 Neil Evans, 'Urbanisation, elite attitudes and philanthropy: Cardiff, 1850–1914', International Review of Social History xxvii (1982), 308.
134 Nursing Record, 5 Mar. 1898, 199.
135 Lancet ii (1866), 730.
136 Prochaska, Voluntary impulse, 47.
137 St Bartholomew's, minutes of the board of governors, 14 Jan. 1862, SBH, Ha 1/22.
138 Charity Record & Philanthropic Messenger, June 1868, 138; Charity, Apr./May 1891, 285–7.
139 Times, 9 June 1868, 12.

reflected a widespread opinion when they noted in 1858 that without an annual dinner and the influx of donations it produced, they would not have been able to meet the hospital's 'liabilities'.[140]

The dinner was an important occasion that demanded long and careful planning, and invariably a special subcommittee was formed to relieve the main managing body of the work. Governors were anxious that everything should go to plan as the event reflected on the hospital. When the governors of the London felt they had been treated badly by the Hotel Cecil in 1868 they demanded a 3s. reduction per head.[141] Planning was meticulous and expensive. At the Royal Hospital for Diseases of the Chest the 1883 dinner cost £481 to organise, but it was worth it as it raised a total of £4,384.[142] Many hotels and meeting rooms offered special rates as a successful event often brought hospitals back to the same venue year after year. To meet some of the initial organisational cost tickets were sold and guests were invited to attend. University College Hospital, for example, sold tickets in 1897 for one guinea per head; the only free invitations went to 'various newspapers' for publicity purposes.[143] Prominent members of civil society were invited to speak, and governors initially aimed high before dropping their sights until a speaker was found. Lord Shaftesbury and the prince of Wales regularly had to decline invitations because of the sheer number of dinners they were invited to address. Speakers were called upon to praise the crown, the country, the army and the hospital. They were followed by rousing speeches made by the hospital's governors and doctors that praised the institution's good work and lamented its financial difficulties. Once the annual report and the financial statement had been read, thanks were given to the hospital's medical staff, and finally the 'plate' was passed round. The intention was to motivate a captive and well-wined and dined audience to new heights of generosity. The annual dinner became an institution that was carefully manipulated for funding purposes.

Sermons on a hospital's behalf were a more sombre and thoughtful way of raising money. The charitable sermon fitted easily with many Victorian churches' interest in the 'civilising mission' and need to provide or encourage social services.[144] By lending their support to a local hospital both these interests could be served at once while at the same time demonstrating that the church could be a broker between rich and poor and a solution to fears about a breakdown in social harmony. The hospital sermon in many ways 'articulated the hopes and motives of their audiences'.[145] The activities of the Met-

---

140 German Hospital, annual report 1858, SBH.
141 London Hospital, minutes of the house committee, June 1868, LH, A/5/34.
142 RCH, council minute book, 15 Mar. 1883, LMA, H33/RCH/A1/5.
143 UCH, subcommittee minutes, 2 Dec. 1897, UCL, A1/5/2.
144 Jeffrey Cox, *English churches in a secular society: Lambeth, 1870–1930*, Oxford 1982; Yeo, *Religion and voluntary organisations*.
145 Andrew, *Philanthropy and police*.

ropolitan Hospital Sunday Fund in 1873 (see below) did serve to reduce the number of hospital sermons, but church collections for individual hospitals continued. Governors persuaded prominent bishops to preach on the hospitals' behalf and local clergy were constantly reminded of their duties to the local hospital. The London in 1869 wrote to 'all the clergy of the neighbourhood' to remind them that they should give 'an Annual Sermon on behalf of the London Hospital'.[146] At a local level hospital sermons became a regular, even annual feature of the local community, but the amounts collected were invariably small. The largest amount raised by a sermon for University College Hospital was £100 11s. 9d. in 1852 at St Pancras church, but in general collections were rarely over £20.[147]

Variations existed on these active forms of fundraising. Philanthropists put on musical programmes, recitals and plays for the hospital and gave the profits as a donation. Organisation and responsibility remained with the hospital's supporters and governors preferred to keep their distance. When the governors of the Royal Hospital for Diseases of the Chest accepted an offer from an amateur dramatics club for their fundraising programme of performances, they did so only with the proviso that it would involve no additional cost to the hospital. It was a realistic request as one play for the German Hospital in 1887 made a loss of £20 which the governors were asked to meet.[148] The nature of entertainments varied widely and most were of an amateur nature. University College Hospital benefited from a play, a recital and a concert held on its behalf in 1883 alone, while Guy's welcomed the £130 raised by the Anomalies Amateur Dramatics Club in 1896.[149] Not all offers were accepted. The German Hospital resisted any attempt to hold an event in its name after 1887, while the governors of the Hospital for Sick Children disapproved of amateur dramatic performances and preferred the more professional offer of the West End play 'Sweepstake' in 1891.[150] These rebuffs did not discourage philanthropists. There was always one hospital glad to accept any money raised by these means.

The most innovative and widely criticised form of active fundraising was the charity bazaar. Modelled on the commercial bazaars that had become popular in the 1820s as an urban variant on the rural market, the number of charity bazaars increased in line with the urban population and competition between voluntary organisations eagerly trying to find new fundraising activities. Popularity and fashion were not enough to prevent bazaars from being criticised and ridiculed. Churches warned of 'a vigorous inconsiderate benevolence, which is not indeed benevolence, but only a more specious

---

146 London Hospital, minutes of the house committee, 27 Apr. 1869, LH, A/5/34.
147 UCH, annual report 1897, UCL.
148 RCH, council minute book, 9 Jan. 1879, LMA, H33/RCH/A1/5; German Hospital, minutes of the house committee, 12 May 1887, SBH, GHA 2/8.
149 UCH, minutes of the finance committee, 2 Nov. 1883, UCL, A1/3/3; Guy's Hospital, minutes of the court of committees, 22 Feb. 1896, LMA, H9/Gy/A3/11.
150 Hospital for Sick Children, press cuttings, GOSH, 8/153.

form of selfishness', while organisers of commercial bazaars saw them as unfair competition and an attack on their livelihoods. Hospitals ignored these slights and energetically embraced the bazaar as part of their fundraising activities; even the godly had to admit that 'large sums are frequently raised by these means'.[151]

Bazaars fitted within the practice of active fundraising and fulfilled subscribers' desires 'to have something to show for [their] money'.[152] The benevolent were encouraged to donate a wide range of gifts and then attend the bazaar to buy articles of a similar nature. In some cases an internal economy was created and goods purchased at one bazaar were given to another. Subcommittees that had been formed to organise dinners were converted into bazaar committees and their accumulated experience was transferred into this new flexible fundraising format. Bazaars capitalised on their entertainment value, synthesising duty with shopping, so that in Robert Louis Stevenson's words they gave 'a direct and emphatic sense of gain'. It was an ideal entertainment for the leisured classes and organisers spared no effort in devising new attractions to create a carnival atmosphere 'to make the exercise of charity entertaining in itself'.[153] Cornhill Magazine described a typical bazaar in 1861:

> the bazaar is held in a large marquee which is surrounded by stalls and gaily decked out with ribbons, wreaths and flags, and covered with merchandise; and numberless young ladies preside at the stalls, dressed in the height of fashion, and never cease to attract public attention to the goods with the most winning, coaxing, insinuating, and, if one may be allowed the expression, wheedling ways.[154]

When the German Hospital held its first bazaar in 1848 dignitaries were invited from Germany and England and the items that were put on sale were collected through donations from across Europe. A subcommittee had been formed in 1846 to plan the bazaar, but the work strained the hospital's management resources and a special ladies committee was appointed in 1847 to help in the final arrangements. The bazaar, initially scheduled for 1847, was postponed until 1848 after the Irish famine aroused fears that money might not be forthcoming. The governors' meticulous organisation was not unusual, though the European scope of the hospital's appeal was indicative of the institution's immigrant character.[155] Planning was beset with problems and often frustrated by unforeseen obstacles, but in later years the hospital's bazaars were arranged with greater speed as experience was accumulated. University

---

[151] Frank K. Prochaska, 'Charity bazaars in nineteenth-century England', *Journal of British Studies* xvi (1976/7), 63, 81–4.
[152] *Hospital*, 17 Aug. 1895, 349.
[153] Robert Louis Stevenson, *Charity bazaar: an allegorical dialogue*, London 1868.
[154] Anon. [Robert Louis Stevenson], 'A charity bazaar', *Cornhill Magazine* iv (1861), 339.
[155] German Hospital, minutes of the bazaar committee, 18 Mar. 1847, SBH, GHA 14/1.

College Hospital's bazaar in 1886, after three decades of experience, took only four months to organise, though the bazaar committee met nearly every week. Plans quickly escalated. To the 135ft run of stalls draped in yellow and white and banners proclaiming 'Success to the University Hospital', marionettes, a Punch and Judy show, fortune tellers, light refreshments, artistic performances by the college's Amateur Dramatics Society and a fish-pond were added. Police were positioned inside and outside to maintain order, though the entrance fee of 5s. on the first two days ensured that only the most respectable gained admission.[156] The governors of the German Hospital felt that such an atmosphere was unwise. In 1869 they rejected solo performers as 'they would too greatly attract the attention of the public and consequently stop the progress of the sale'.[157] Bazaars were after all designed to raise money, not solely to provide charitable entertainment, as this was merely a means to an end.

The financial rewards were invariably worth the organisational effort: in 1898 the London's Press Bazaar added some £12,000 to the hospital's ailing funds and the German Hospital's 1867 bazaar was important in removing the debt that had burdened the institution since rebuilding.[158] In combining commerce with amusement, charity bazaars were popular, fashionable and highly profitable. More time was devoted to the organisation of them than to the hospitals' day-to-day management and in comparison the arrangements for the annual dinner seemed trivial. Royal and aristocratic patronage gave these events a patina of respectability and provided an important attraction. Strenuous efforts were made to have a member of the aristocracy open the bazaar, though for the London hospitals, with their high profile and aristocratic support, this was less of a problem than for smaller charities. At the German Hospital this was utilised to the full and personal contacts created a network of support that extended across Europe. However, the organisation and publicity needed ensured that though bazaars became a regular feature of the benevolent economy, for individual institutions they remained a periodic spectacle. Given philanthropy's competitive nature, it was often easier to organise a charitable ball or dinner where the appeal could be directed to existing supporters, leaving bazaars as an important but infrequent source of funding.

Collections provided a more regular source of charitable income. Governors aimed to stimulate donations by placing collection boxes in the hospital and throughout London. Boxes in out-patients' departments generated much interest as it was believed that they reflected contributions from the grateful

---

156 UCH, subcommittee minutes, UCL, A1/5/1: five shillings seems to have been a standard entrance fee for bazaars, helping to maximise the hospitals' income even if nothing was bought, though this was difficult in itself as 'customers' were assailed from every quarter and stall holders were not above a certain element of dishonesty.
157 German Hospital, minutes of the bazaar committee, 29 Apr. 1869, SBH, GHA 14/2.
158 London Hospital, minutes of the house committee, 11 July 1898, LH, A/5/47.

and 'deserving' poor. By 1888 the Royal Hospital for Diseases of the Chest had some 1,027 boxes in London, but they raised little money.[159] Outside the hospital individuals arranged collections; plates were passed around at meetings and Catherine Gladstone, whose husband was to become prime minister, even extended this to her breakfast parties. Most were on a more organised basis. Although governors did not adopt the door-to-door techniques of the Bible Society, they did try to encourage collections, especially at a local level. Contemporaries disapproved of noisy street collections, but the governors of the Royal Hospital for Diseases of the Chest had no qualms in taking money collected in the local public houses.

The London and University College Hospital attempted to organise these collections on a systematic basis. Unlike the Sunday Fund and Saturday Fund (discussed below) these collections were highly localised and limited to one hospital. The first systematic hospital collection scheme was started in 1868 in Whitechapel to aid the London. In April an independent organisation called the People's Five Shillings Subscription Fund started to make inquiries about the admissions' rights that could be given to 'small' subscribers. The governors agreed to allow three out-patient admissions for every annual subscription of one guinea from the organisation.[160] The fund aimed to allow those 'who may come to the Hospital for Medical or Surgical aid' to 'subscribe directly through their Firms or their Clubs to the maintenance of the Institution' and it set about organising collections in the surrounding factories and firms and among local working-class organisations.[161] The People's Subscription Fund became a semi-autonomous body with an organisation separate from the hospital, though the governors paid the collector 25s. per week from 1870 onwards.[162] At first the amounts raised were small, but after 1878 the fund's contributions began to increase, mirroring the rising popularity and success of the Saturday Fund. The governors, however, only ever found the work of the fund 'satisfactory' and made few references to it in their minutes, though they acknowledged its support in their annual reports.

University College Hospital developed a similar scheme in 1877, but here the governors and chiefly Newton Nixon, the hospital's secretary, retained the guiding influence. Nixon had gained his administrative experience at the London School Board before he was appointed to University College Hospital. Both ambitious and dedicated to the hospital, which he visited daily, he was in favour of any scheme that would increase the hospital's income and make it more efficient. Nixon's recommendations to the governors in November 1877 presented the scheme as one that would encourage self-help, allowing workers to contribute towards the cost of their own future medical

---

[159] RCH, minutes of the finance committee, LMA, H33/RCH/A5/1.
[160] London Hospital, minutes of the house committee, 26 May 1868, LH, A/5/34.
[161] London Hospital, annual report 1899, LH.
[162] London Hospital, minutes of the house committee, 13 Dec. 1870, LH, A/5/35.

care.[163] The People's Contribution Fund aimed to facilitate the 'appointment of annual and life governors amongst the tradesmen and the working classes, in order to place in their own hands the facilities for obtaining hospital treatment'. It also hoped to 'increase the annual income of the charity, by creating an interest in the prosperity of the hospital amongst those for whose benefit it is intended'.[164] An altruistic rhetoric did not conceal a desire to reduce social tension. The intention behind the fund was purely financial, an opportunity carefully controlled by the governors to raise money from the working classes that did not offend the subscription rights of middle-class supporters. Local groups under middle-class leadership were set up throughout London to stimulate working-class contributions and collection boxes were widely distributed. No contribution was too small and the fund proved highly successful.

Attempts to organise such schemes at a metropolitan level produced a new type of giving that partially redefined the role of individual benevolence. The foundation of the Metropolitan Hospital Sunday Fund in 1873 signified a new departure in hospital funding; it was the first in a series of benevolent funds that culminated in the Prince of Wales Hospital Fund for London. The Sunday Fund set the pattern for others to follow. Of these the Metropolitan Hospital Saturday Fund proved the most successful. Others like the Football Fund never progressed beyond the planning stage. Together they represented the most innovative source of hospital funding and a new form of benevolence through 'indirect' philanthropy, where the individual ceded the right to control the destination of the gift to an investigating organisation. The work of the Saturday Fund is discussed in the following chapter along with the fund's financial contribution to the London hospitals, but to illustrate the aims and ambitions behind the benevolent funds the Sunday Fund is explained here.

The Sunday Fund was not unique. It fitted within an existing pattern of charitable societies and provincial collecting schemes. Despite the rival claims of the unknown Mr Henn, the movement was inspired by Thomas Barber Wright in Birmingham.[165] As proprietor of the *Midland Counties Herald* he used the paper to launch a public fund in 1859 to aid the Birmingham General Hospital.[166] Wright's scheme was pioneering in that he subtly changed the nature and intention of the appeal. The idea was simple: one Sunday a year was to be set aside to collect money from every place of worship in the locality. The income raised would then be distributed according to the 'needs and merits' of the local medical charities.[167] Sympathetic clergy had traditionally dedicated church collections to individual hospitals, but under a

163 UCH, minutes of the general committee, 21 Nov. 1877, UCL, A1/2/4.
164 *BMJ* i (1880), 903.
165 *Hospital*, 13 Oct. 1894, 33.
166 Ibid. 17 Nov. 1888, 99.
167 Owen, *English philanthropy*, 485.

fund these contributions were redirected away from a single institution to an organisation that co-ordinated sermons, universalised support and redistributed collections as a solution to the medical charities' perceived financial difficulties. The pulpit was co-opted to preach the gospel of hospital funding, systematically publicising medical relief to motivate benevolence. It was envisaged that a fund would encourage reform, as distribution was to be placed in the hands of a scrutinising committee that would identify any problems and penalise hospitals accordingly. Hospitals, it was hoped, would reform, if only to improve the size of their awards.

James Wakley, editor of the radical *Lancet*, recognised in the Birmingham scheme a system through which the London hospitals' endemic financial crisis could be resolved within a framework that encouraged wider reform. From 1869 he called for the national extension of the Birmingham movement, stressing the moral benefits of community action and the practical advantages of ensuring that hospitals remained adequately funded. Donations to such a fund, it was argued, removed the sick poor from those 'permanently chargeable on the poor rates' by guaranteeing effective hospital treatment and a quick return to work, thus playing on one of the hospital's main attractions.[168] Wakley's agitation initially had no immediate impact in London, but spurred further provincial collections. When representatives from the London hospitals finally met they were uncertain and inclined to believe that a fund would 'lead to a falling-off in annual subscriptions and dinner collections'.[169] Hospitals jealously guarded their independence and no governor was prepared to propose a plan that would potentially benefit another institution over his own. It was also widely doubted whether Christianity could make such a firm commitment when London faced spiritual destitution. An increased awareness of social inequality, a growing desire to be free from puritan restraints and a revulsion against orthodox theology were prompting a transformation in religion. Simultaneously there was a fall in the size of congregations and many felt that the Church itself needed reforming before religion could help the hospital.[170] However, congregations did offer their support, whether enthusiastically or not, and in doing so ensured the success of the Sunday Fund. This can be explained by the moves churches and chapels made to secularise their appeal. They moved into the community and reoriented recreation on moral grounds through leisure activities, clubs and associations in which the religious meaning was subverted by the need to hold the congregation together.[171] The Sunday Fund was part of this attempt to place organised religion on a new and popular footing. Church and Chapel benefited by associating themselves with practical benevolence in an 'irreve-

---

[168] *Lancet* ii (1869), 781.
[169] Ibid. i (1872), 624.
[170] Hugh McLeod, *Class and religion in the late Victorian city*, London 1974, 285.
[171] See Yeo, *Religion and voluntary organisation*; Brian Harrison, 'Religion and recreation in nineteenth-century England', *Past and Present* xxxviii (1967), 98–125.

rent age' and the fund acted as an additional means of involving the church in the neighbourhood while upholding the sanctity of the Sabbath for the good of the community.[172]

The Sunday Fund served another purpose for Church and Chapel. According to Kent, urban Anglicanism was moving towards a common identity with other religious institutions.[173] The fund could be projected by more enlightened ministers as a means of establishing interdenominational co-operation to counter the heated debates within Christianity that threatened the social power of religion. Benevolent societies such as the British and Foreign Bible Society had been used to create a consensus for religious co-operation, but charity to the sick poor had a wider appeal.[174] It was uncomplicated, fitted within established Christian doctrines and was easy to support. By common association in a benevolent fund without political connotations and sympathetic to all denominations, co-operation could be seen as an attempt to jettison differences and provide a modicum of ecumenical collaboration in dealing with one of society's more pressing problems.

How much these views influenced the participating congregations is uncertain. Sir Sydney Waterlow, the then lord mayor of London and treasurer of St Bartholomew's, certainly believed that part of the motivation behind the Fund was to 'help people to believe that, though there were religious differences, they had still a common ground of action and a common object which all might promote'.[175] Waterlow was ideally placed to express this conviction. From an unsectarian background and with considerable connections to London's churches, he had already established himself as a hard but influential London philanthropist. Waterlow was obstinate and wilful from youth. From an apprenticeship to the Stationers' Company he had built up the family printing firm by exploiting the railway companies' demand for printing. Aware of the need for sound management he associated philanthropy with business, arguing that practical schemes were vital because charity was not 'the thing British working men will ask for, nor, save in the last extremity, accept'. With an unwavering faith in voluntarism, he liked to deal with suffering on a grand scale and the Sunday Fund fulfilled this interest. According to the prince of Wales, few men had done more for the London poor 'and none have asked or expected less in recognition of their service'.[176]

Waterlow's first interest was not hospitals but the philanthropic housing movement. He quickly became an authority on working-class housing needs

---

172 *Hospital*, 21 Jan. 1893, 260.
173 J. Kent, 'The role of religion in the cultural structure of the late Victorian city', *Transactions of the Royal Historical Society* xxiii (1973), 159; Currie, *Methodism divided*, 176–85.
174 See R. H. Martin, *Evangelicals united: ecumenical stirrings in pre-Victorian Britain, 1795–1830*, London 1983.
175 *Times*, 17 Jan. 1873, 8; Morris, *Class, sect and party*, argues that voluntary organisations served as a class unifier and even when divided on religious grounds they created parallel organisations which provided common experiences.
176 G. Smalley, *The life of Sir Sydney H. Waterlow*, London 1909, 9–85, 199, 3.

and was included at a parliamentary level in discussions on housing. His enthusiasm for housing and practical benevolence combined in the Improved Industrial Dwellings Company, founded in 1860 in the wake of his work to house some eighty families in Finsbury where he had been born. Through his political influence, the 1866 Labouring Classes Dwellings House Act empowered the Public Works Loans Commission to lend money for labourers' dwellings and Waterlow secured preferential funding for his company in his bid to provided oases 'of wholesomeness in some dirty desert of dingy and rickety buildings'. Wohl estimates that Waterlow's Company housed some 30,000 people where it was most needed, though he was primarily interested in only helping the 'deserving' poor.[177] Hospitals proved his second passion. His position as treasurer of St Bartholomew's, a sickly childhood and early wish to become a doctor may have encouraged his interest, though he was already familiar with the problem of healthcare having served as a member of the central London Sick Asylums District. Waterlow was also an ambitious man who wanted to promote great causes and the Sunday Fund represented an ideal organisation that built on his business and religious contacts. Of all the organisations he was involved in, he claimed to be most satisfied with the fund.[178] Wakley provided the journalistic support; Waterlow the organisational effort. His forceful character and desire to get his own way overcame the hospitals' practical opposition and established the Sunday Fund in London.

It was not until November 1872 that a meeting of hospital representatives was convened. This established a provisional committee to test the practicality of founding a fund in London. By this point a consensus had started to develop as governors became aware that their increasingly insecure economic position was not a temporary phenomenon. Waterlow's view that the movement 'had not heard a single objection against it' was, however, clearly erroneous. Considerable animosity surrounded these early efforts and Waterlow worked tirelessly to organise an administration committee, which was finally established in January 1873. The committee's discussions and Waterlow's control established in advance the basic organisational principles. Hospital governors were consulted, but much to the BMJ's annoyance the medical profession was excluded, a reflection of doctors' marginal role in the debate over hospital funding. The members of the committee, who were among London's leading financiers, businessmen, politicians and philanthropists and often friends of Waterlow, ensured that organisation was on strict commercial grounds. 250 invitations were issued to the clergy for a conference on 16 January 1873 to launch the fund and each minister was asked to invite a layman to avoid clerical dominance. The conference was a success

---

[177] Enid Gauldie, *Cruel habitations: a history of working-class housing*, London 1974, 259–61; Anthony S. Wohl, *The eternal slum: housing and social policy in Victorian England*, London 1977, 175, 149–51.
[178] Smalley, *Waterlow*, 194.

and endorsed all of the provisional committee's plans, re-appointing it as a management committee to organise the first collection.[179] A few West End parishes complained that the administrative task was too large and the bishop of London made last-minute recommendations to postpone the collection after fears were raised that the fund might damage parish collections. The fund, however, having already set the date for the first collection was determined not to make any alterations.[180]

The first collection was not as impressive as the organisers had envisaged, raising £27,700, a sum far below the *Spectator*'s estimate of £80,000. The result was nevertheless heralded as a triumph. *The Times* congratulated the fund, but *The Lancet* was disappointed. It continued to campaign ardently for the movement, establishing a special supplement in 1886 to publicise the fund, but the anticipated collection of £50,000 *per annum* proved elusive and the journal periodically lamented that more could not be achieved. Other contemporaries were more caustic. Critics saw in the fund a challenge to the role of the active citizen and predicted that consequently hospitals' charitable resources would fall. To discredit the movement, the *Saturday Review* labelled it 'bastard benevolence', arguing that the Sunday Fund allowed contributors to ease their conscience while giving no thought to the object. It went on to claim that the fund's managers were an 'irresponsible body of administrators'.[181] The *Charity Record & Philanthropic News* proved a more constant antagonist. It believed that the Sunday Fund produced no real benefit and deemed it a 'failure', despite publishing contradictory statements.[182] Antagonism stemmed partly from the fact that the journal was a firm supporter of the fund's competitor, the Saturday Fund, and although it was sympathetic to the Sunday Fund's intentions, nothing it did met with its approval.

By 1881 criticisms had largely abated. Subscriptions and donations had not fallen as feared but continued to rise. For hospitals, as long as administration and expenditure were kept within pre-defined boundaries, a grant was almost guaranteed. The Sunday Fund universalised support and *The Lancet* believed that it transcended the 'exclusive care of the wealthy and aristocratic classes of society'.[183] The fact that the fund could be projected as a solution to social tensions was a useful by-product that was not part of the original founders' intentions. However, it was used to improve the fund's status. In effect the Sunday Fund had succeeded in making hospitals more visible to the public and became 'one of the most important sources of income that many of the London hospitals possess'.[184] It allowed a greater

---

179 *Times*, 11 Jan. 1873, 6; 17 Jan. 1873, 8.
180 *Lancet* i (1873), 280.
181 Ibid. 882.
182 *Charity Record & Philanthropic News* vii (1887), 120; viii (1888), 200.
183 *Lancet* ii (1882), 126.
184 Ibid. i (1896), 1613.

number to contribute, but removed the traditional benefits of subscription. This is perhaps why indirect philanthropy could never replace direct philanthropy's financial contribution. Many subscribers wanted more than a feeling that they had helped the sick poor and the fund failed to offer rights to individual subscribers though it extended a limited number of letters to congregations.

The stimulants to charity, the balls, the bazaars and the Sunday Fund, were designed to raise money, but benevolence was not limited to acts of materialism. Where the majority were content to ease their philanthropic conscience by giving a few shillings, others donated their time. The Hospital lamented in 1887 that more people could not be encouraged to take an active interest in hospital management, but explained that those who did gave their time with energy and enthusiasm.[185] The donation of time is not easy to quantify, but like monetary support it had its material benefits. Men like Waterlow, Sir Francis Goldsmid, Jewish financier and chairman of University College Hospital, Samuel Whitford, secretary to the Hospital for Sick Children, and Edmund Lushington, the headstrong treasurer of Guy's, were indefatigable. Similar figures could be found in every London hospital. For example, at the German Hospital between 1845 and 1898, 135 men served on the management committee. Levels of involvement varied, though after 1855 the length of active participation increased and most sat on committees for at least three years, often longer. Some were more noticeable than others: Arthur Allen served on the board of management from 1863 to 1910; J. Satow, during his appointment from 1848 to 1872, constantly visited the wards and attended meetings. Adolphus Walbaum matched Satow's commitment. Pastor of the Hamburg Lutheran Church in Trinity Lane, from 1845 to 1890 he was also the hospital's chaplain and house secretary, present at almost every meeting and a guiding influence in the administration.[186] Long and active service was not unique to the German Hospital. It could be found at the Hospital for Sick Children or the Royal Hospital for Diseases of the Chest. Without these men many London hospitals would not have been founded, and certainly would not have been able to function at the level they did. Philanthropy in this respect remained crucial.

Philanthropy was no simple phenomenon. The motivations for supporting a medical charity were made up of a number of inspirations that could exist simultaneously in the philanthropists' act of giving, combining altruism with self-interest and duty. No two philanthropists were inspired by the same concerns or the same set of circumstances, and each gave of his own accord. Hospitals responded with an equally diverse range of fundraising activities that were designed to stimulate charity, make benevolence enjoyable and direct it to the hospital. Governors sought to combine activities, relying on

---

[185] Hospital, 26 Mar. 1887, 429.
[186] German Hospital, list of committee members, 1845–1918, SBH, GHA 21/1.

no single tactic, as often novelty was the key to success. Other charitable societies adopted similar techniques, but hospitals were one of the most effective at generating support. The result was an endless stream of fundraising activities.

This activity raises important questions about the extent of charitable support. How important was direct philanthropy in funding the hospital? Did all hospitals rely on charity for their income? How did charity's contributions change over time? What other resources could hospitals draw on? It is to these questions that the next chapter turns in a discussion of charity and hospital finance.

3

Paying for the Sick Poor

Victorians were convinced that theirs was a 'land of charity'.[1] Sydney Waterlow, from his position as chairman of the Metropolitan Hospital Sunday
Fund, felt that the potential for charitable contribution was limitless, but
hospital governors were all too aware that benevolence was a finite resource.
They continued, however, to hope that philanthropy would meet all their
financial needs. When the governors of the Royal Hospital for Diseases of the
Chest launched a special building appeal in 1893, it was expected that 'charity would put [its] shoulder to the wheel'.[2] The governors of University College Hospital shared a similar faith, believing that their £14,000 deficit would
be cleared by Queen Victoria's golden jubilee in 1887.[3] However, there was 'a
limit to the generosity of even the most benevolently disposed persons' that
even the most vigorous fundraising could not overcome.[4] A survey in the
Medical Times & Gazette in 1864 found that 46 per cent of the London hospitals' income came from voluntary sources.[5] A similar investigation by the
Charity Organisation Society (COS) in 1910 reported that the level of philanthropic support had only risen by 1.7 per cent.[6] Other contemporaries
reached similar conclusions and illustrated that London's hospitals were not
entirely supported by voluntary contributions.[7] Governors, preoccupied with
the problems of finance, knew that charitable income was at best precarious
and they erratically supplemented philanthropy with other sources of
funding.

Each hospital's financial structure was strongly influenced by the resources
available to it within London's benevolent economy and by the accepted
notions of hospital funding. Rarely did institutions step outside these
boundaries to solve their economic problems. Unlike the National Society
and the British Foreign School Society (which had accepted building grants
from Grey's Whig government), hospitals retained their firm faith in an undi-
luted voluntarism and saw government assistance as anathema. Even when
they appeared to face considerable economic problems from the 1880s
onwards only those on the margins of reform suggested that the state should

1 *Hospital*, 2 Feb. 1889, 278.
2 *Charity Record & Philanthropic News* ii (1882), 13; xiii (1893), 102.
3 *Charity*, Aug. 1887, 60.
4 *Charity Record & Philanthropic News* iii (1883), 40.
5 *Medical Times & Gazette* ii (1864), 98.
6 Loch, *Charity and social life*, 487–8.
7 See appendix on classification and the method of calculating hospital income.

intervene. In the Victorian hospital sector the boundaries between civil society and the state were firmly drawn. It was not until the 1920s that the possibility of limited state funding became a temporary reality. Every other available resource, however, was exploited, though funding remained 'to a great extent a matter of chance and speculation'.[8]

There were 'great differences in [hospitals'] modes of raising income' and each institution's financial make-up was partly conditioned by its location, age and nature.[9] However, using the evidence available from individual hospitals it is possible to reconstruct their finances. Hospitals drew their income from five principal types of funding: from direct and indirect philanthropy, from property and investments, from the hospitals' function as a medical institution, and from loans. Hospital finance was not a matter of dependence on any one type of funding, but a reliance on several related sources of income that together made up an individual hospital's structure of funding.

Funding the hospital: charitable income

All hospitals, even those with a large endowed income, received some money from charity. A tension, however, existed between the governors' incessant fundraising and the amount of money available from within London's benevolent economy. Although contemporaries worried about annual fluctuations in subscriptions and donations, the charitable resources available to London's voluntary sector in theory expanded with an increase in Britain's GNP, which stood at £642m. in 1855 and £1,459m. in 1895.[10] An expanding economy was just part of the reason why more money was being made available for philanthropy. A rise in the standard of living, caused by falling prices, a reduction in family size and an increase in middle-class incomes, freed more money for charity, though donations failed to rise as fast as national income.[11] All sections of society gave, but some contributed more than others. The 'insecurity of working-class income' and the importance of middle-class and professional occupations in London ensured that voluntary societies were funded mainly by the middle classes. The same was true outside London and where there was a small middle class, as in Cardiff, philanthropic activity could be stunted.[12] On average middle-class families spent 10.7 per cent of their income on charity by the 1890s, a larger proportion of their income than that

8 *BMJ* ii (1892), 31.
9 *Times*, 26 Apr. 1878, 9.
10 Charles H. Feinstein, *Statistical tables of national income, expenditure and output of the United Kingdom, 1855–1965*, Cambridge 1976, table 1, T4–5.
11 J. A. Banks, *Prosperity and parenthood: a study of family planning among the Victorian middle classes*, Aldershot 1954, 104–13, 132–4.
12 Paul Johnson, *Saving and spending: the working-class economy in Britain, 1870–1939*, Oxford 1985, 219; Richard H. Trainor, 'Peers on an industrial frontier: the earls of Dartmouth

Table 1: Income from charity by institution, 1892

Type	No.	Total income	Charitable income	%
General	21	£185,137	£139,151	75.2
Chest	5	£31,445	£25,842	82.2
Children's	11	£28,002	£20,235	72.3
Lying-in	4	£9,203	£2,757	29.9
Women's	6	£13,373	£13,263	99.2
Other specialist	20	£40,624	£25,873	64.7
Convalescent	15	£21,154	£8,251	39.0
Cottage	6	£2,180	£825	37.8
Other	5	£13,432	£5,425	40.4
TOTAL	93	£344,550	£241,622	70.1

Source: Hake, *Suffering London*

contributed by mid Victorian provincial aristocrats.[13] Their stable commitment to voluntarism was reflected in the amounts middle-class families left to charity. Small charitable bequests in the late seventeenth and early eighteenth century were replaced by gifts to Victorian hospitals of a larger average size.[14] The unpredictable nature of bequests makes them an inaccurate barometer of wealth, but they do reflect an increase in middle-class charitable expenditure. For the middle classes, charity came to represent a form of voluntary 'taxation' that was less controversial and seemed less oppressive than the state's fundraising. The trend towards more support for London's benevolent organisations was not a smooth one however. If the amount contributed to charitable organisations rose from £1,022,846 to £2,150,000 between 1850 and 1910, an increase in the number of charities ensured that it was spread between a greater number of voluntary organisations, reducing the impact of this rise for individual societies.[15]

A rise in charitable income within the benevolent economy benefited individual institutions in different ways according to their ability to attract direct philanthropy. Hake's survey (see table 1) illustrates how different types

and of Dudley in the Black Country, c. 1810–1914', in Cannadine, *Patricians, power and politics*, 104; Martin Daunton, *Coal metropolis: Cardiff, 1870–1914*, Leicester 1977, 112.

[13] *Statistics of middle-class expenditure*, British Library of Political and Economic Science, pamphlet HD6/D267, table ix, cited in Prochaska, *Women and philanthropy*, 21; F. M. L. Thompson, *English landed society in the nineteenth century*, London 1963, 210.

[14] Peter Earle, *The making of the English middle class: business, society and family life in London, 1660–1730*, London 1989, 315–19.

[15] Sampson Low, *The charities of London, comprehending the benevolent, educational and religious institutions: their origins, progress, and present-position*, London 1850; Loch, *Charity and social life*, 487–8.

of hospital had a distinct appeal to charity, but his assessment does not tell the whole story. Contemporaries complained that the specialist hospitals, with their 'increased energy and continuous and extensive appeals', attracted a greater amount of charitable income than other institutions.[16] The exaggerated claims made by the Lord Mayor of London in 1892 that the Royal Hospital for Diseases of the Chest was 'almost entirely dependent for its support on voluntary contributions' contained an element of truth.[17] Both the Royal Hospital for Diseases of the Chest and the Hospital for Sick Children did have a higher level of philanthropic support than many of their general counterparts at a time when charity was assuming a less prominent role in hospital funding. At the Royal Hospital for Diseases of the Chest direct philanthropy increased its financial importance, rising from just over 67 per cent of the total income between 1850 and 1855 to 86 per cent between 1890 and 1895.[18] The reasons for this difference are explained in the following chapter, but are linked to the specialist nature and age of these hospitals.

Subscriptions were seen as the only 'reliable' source of charitable funding and for the prince of Wales they were 'the true test of a charity's repute'.[19] During the eighteenth century subscriptions for most voluntary hospitals had, on average, provided between half and three-quarters of their income.[20] In the nineteenth century it was felt that the situation had not dramatically changed. One speaker at the Social Science Association (SSA) conference in July 1883, explained that subscriptions still represented provincial hospitals' most important source of funding.[21] At the Royal West Sussex Hospital, Chichester, for example, subscriptions generated 63 per cent of the total income between 1850 and 1855 and even by the 1890s they remained the hospital's most significant source of funding, representing 31.4 per cent of the income.[22] The same was not true of London (see table 2). Henry Burdett, now firmly established through the Hospitals Association as an expert on hospital finance, estimated in 1890 that subscriptions provided only 12 per cent of the income of London's general hospitals.[23] An explanation for this difference can be found in the relative amounts of income subscriptions generated and in the nature of London's civil society and the structure of its benevolent economy. Although London's hospitals collected more from sub-

---

[16] *Hospital*, 3 Sept. 1892, 381.

[17] *Charity Record & Philanthropic News* xii (1892), 108.

[18] RCH, annual reports 1850–95, LMA.

[19] *Lancet* ii (1883), 72–3.

[20] Guenter B. Risse, *Hospital life in enlightenment Scotland: care and teaching at the Royal Edinburgh Infirmary*, Cambridge 1986; William Brockbank, *Portrait of a hospital, 1752–1948*, London 1952. Differences did exist and at the Bath infirmary subscriptions represented under a quarter of the total income: Borsay, 'Cash and conscience', 211–12.

[21] *BMJ* ii (1883), 32.

[22] Royal West Sussex Hospital, annual reports 1850–1900, West Sussex County Record Office, Chichester, RWSH/26–28.

[23] *Hospital*, 8 Mar. 1890, 353.

Table 2: Income from direct philanthropy, 1850–95
(% of total income)

Hospital	Income source	1850–5	1863–5	1870–5	1890–5
German*	Subscriptions	23.5		13.2	18.0
	Donations	39.9		37.4	34.4
	Legacies	2.1		2.5	6.3
	Collections	8.3		0.2	0.5
Guy's**	Subscriptions	0.0		0.0	0.0
	Donations	0.4		0.2	23.0
	Legacies	0.0		2.1	0.0
Hospital for Sick	Subscriptions	28.8		19.9	16.6
Children	Donations	26.8		39.2	22.4
	Legacies	4.8		9.8	23.7
	Collections	8.6		0.7	0.4
	Entertainment	0.0		0.0	0.2
	Endowment funds	0.0		0.0	4.8
London	Subscriptions	5.0		3.5	4.7
	Donations	11.0		17.3	11.2
	Legacies	5.6		6.3	19.9
	Collections	0.3		0.2	0.8
	Special fund	0.0		12.3	1.3
Royal Hospital for	Subscriptions	46.5		27.8	26.2
Diseases of the Chest	Donations	20.6		54.6	39.9
	Legacies	0.0		0.3	18.8
	Collections	0.0		1.3	0.9
	Entertainment	0.0		0.0	0.5
St Bartholomew's#	Donations	0.0	1.5	0.9	0.5
	Legacies	0.0	0.2	2.1	2.7
University College	Subscriptions	15.6		8.4	7.9
	Donations	27.7		30.4	21.5
	Legacies	12.4		16.2	24.4

* Figures for the German Hospital start from 1851, the first year in which detailed accounts were published
** Figures for Guy's start from 1853, the first year in which detailed accounts were published
# No ledger exists for 1850 to 1855
Source: Annual reports 1850–95; Guy's, financial abstracts, LMA, H9/Gy/D/1–3, A/94/1; St Bartholomew's, general account books, SBH, Hb/23/3–4

scriptions than many provincial institutions, their overall contribution was reduced by the amount of money raised from other sources. Equally, hospitals in London were only one of a number of charitable institutions competing for funds and, whereas competition existed outside London, the number of voluntary organisations in the capital stretched the amount that could be raised by individual societies.

Subscriptions were vital for hospitals in the first decade after their foundation, but as a hospital aged other sources of philanthropy came to dominate, so reducing subscriptions' relative financial contribution. For established hospitals (i.e. those more than ten years old) donations came to replace subscriptions as the main means through which the philanthropic public expressed their support. Donations also generated more money: at Guy's, for example, the 1886 appeal collected £15,000 in donations, which the governors used to cover the hospital's overdraft.[24] Governors tailored their fundraising accordingly and directed it to stimulating and collecting donations. It was not an experience limited to the London hospitals. The NSPCC (even with its 46,000 subscribers in 1899) and many other large charities were equally dependent on donations.[25] Legacies were more erratic but provided a permanent feature of hospital funding. Bequests, it was noted in 1895, kept hospitals 'afloat' and this created anxiety for their future.[26] Many governors initially hoped to use legacies as a form of investment to increase their hospital's reliable income, but as expenditure rose bequests were increasingly diverted to the general fund. For the governors at University College Hospital this became an essential part of their financial strategy and bequests were used to pay debts, leaving little room for manoeuvre. Few other hospitals depended on the 'dead hand' of charity to this extent, but even the most carefully managed felt that without bequests their finances would be in a 'deplorable condition'.[27] Legacies, if not reliable, were seen as an important and often fortuitous source of funding.

Income from direct philanthropy and the hospitals' fundraising tactics attracted the most public attention, publicity and criticism. Charitable contributions characterised hospitals as benevolent and voluntary institutions, but even in the eighteenth century philanthropy had been unable to meet the hospitals' running costs. As a result, other sources of funding were used to fund the gap between income and expenditure that charity could not fill.

[24] Guy's to Charity Commission, Apr. 1884, LMA, H9/Gy/A172/2. Historians have seen the Charity Commission as a weak body which gradually lost its initial momentum in the face of its inability to rationalise charitable endowments, citing contemporary dissatisfaction with the extent of the commission's powers (see Owen, English philanthropy, 299–329, and Richard Tompson, The Charity Commission and the age of reform, London 1979, for the commission's foundation). Perhaps this view is too pessimistic. The commission could only influence the endowed hospitals, but governors of other hospitals wrote to it for information and advice on legacies. At the endowed hospitals the Charity Commission had more influence on a practical level than has been assumed. It used its power to sanction developments (particularly loans) as a handle on policy. At Guy's and St Thomas's the commission was able to encourage the governors to adopt new financial policies in the 1880s, particularly the introduction of patient payment schemes (see below). There was no intervention to alter the pattern of endowments, perhaps because they continued to produce a sizeable income even after 1880. However, the commission exerted influence to manoeuvre both hospitals into action. It could be said that the commission persuaded Guy's and St Thomas's to address their position in a positive manner and they responded accordingly.

[25] Behlmer, Child abuse, 143.

[26] Burdett, Hospitals and charities annual, 99.

[27] Daily Mail, 16 Oct. 1897, 4.

Figure 2: Sunday Fund: total collections, 1873–95

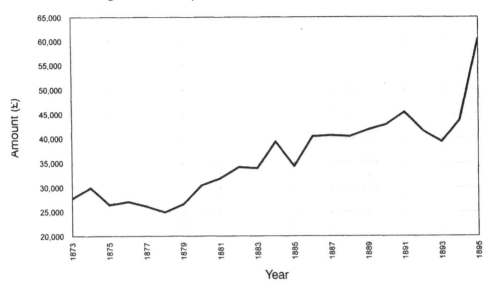

Source: *Lancet*, 1873–95

'Indirect' philanthropy

The foundation of the Sunday Fund in 1873 created a new channel for voluntary contributions that aimed to encourage the middle classes to abandon subscriptions as a means of support for London's hospitals. In the following year, the creation of the Metropolitan Hospital Saturday Fund extended the amount collected from indirect philanthropy. Between them they provided a new and valued source of funding. Governors made positive attempts to ensure that they received the maximum grant they were entitled to, viewing any fall in their grant with concern. The funds could not solve the London hospitals' financial problems, but they went some way to ensure that their precarious economic position was moderated.

The Sunday Fund was not initially an unwarranted success and disappointed many of its supporters. However, after 1878 the fund gathered momentum, raising as much as £43,679 in 1894 and distributing 96 per cent of the collection to 127 hospitals and fifty-five dispensaries.[28] From 1873 to 1894 a total of £725,647 was raised (see figure 2), but not all were entirely satisfied as the need for an additional £100,000 *per annum* became apparent. In 1881 the ever critical and blunt Burdett expressed a growing opinion that the collections were 'lamentably small'. Thirteen years later the *Charity Record & Philanthropic News*, after what later proved to be a temporary fall in

[28] *Lancet* ii (1894), 1509.

Figure 3: Sunday Fund's grant to University College Hospital, Royal Hospital for Diseases of the Chest, and Guy's, 1873–95

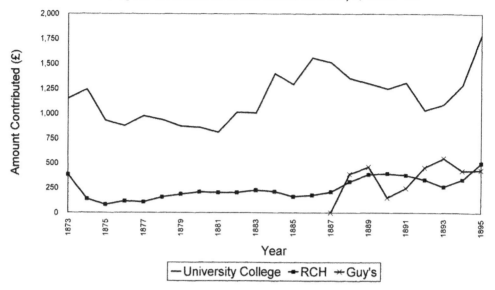

Source: Annual reports 1873–95; Guy's, abstract of accounts, LMA, H9/Gy/D191–42

collections, worried that the fund was on the 'wane'.[29] This should not belittle the fund's development. Support was mobilised through incessant publicity and the fund's low administrative costs created a favourable image of efficient management that contrasted with the running of other metropolitan charities. It was successful in attracting a large body of support and its collections reflected the trade cycle and wider ebb and flow of metropolitan charity, which had a direct bearing on the amounts awarded to individual hospitals (see figure 3). A sharp rise in the fund's income in 1883 coincided with the publicity surrounding the *Bitter cry of outcast London*, which heightened concerns over poverty and encouraged philanthropy.[30] The gradual increase during the 1880s, only interrupted when benevolence was diverted to a special Mansion House Fund in 1885–6 after worker demonstrations in the West End aroused public concern, was a product of this emerging awareness of poverty combined with a growth in national income. The fund received a further boost in 1895 when profits from the 'South African Boom' in the City were partially redirected into it. Here Waterlow's business contacts and the efforts of Burdett, who had been appointed secretary to the Shares and Loans Department of the London Stock Exchange in 1881, proved crucial. The liberality of Messrs Burdett and Harris, Messrs Pym and

29 *Charity Record & Philanthropic News* xiv (1894), 235.
30 E. P. Hennock, 'Poverty and social theory in England: the experience of the eighteen-eighties', *Social History* i (1976), 67.

Vaungham of the Stock Exchange, 'and other City friends' pushed receipts to a total of £60,000.[31] The City plutocracy had aligned itself behind London's hospitals, a tendency that was strengthened with the foundation of the Prince of Wales Hospital Fund in 1897.

To maintain support poor collection returns were explained by short-term economic problems, epidemics (particularly influenza in 1892 and 1893), the weather and even the death in 1891 of Archbishop Magee, a prominent supporter of the NSPCC. The Prince of Wales Hospital Fund had a longer-term effect. At a meeting in 1898 the chairman of the Sunday Fund explained that 'many of their large contributors, who used to give £500 or £1,000 had either transferred to the Prince of Wales Fund or had divided it'.[32] The fund's organisers hoped to find another explanation for its declining success; some even blamed Waterlow's prejudice against the specialist hospitals, but in reality both funds competed for the same charitable resources.[33] From the outset, the Prince of Wales Fund was more effective in mobilising philanthropic support.

The Sunday Fund drew most of its collections from a Sunday collection in June, which became the focus of the movement. Contributions were generally small, averaging 2d. per head. Not all gave. It is impossible to determine how many went as far as Jack Brown, a fictional character in The Lancet who remained 'blind drunk' for the entire day to avoid making a contribution, but evasion was difficult, at least for those attending church.[34] None could rival Canon Flemming, vicar of St Michael's, Chester Square, for encouraging his congregation to give generously; in 1894 he collected a record amount of £1,202 15s.[35] Flemming was an Anglican minister, reflecting the Church of England's social prominence, wealth and importance in the fund's collections. Anglican congregations contained the highest proportion of middle- and upper-class citizens in London, ensuring that collections in Anglican churches drew on those social groups that could most afford the fashion of philanthropy. It was also the largest religious body: in 1886/7 13.5 per cent of Londoners attended a Church of England service and despite a fall in attendance to 9.4 per cent by 1902/3 no other denomination could rival its influential position (see table 3).[36] This does not completely explain why other denominations contributed comparatively smaller amounts. All denominations faced problems of attendance, but the Church of England retained its position in the fund, not because of its disproportionate stress on the merits of benevolence, or the wealth and size of its congregations, but because it had few other outlets for charitable action. Other denominations had their own charitable tendencies and patronised voluntary societies that matched their

31 Lancet i (1895), 1052–3.
32 Times, 4 Aug. 1898, 7.
33 Hospital, 13 Aug. 1898, 343.
34 Lancet i (1886), 1195.
35 Ibid. ii (1894), 1509.
36 McLeod, Class and religion, 314.

Table 3: Sunday Fund: contributions from congregations, 1884, 1894

Denomination	1884	%	1894	%
Church of England	£25,127	81.0	£28,368	84.3
Congregationalist	£2,102	6.8	£1,499	4.5
Baptist	£1,102	3.5	£836	2.5
Wesleyan	£1,057	3.4	£979	2.9
Presbyterian	£708	2.3	£1,064	3.2
Roman Catholic	£523	1.7	£484	1.4
Unitarian	£245	0.8	£278	0.8
Other	£162	0.5	£126	0.4
TOTAL	£31,036	100.0	£33,634	100.0

Source: Henry Burdett, *Hospitals and charities annual*, London 1895, 211

religious nature. Nonconformists had their Dorcas meetings, at which ladies of the chapel met to drink tea and make clothes for the poor; Catholicism tried to dominate the whole non-working life of its believers. The Catholic Church provided clubs for each distinctive group and a host of welfare services, including loans at a low rate of interest. Aid to the Irish, education and the work of the Society of St Vincent de Paul (which had few active members but an income of £1,461 5s. 7d. in 1895), dominated its philanthropic activities.[37] Within this established network of church charity the Sunday Fund was an intruder and consequently assumed a peripheral importance.

The Saturday Fund, founded in 1874, was the working-class equivalent of the Sunday Fund and drew its name from the day of the week when most workers were paid. The movement built on provincial initiatives started in Liverpool and aimed to 'aid in every possible way to perfect the system of Medical relief in the Metropolis by supporting the Hospitals and kindred institutions'.[38] Both funds shared a common concern to raise the income of the London hospitals, but from the start the Saturday Fund aroused hostility. Burdett, as a firm advocate of economic management and supporter of the social elite's active participation in hospital affairs, was critical of the fund, especially given its working-class nature. He attacked it as injurious and extravagant, and as a movement that did not have the sympathy of the working classes. Others criticised the fund as a misguided provident scheme with

[37] Society of St Vincent de Paul, annual report 1895.
[38] Henry Burdett, *Hospital Sunday and Hospital Saturday: their origin, progress and development together with suggestions for making both funds more useful to hospitals*, London 1884, 8–9; *Hospital Saturday Fund Journal*, Dec. 1897, 8. Yeo, *Religion and voluntary organisation*, 216–18, describes the evolution of a similar movement in Reading, while Marland, *Medicine and society*, 158–9, shows the development of a Saturday Fund in the Huddersfield area.

Figure 4: Saturday Fund: total collections, 1874–98

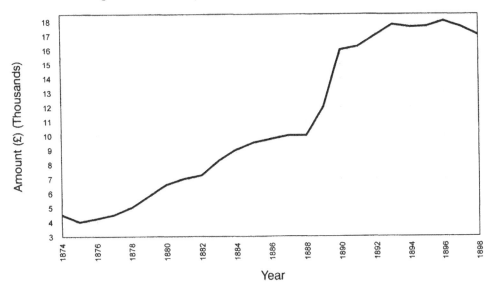

Source: *BMJ* and *Lancet*, 1874–98

exorbitant expenses that was a waste of charitable resources and a threat to general practitioners. Socialists saw it as a capitalist dupe. The fund's inauspicious beginnings only fuelled opposition. The first collection was a disappointment and the movement blamed its lack of support on the press's unenthusiastic reception.[39] For the *Morning Post*, however, the Saturday Fund's poor results was due to the working classes' refusal to accept its responsibilities.[40] The fund's apologists dismissed these claims and sought other explanations that included the weather and competition from other collection schemes. The next three collections were no better, but from 1878 onwards confidence in the fund increased. As experience was accumulated, the fund managed to cut its expenses from 35.2 per cent of the amount collected in 1874, to 14.5 per cent in 1885, enabling it to project a more realistic impression of its usefulness.[41] A change in the fund's fortunes saw a rise in collections (see figure 4). The golden jubilee produced a patriotic upsurge in the organisation's activities as 'monster demonstrations' and collections were organised in Victoria Park, but this had little influence at a time when competition for charitable resources was intense.[42] The sudden rise in collections from 1889 was helped by the introduction of a 'penny-a-week' collection scheme that aimed to raise £100,000. The new scheme attracted widespread

39 *Medical Times & Gazette* ii (1874), 662.
40 *Lancet* ii (1874), 705.
41 *BMJ* i (1886), 455.
42 *Hospital*, 11 June 1887, 177.

interest and opposition and though it did not generate the amount expected, it served to boost the fund's collections and maintain them at a higher level.[43] By 1894 the Saturday Fund was dividing £17,500 between 165 participating institutions.

From the start, the Saturday Fund was heralded as a working-class collection scheme, an 'appeal to the "pence of the workman" '.[44] Collections were centred on the capital's workshops and by 1884 the fund was sending out 20,000 collection sheets to businesses in London.[45] Members of the workshop and streets collection committee worked hard to increase the fund's support, visiting every business that wanted to hold a collection and insisting that £5 had to be contributed annually for it to remain in the scheme.[46] In exchange the fund attempted to acquire from the hospitals it supported the right to admit patients and then distribute these rights to participants in the fund. Hospital governors did not welcome the move. They resisted the distribution of admission rights, hoping to balance the financial support received from the Saturday Fund with their own subscribers' interests. Critics inevitably saw the fund's efforts as a misguided attempt at working-class self-help, arguing that small contributions to the fund created the erroneous impression that participants had a right to treatment. Such opposition damaged the fund's activities, but by 1897 it was estimated that the Saturday Fund was giving back the equivalent of 30 per cent of its collections in services to its supporters.[47]

The Saturday Fund was, however, never entirely a working-class organisation; from the start its character was transcended through a number of fund-raising activities that aimed to collect money from all classes. Collection boxes were placed in railway stations and post offices, while street collections, run and staffed by 'ladies', were organised on one Saturday every year. From the 1890s onwards, sport and cycling clubs organised special events to raise money, capitalising on the movement towards recreational sport and working-class leisure.[48] Individuals gave their effort voluntarily and London was divided into thirty districts, each with an organisational committee composed of local working men, employers and middle-class activists.[49] A carefully regulated and audited management could not prevent fraud, which remained a major problem for the fund. The theft of thirteen collection boxes in the Norwood district in 1893 generated widespread public concern and minor cases of fraud were common.[50] The fund, however, persisted. Camberwell, St George's and Westminster, Southwark and Woolwich consistently

43 BMJ i (1889), 50.
44 Charity, June 1887, 15.
45 Charity Record & Philanthropic News iv (1884), 278.
46 Hospital Saturday Fund Journal, Dec. 1897, 6.
47 Charity Record & Philanthropic News xvii (1897), 470.
48 Hospital, 14 Jan. 1893, 250. See also Helen E. Meller, Leisure and the changing city, 1879–1914, London 1976, or R. Holt, Sport and the British: a modern history, Oxford 1989.
49 Charity, July 1887, 40.
50 FWA, correspondence on the Metropolitan Hospital Saturday Fund, 1875–1934, LMA,

Table 4: Institutions assisted by the Sunday and Saturday Fund, 1897

Type							
	No.	%	Sunday Fund amount	No.	%	Saturday Fund amount	
General	26	51.2	£22,086 15s. 1d.	28	36.5	£6,566 5s. 0d.
Special	57	31.7	£13,650 6s. 8d.	64	34.9	£6,289 1s. 0d.
Convalescent	23	6.8	£2,950 14s. 2d.	25	12.3	£2,209 18s. 0d.
Cottage	12	1.2	£511 17s. 4d.	5	0.8	£140 0s. 0d.
Dispensaries	55	2.8	£1,190 19s. 0d.	37	5.4	£982 19s. 0d.
Misc.	7	1.2	£517 5s. 0d.	22	4.5	£812 8s. 8d.
Surgical appliances	3,632	5.9	£2,140 16s. 11d.	2,782	5.6	£1,009 7s. 0d.
TOTAL			£43,046 3s. 0d.			£18,009 18s. 8d.

Source: *Hospital Saturday Fund Journal*, Dec. 1897, 2

contributed the largest collections, but despite the obvious success of the scheme street collections increasingly attracted staunch opposition. The *BMJ* attacked street collections as 'organised begging' and in 1895 the COS arranged a conference to discuss how they might be stopped.[51] The fund's organisers were aware of the hostility their street collections created. After lengthy discussion in 1897 they finally decided to abandoned them after the metropolitan police had protested against the disruption they caused. The decision was partly an attempt to counter criticism, but also reflected a fall in the sums street collections were raising. From a high point in 1892 when £5,925 was collected, the amount raised by street collections had fallen to £4,642 17s. 4d. in 1896. A new strategy of fundraising was adopted. Private collections were organised, meetings were held and the Saturday Fund started to advertise for donations.[52] Many consequently feared that the 1898 collection would be a disaster. Although the fund did raise £2,000 less than in 1897, the collection was deemed 'satisfactory' and even the fund's critics felt that it had acted with sensitivity and courage to abandon its traditional practices.[53]

The distribution of grants by the Sunday Fund and the Saturday Fund (see table 4) was carefully controlled by a distribution committee and elaborate rules and procedures were established to work out each hospital's grant. The Sunday Fund distributed grants according to the hospital's expenditure, while the Saturday Fund assessed hospitals on the amount of relief they provided.[54]

A/FWA/C/D61/1. Most cases of fraud were similar to the £4 stolen in 1893 by a man disguised as an official collector and the fund was always keen to show that it was a responsible organisation by pressing for prosecution: *Hospital Saturday Fund Journal*, Dec. 1893, 2.
51 *BMJ* ii (1874), 468; *Charity Record & Philanthropic News* xv (1895), 60.
52 *Hospital Saturday Fund Journal*, Mar. 1898, 2; Sept. 1894, 53.
53 *Charity Record & Philanthropic News* xviii (1898), 389, 416.
54 *Hospital Saturday Fund Journal*, Dec. 1898, 1; Dec. 1895, 31.

Table 5: Contributions from benevolent funds to indvidual hospitals (% of total income)

Hospital	Fund	1875	1895
German	Sunday Fund	5.6	5.8
	Saturday Fund	1.1	1.4
Guy's	Sunday Fund	–	2.2
	Saturday Fund	–	0.0
Hospital for Sick	Sunday Fund	2.1	5.5
Children	Saturday Fund	0.3	1.2
London	Sunday Fund	5.3	8.4
	Saturday Fund	–	1.5
	People's Fund	1.4	2.7
Royal Hospital for	Sunday Fund	2.5	5.9
Diseases of the Chest	Saturday Fund	1.6	3.6

Source: Annual reports 1870–95; Guy's, financial abstracts, LMA, H9/Gy/D/19/1–2, A/94/1

The main emphasis of the Saturday Fund remained on the general and specialist hospitals, but with a broad definition of 'kindred institutions' it provided surgical appliances and assisted dispensaries, ambulance services and convalescent homes. The Sunday Fund avoided this style of distribution. Most of its grants went to the non-endowed general hospitals on the grounds that they treated the largest number of patients and had the most significant impact on suffering. Wider hostility to specialist hospitals and Waterlow's opposition to them ensured that they were reluctantly supported.

Individual hospital collection schemes were of a more localised benefit. The London Hospital's People's Five Shillings Subscriptions Fund and University College Hospital's People's Contribution Fund subscribed to a similar rhetoric of indirect philanthropy, but remained more organised collection schemes than benevolent funds. The difference rested on the nature of the two types of collection. Organised collection schemes were designed, unlike the benevolent funds, to raise money only for the London or University College Hospital. Income was not distributed on merit, merely assigned to each hospital. Between 1871 and 1898 the People's Five Shillings Subscriptions Fund collected over £45,085 and annually provided more income for the London than the Saturday Fund.[55] A similar situation existed at University College Hospital (see figure 5). As organised metropolitan collection schemes for individual hospitals they proved highly effective.

Yearly figures disguise the relative importance of the grants made by the Sunday Fund and the Saturday Fund to individual hospitals (see table 5). The

[55] London Hospital, annual reports 1871–98, LH.

Figure 5: University College Hospital: contributions from funds,
1873–95

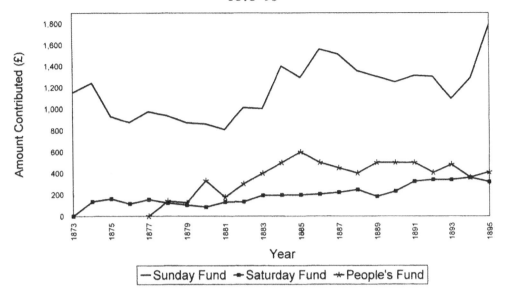

Source: Annual reports 1873–95, UCL

Sunday Fund, because it collected more than the Saturday Fund and had lower running costs, had a greater impact on hospital finance. For example, at University College Hospital the Sunday Fund contributed, on average, twice as much to the hospital as the Saturday Fund (see figure 5). Fluctuations in the relative amounts contributed by each fund matched University College Hospital's financial fortunes and the general level of support for each movement. Outside London the impact of working-class collection schemes was greater; increasing to 24–99 per cent of provincial hospitals' income by the 1920s.[56] Not all governors welcomed the benevolent funds or their methods, but many feared that a withdrawal of their support 'would mean the closing of their hospitals'.[57] They regarded the funds' grants as reliable and saw them as an important source of income. However, in 1887 the BMJ delivered a telling verdict on their activities: 'the Hospital Sunday and Hospital Saturday Funds are well-meant efforts to meet the [hospitals' financial] difficulty; but their most sanguine friends cannot pretend that they have solved it'.[58] Even indirect philanthropy had its limits, partly because it could not be separated from the constraints operating on London's benevolent economy.

56 Cherry, 'Before the National Health Service', 319.
57 *Charity Record & Philanthropic News* xiv (1894), 74.
58 *BMJ* ii (1887), 474.

Funding the hospital: non-charitable income

The editor of the *Hospital Saturday Fund Journal* was aware that 'what the Hospitals want is a regular income' that was free of the 'perpetual straining' entailed by raising money from philanthropy.[59] Fear of a 'general falling off in the contributions of the benevolent' heightened concern about hospital funding so that by the 1890s charity was seen to be '*in extremis*'. After the 1911 National Insurance Act extended general practitioner care calls became shriller with a decline in subscription income.[60] New schemes of raising money from charity were suggested, but governors had always sought money from non-charitable sources to cover the deficit that philanthropy left. As the governors of University College Hospital explained in 1861, governors were 'bound to use every means to continue . . . the good work which [their] Hospital has done hitherto'.[61] Non-charitable income supplemented the money available from within the benevolent economy and in the endowed hospitals it provided the main source of funding.

Income from non-charitable sources was generated in several ways, but money from land and investments provided a reservoir of funding for all London's hospitals. Income of this type invariably had a charitable origin, especially when most of a hospital's property came from past bequests. Over time the original nature of these gifts was submerged. Charitable contributions were converted via the purchase of land, houses or investments into a 'reliable' source of funding with an income separate from the benevolent economy. In hospital account books such resources were always recorded separately from the revenue generated by philanthropy. According to Pinker, in 1891 'investments' represented 43.7 per cent of hospital income in London and their importance as capital funding only increased during the twentieth century.[62] In endowed hospitals this proportion was higher and *The Lancet* rightly pronounced them an 'anomaly' in a society generally opposed to posthumous benevolence.[63] In financial terms St Bartholomew's, Guy's and St Thomas's existed outside the benevolent economy.

St Bartholomew's was the archetypal endowed hospital. Although never entirely dependent on its endowments, income from property remained central. Land had been slowly acquired from 1123 onwards and a series of bequests had added to the hospital's acquisitions.[64] By the nineteenth century, after seven centuries of accumulation, St Bartholomew's had become a major landowner, a position that guaranteed a large rental income. By the

---

59 *Hospital Saturday Fund Journal*, Dec. 1895, 28.

60 *BMJ* ii (1885), 1174; Cherry, 'Before the National Health Service', 314–15.

61 UCH, annual report 1861, UCL.

62 Robert Pinker, *English hospital statistics, 1861–1938*, London 1966, 152; Cherry, 'Before the National Health Service', 313–14.

63 *Lancet* ii (1879), 738.

64 *Thirty-Second Report of the Charity Commission*, 13–15.

Figure 6:   St Bartholomew's Hospital – rental income, 1863–95

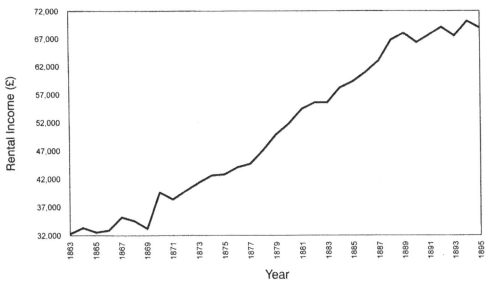

Source: General account books, SBH, Hb/5/3–4

1890s the hospital's treasurer estimated that St Bartholomew's owned 13,000 acres outside London, mostly in country estates and farms in Essex and the south.[65] From the thirteenth century onwards, however, the emphasis had been on metropolitan real estate, freeing St Bartholomew's from the financial problems experienced by other endowed institutions during the agricultural depression of the last quarter of the nineteenth century.[66] Metropolitan property was favoured purely on economic grounds. Urban land values rose rapidly during the late 1850s and there was an upward swing in house building at a national level from the mid-1860s to 1876 (which continued in London until 1881/2), followed by a further boom in the mid 1890s. London's 'appetite for increase', combined with an incessant demand for urban property, ensured that St Bartholomew's possessed an asset that only accumulated in value (see figure 6).[67] Throughout the nineteenth century the governors invested in urban property, aware that the return was consistently higher than that provided by rural estates. For example, Mayland Hill farm could be leased to George Partridge for £80 *per annum* in 1891, while three houses in Warling Street were let to the bookseller W. H. Smith for £1,000.[68] Contem-

65 *SC on Metropolitan Hospitals, First Report*, 169.
66 Medvei and Thornton, *Saint Bartholomew's*, 32.
67 S. B. Saul, 'House building in England, 1890–1914', *EcHR* xiii (1962), 120, 135; cited in Donald J. Olsen, *The growth of Victorian London*, London 1976, 28.
68 St Bartholomew's, view and survey books, SBH, Hc 9/4–6.

poraries associated St Bartholomew's 'with resources of finance which are almost inexhaustible', though critics wrongly assumed that this encouraged extravagance.[69] Under these conditions, the hospital prospered, though arrears, amounting to £30,000 in the 1870s, impeded the smooth flow of income.[70]

At Guy's income from endowments dominated the hospital's finances until 1879 to a degree not experienced at St Bartholomew's. Thomas Guy, having launched the scheme to found the hospital in 1721, left his hospital a total of £220,124 2s. 7d. from the fortune he had made in the South Sea bubble when he died in 1724.[71] His will stipulated that this had to be invested in land to endow the hospital; any income raised from the sale of this property had to be reinvested in land, tying the hands of future governors and ensuring that most of the hospital's income would always be from rural estates. The governors were anxious to find bargains. After the main agricultural estates had been purchased between 1724 and 1754 neighbouring property was bought when it became available, saddling Guy's with some dubious holdings.[72] A third of the property was held in Essex with other substantial estates in Herefordshire and Lincolnshire. Urban property was limited to the immediate area surrounding the hospital in Southwark to allow for the institution's growth. 'Till the year 1875', the hospital's treasurer explained in 1887, this had created few problems because 'the income from the joint bequests, mainly derived from their landed estates' was sufficient to fund a hospital of 650 beds.[73]

According to Spring an un-businesslike approach to land management was unusual for most landowners.[74] Most noble and large landowners pursued an enlightened policy of estate control, improving or developing property.[75] Like all major landowners, St Bartholomew's and Guy's employed a professional land agent to manage their affairs at a local level, but the governors retained absolute control over the hospital's finances. The land agent dealt with the day-to-day management of the estates and reported to an estates committee appointed by the governors. The hospitals' president and treasurer were *ex officio* members, but it was generally the treasurer, as the most

[69] *Lancet* i (1861), 518.

[70] St Bartholomew's, minutes of the board of governors, SBH, Ha 1/22.

[71] Guy's Hospital, will and Act of Incorporation, LMA, H9/Gy/A48/5.

[72] B. E. S. Trueman, 'The purchase and management of Guy's Hospital estates, 1726–1806', in C. Chalkin and J. R. Wordie (eds), *Town and countryside: the English landowners in the national economy*, London 1989, 52–82.

[73] Guy's Hospital, treasurer's report 1887, LMA, H9/Gy/A93/1.

[74] D. Spring, *The English landed estate in the nineteenth century: its administration*, Baltimore 1963, 19.

[75] S. Wade Martins, *A great estate at work: the Holkham estate and its inhabitants in the nineteenth century*, Cambridge 1980, 57; Cannadine, *Lords and landlords*, 81–225, 229–381. See also F. M. L. Thompson, 'The English great estate in the nineteenth century', *Contributions and communications to the first international conference of economic history*, Paris 1960, for a discussion of aristocratic investment.

Table 6: Rental income (% of total income)

Hospital	1850–5	1870–5	1890–5
German*	0.0	0.0	2.0
Hospital for Sick Children	0.9	0.8	0.0
London	11.9	5.5	17.5
Royal Hospital for Diseases of the Chest	3.3	0.5	0.0
University College	0.0	0.0	1.6

* Figures for the German Hospital start from 1851, the first year in which detailed accounts were published
Source: Annual reports 1850–95

active governor, who remained the main force behind all the decisions. Contemporaries had a low opinion of how the old endowed charities in London were managed and in 1883 the City Parochial Foundation was established to promote reform.[76] Although the endowed hospitals were not included in the Foundation's remit, they were also accused of mismanaging their estates and funds, but these attacks were often ill-founded, the product of the closed administrations of endowed hospitals. St Bartholomew's adopted policies that matched the efforts of other improving landowners. Careful management and judicious expansion increased the hospital's aggregate income from its estates. Strenuous efforts were made to raise the value of the hospital's property and from 1893 all the London holdings were gradually improved.[77] Guy's, however, managed its estates differently, partly because Thomas Guy's will limited the governors' field of action. Surpluses were infrequently invested, property was not developed or urbanised, and high-farming techniques were ignored until the 1880s. Part of the reason must be found in the nature of the estates, which remained essentially suited to farming and presented few opportunities for improvement. The hospital's endowed nature produced a quasi-autocratic framework of management where the governors had no financial commitment to the institution and, as explained in chapter 5, this discouraged an active policy. Meetings were poorly attended, leaving the treasurer to make all the major decisions. Until the appointment of Edmund Lushington in 1876, weak treasurers ensured that no concerted policy was pursued and that Guy's remained a charity with urban responsibilities, but with an income dependent on the fortunes of agriculture. This stored up financial problems for the future and encouraged a series of financial innovations discussed below.

Non-endowed hospitals did not hold such large amounts of land, but most

76 See Victor Belcher, *The City Parochial Foundation, 1891–1991: a trust for the poor of London*, Aldershot 1991.
77 St Bartholomew's, minutes of the board of governors, SBH, Ha 1/26–7.

Table 7: Income from investments (% of total income)

Hospital	1850–5	1870–5	1890–5
German*	2.0	24.1	18.6
Hospital for Sick Children	2.7	4.5	9.8
London	45.2	24.2	18.1
Royal Hospital for Diseases of the Chest	24.7	5.6	1.3
University College	0.5	14.4	12.4

* Figures for the German Hospital start from 1851, the first year in which detailed accounts were published
Source: Annual reports 1850–95

continued to draw part of their income from rents (see table 6). Even the Middlesex, where the governors avoided any investment in land, still raised 9.5 per cent of its income from rent in 1890 after it had been left several properties.[78] The London had the opposite policy to the Middlesex. It was one of the few non-endowed hospitals to manage substantial estates. Located in the East End, property was owned locally. Houses were rented out and carefully maintained and from the 1880s onwards an average of £4 per house was spent on renovations.[79] Rents varied, but when the governors redeveloped their property in New Panfelt Street, rent for a three-room tenement with scullery was set at 8s. 6d. per week. The governors gradually increased the value of their holdings, which generated a rental income of £2,229 0s. 4d. in 1850 (12.8 per cent of the income for that year) rising to £8,933 5s. 8d. in 1895 (16.2 per cent of income) as urban land prices soared.[80] Most other non-endowed hospitals did not own such extensive estates and where property was held money raised from rent generally formed only a small part of the income. For example, at the Hospital for Sick Children rental income rose from a mere £15 in 1853 to only £195 13s. 6d. by 1875.[81] Property in the form of stocks and shares was a different matter and represented an important source of funding. Hospitals did not share the RSPCA's hostility to 'funded property'. They looked upon investments as a permanent source of revenue

[78] SC on Metropolitan Hospitals, Second Report, 123.
[79] Monica Paton, 'Corporate East End landlords: the example of the London Hospital and the Mercers' Company', London Journal xviii (1993), 117–18, discusses how the hospital managed its estates until the 1940s, representing a successful provider of working-class housing.
[80] London Hospital, minutes of the estates subcommittee, 18 July 1892, LH, A/9/41; annual reports 1850, 1895, LH.
[81] Hospital for Sick Children, minutes of the committee of management, GOSH, 1/2/1–19.

when other resources were essentially unreliable (see table 7); for the governors of the Brompton Hospital they were the only 'reliable' form of funding.[82]

A writer in *The Lancet* in 1886 recommended that hospitals should invest 75 per cent of their income. Though this was clearly impractical for many governors starved of funds, they did invest any surplus income, favouring government securities and profitable railway stock for their stability and high interest rates.[83] A period of institutional stability at the Royal Hospital for Diseases of the Chest in the early 1870s saw the governors investing most of the hospital's legacies and large donations, but by 1877 a deteriorating financial situation had ended this policy.[84] The governors of the German Hospital had always attempted to invest some of their annual income. However, the rebuilding of the hospital between 1863 and 1865 left a legacy of financial problems that saw the governors placing a new emphasis on investments when Baron Diegrad's gift of £10,000 in 1869 reversed the previous six years financial problems. A special subcommittee decided to invest £6,000 and in 1873 a firm decision was made to increase investments to prevent a further financial crisis.[85] The previous policy of investment was elevated into the hospital's main financial strategy, removing its reliance on, but not enthusiasm for, philanthropy. The governors of the Hospital for Sick Children, after a period of uncertainty that lasted from 1852 to 1865, also carefully managed their investments. With a preference for Indian Bonds, the governors increased the hospital's invested property when funds were available. Unprofitable stock was sold and the money raised was reinvested: in 1899 the governors sold £15,000 of Indian 3 per cent stock for £15,898 5s. 3d. and used the money to buy securities that yielded a higher rate of interest.[86] The governors' provision of endowed beds was part of this strategy in a move to attract legacies for investment purposes. Other hospitals, on the advice of the *BMJ*, followed the lead of the Hospital for Sick Children, but they needed little encouragement to invest surplus capital.[87]

The governors of the London modified the structure of their investments in 1863 in a move that introduced a new variant on invested income. To increase the hospital's level of funding, the governors decided to reinvest some of the hospital's stock and use the income to provide mortgages that would yield a higher rate of interest. Initially £30,000 was allocated, but after two years of deliberation the house committee, which was responsible for all the main decisions in the hospital's administration, recommended that

---

82 Harrison, 'Philanthropy and the Victorians', 366; P. Bishop and others, *The seven ages of the Brompton*, Guildford 1991, 68.
83 *Lancet* i (1886), 26.
84 RCH, council minute book, 19 Oct. 1877, LMA, H33/RCH/A1/4.
85 German Hospital, minutes of the annual general court, 27 Jan. 1873, SBH, GHA 5/2.
86 Hospital for Sick Children, miscellaneous financial records, GOSH, 3/4/7.
87 *BMJ* i (1872), 617.

£100,000 should be reinvested.[88] The committee, however, could not act on its own recommendations. Such a large change in the hospital's financial policy required the approval of a special meeting to which all the governors were invited. Legal advice was sought, a special governors' meeting was held, and the house committee was finally authorised to sell part of the hospital's securities for this purpose. In August 1865 the house committee considered providing a mortgage of £95,000 for a property in Lincolnshire, but they did not act until December during which time the owner, Mr Augustine, was investigated. Once the investigation had been completed and the property was found to be worth £200,000 and have an annual income of £7,640 16s. 4d., a mortgage of £100,000 was agreed at 4 per cent (1 per cent higher than most of the other investments).[89] The move represented the London's largest investment. With rising land prices and the hospital drawing approximately 10 per cent of its income from property, the decision was a rational one given the incessant need for funds. Further mortgages were arranged, but by the late 1860s the initial enthusiasm had waned and invested property was increasingly sold to meet expenditure, leaving little room for further experimentation. The governors' flirtation with lending on mortgage had ended with £182,750 tied up in land.[90]

By the late 1880s falling land prices strained repayment and in February 1897 it seemed that the hospital would lose the investment it had made in Augustine's property. The London was already facing financial problems. Income barely covered recurrent expenditure and pressure was mounting for the hospital to add new wards and an out-patients' department. Sydney Holland was appointed chairman to reverse the London's financial fortunes following his success at East and West India Dock Company and the Poplar Hospital. From a wealthy and influential family, Holland was not just the 'Prince of Beggars' and a charming self-publicist. Having acted as a director of London's first Coffee Tavern Company and of the East and West India Dock Company during the 1889 dock strike, Holland was a shrewd administrator who had become involved in hospital management through his work at the dock company.[91] After Holland had instructed his solicitor to investigate, half the mortgage was repaid in September followed by a further £18,000. With a solid understanding of the financial problems facing the hospital he rapidly realised that mortgages were not the secure investment initially hoped for and now proved a liability. Under his stewardship a more conventional investment policy was encouraged and when further mortgages were suggested in August 1897 no action was taken.[92] The change in policy did not

[88] London Hospital, minutes of the court of governors, 4 Mar. 1865, LH, A/2/12.
[89] London Hospital, minutes of the house committee, 26 Dec. 1865, LH, A/5/32.
[90] London Hospital, annual report 1875, LH.
[91] See Gore, Lord Knutsford; Barnes, 'The Docker's Hospital'.
[92] London Hospital, minutes of the house committee, 1 Nov. 1897, LH, A/5/47.

Table 8: Income from sale of invested property
(% of total income)

Hospital	1850–5	1863–5	1870–5	1890–5
German*	1.6		13.6	0.1
Hospital for Sick Children	0.0		0.6	0.1
London	0.2		4.5	2.3
Royal Hospital for Diseases of the Chest	11.4		15.4	2.6
St Bartholomew's**	–	11.0	12.8	4.5
University College	0.0		15.0	0.0

* Figures for the German Hospital start from 1851, the first year in which detailed accounts were published
** No ledger exists for 1850 to 1855
Source: Annual reports 1850–95; St Bartholomew's, general account books, SBH, Hb/23/3–4

mean that mortgages had been unprofitable. The governors had initially made a careful investment. If not all the initial investments were recovered, interest repayments of approximately £4,250 had raised £136,000 and between 1869 and 1874 mortgages had provided 15.2 per cent of the hospital's income. However, financial problems from the 1860s onwards prevented further mortgages and the policy was not adopted by other hospitals that lacked the London's invested income.

Property and investments not only provided a permanent source of funding, but at times of financial strain were sold to provide an additional source of income (see table 8). As *The Times* noted, property was drawn on 'without compunction in times of need'. Hamilton, author of the 1906 prize-winning essay, *The economical management of an efficient voluntary hospital*, argued that this was safer borrowing.[93] Others feared that it would damage hospitals' long-term financial position. If the governors of the Middlesex reversed their policy of selling invested property in 1888, most other governors periodically took part of their income from this source.[94] Governors remained careful, but a pressing need for funds over-rode all concerns and they used their connections with London's financial centres to good advantage to secure profitable deals. At the London the governors could afford to sell part of the hospital's invested property because of the large amount it had invested. However, they were careful not to drain the hospital's resources too far and ultimately solicited money from direct philanthropy when the financial demands of medical care in the East End became too great. Other hospitals had to be more cautious, but institutions like St Bartholomew's, the Hospital for Sick Children

93 *Times*, 23 Sept. 1871, 11; A. Hamilton, *The economical management of an efficient voluntary hospital*, London 1906.
94 *SC on Metropolitan Hospitals, Second Report*, 128.

and the German Hospital, for all their careful management, were periodically forced to sell small amounts of their invested property to avoid annual deficits. Investments were sold for two reasons: to fund expansion or to meet a deficit. The provision of new wards and clinical facilities imposed a considerable strain on hospital finance. At the German Hospital £5,500 in London and North Western Railway debentures had to be sold in 1868 to meet the debts incurred in building; in 1898 £2,700 in Great Eastern Railway debentures were sold for the same purpose.[95] The short-term nature of these actions is shown by one of the hospital's rules that required all amounts sold to be reinvested when funds permitted. Generally governors found it easier to accept the sale of stock when it was used to meet building costs. Suggestions made at the Royal Hospital for Diseases of the Chest in 1879 to sell £3,000 in 3 per cent consolidated stock to purchase the hospital's freehold met with approval, but in 1889 those governors not involved in the hospital's immediate management resisted the sale of £6,000 in consolidated stock, arguing that the matter be investigated to determine why this was necessary. Pressure on the hospital's funds, however, saw the governors selling invested property to balance the books rather than fund expansion.[96] Other hospitals were equally motivated by financial necessity at different points in their institutional history, given that income from the benevolent economy was not always available to meet their needs.

Land and investments were not just sold to raise additional capital. Hospitals also periodically disposed of those investments that had become unprofitable or a liability. The governors of the German Hospital prudently reinvested their holdings in Europe in 1875 during the Russo-Turkish war as they feared that interest rates would fall.[97] The governors of the London similarly practised a careful investment policy. St Bartholomew's, as a major landowner, had to adopt a commercial approach to its investments. By 1891 the hospital's property in Essex was considered almost worthless; two farms were empty and when 268 acres were sold for £2,000 the governors were 'glad to get the money'. A small plot of land was also sold to the North London Railway Company for £20,000, a figure far greater than its potential rental income.[98] Governors, with the aim of maximising their hospital's income, could not afford to miss such opportunities, especially if it meant disposing of an asset that could prove a liability.

Land and investments were not the only potential sources of income from the sale of 'property'. The *Hospital* believed that money from kitchen waste was 'worth the collecting' as for every 100 in-patients £30 to £50 *per annum*

[95] German Hospital, minutes of the hospital committee, 23 Jan. 1868, SBH, GHA 2/4; 24 Mar. 1898, SBH, GHA 2/10.
[96] RCH, council minute book, 11 Sept. 1889, LMA, H33/RCH/A2/1.
[97] German Hospital, minutes of the hospital committee, 25 Nov. 1875, SBH, GHA 2/6.
[98] SC on Metropolitan Hospitals, Second Report, 34.

could be raised.[99] The sale of waste material, particularly kitchen scraps, rarely amounted to more than 1 per cent of the hospitals' income, but it was a permanent and unglamorous feature of hospital finance that attracted little attention. More controversial was the sale of resources derived from the hospitals' function as a medical institution. Hospitals offered a number of services to their patients, medical students and the public that could be used to raise money. The Royal Hospital for Diseases of the Chest regularly sold its list of subscribers' names to other institutions as well as copies of the *Pharmacopoeia* to doctors and respirators to patients. The amounts raised were invariably small: in 1889 the sale of respirators made 8*d.* while the *Pharmacopoeia* raised a further £1 10s. 8*d.*[100] Amounts of this size did little for the hospital's total income, but it showed an enterprising spirit that was repeated elsewhere. Guy's offered a scheme from 1894 onwards whereby for a charge of 10s. 6*d.* the hospital would find a locum and a similar service was offered at St Bartholomew's.[101] The Royal Hospital for Diseases of the Chest hired out bath chairs, while University College Hospital opened its baths to the public in 1871, a late attempt to capitalise on moves a decade earlier to found public baths in London.[102] Other hospitals preferred to make money out of something they had to provide.

According to Dingwall, Rafferty and Webster hospitals' precarious financial situation forced governors to economise. To save money they discontinued their employment of nursing sisterhoods, who offered a semblance of professional nursing and an occupation for middle-class women, and established their own nursing schools to provide cheap nursing labour.[103] Though this might be an exaggeration, the growth of a body of trained nurses did have economic benefits. Not all hospitals benefited: training schools were generally established only in the general teaching hospitals, working in tandem with medical colleges. St Thomas's, with the foundation of the Nightingale School in 1860, set the pace. By the 1870s most general hospitals, except St Mary's, claimed to train nurses, though a survey in 1875 by Florence Lee, a Nightingale nurse, found little systematic training.[104] Among the specialist hospitals the Hospital for Sick Children proved an exception. It had been Charles West's wish that the hospital would train nurses specifically for the

99 *Hospital*, 21 Nov. 1896, 134.
100 RCH, minutes of the finance committee, 19 June 1888, LMA, H33/RCH/A5/1.
101 *Lancet* i (1894), 438.
102 RCH, minutes of the finance committee, 19 Oct. 1896, LMA, H33/RCH/A5/2; Wohl, *Endangered lives*, 73–6.
103 Robert Dingwall, Anne Marie Rafferty and Charles Webster, *An introduction to the social history of nursing*, London 1988, 59. For a discussion of the role of the nursing sisterhoods see Judith Moore, *A zeal for responsibility: the struggle for professional nursing in Victorian England, 1868–83*, London 1988; Ann Summers, 'The mysterious demise of Sarah Gamp: the domiciliary nurse and her detractors, c. 1830–60', *Victorian Studies* xxxii (1988/9), 365–86; Helmstadter, 'Origins of the modern trained nurse', 283–319.
104 Rivett, *The London hospital system*, 103–4.

Table 9: Income from nursing
(% of total income)

Hospital	1870–5	1890–5
Guy's	0.0	2.6
Hospital for Sick Children	0.6	5.5
London	0.0	4.3
St Bartholomew's	0.0	1.8

Source: Annual reports 1850–95; Guy's, financial abstracts, LMA, H9/Gy/D/19/1–2, A/94/1; St Bartholomew's, general account books, SBH, Hb/23/3–4

care of children, though a training school was not established. Formal nursing schools developed at a slower rate. In 1877 St Bartholomew's established a school with two members of the medical staff providing instruction; the London followed in 1880.[105] Whereas training schools did increase institutional running costs, contrary to Witz's assessment, probationary nurses also provided a cheap source of nursing labour, and could be used to perform other domestic duties.[106] Nurses equally promoted efficient patient care that meant more patients could be treated, increasing individual hospitals' claims to utility. The benefits extended beyond this. In establishing nursing schools hospitals charged probationers for their training, adding an additional source of income. It must be doubted whether this covered the cost of training and accommodation, but it went some way towards making this new function self-funding. Invariably nursing agencies were established through these training schools, placing nurses in private work. The client paid the hospital who then paid the nurse a fixed annual salary. The London had 100 private nurses on duty by 1899, charging £2 2s. per day for 'ordinary cases', £1 1s. for attendance at an operation and 10s. 6d. per visit for leeching.[107] By 1905 over half the general hospitals in England and Wales hired out private nurses and until 1914 private nurses made up three-quarters of the nursing labour market.[108] Such operations, after an initial investment had been made in the nurses' education, were more lucrative. By 1891 income from nurses represented 2.5 per cent of the national hospital income and acted as a 'modest but reliable source of income'.[109] This overall figure obscures the benefit to individual hospitals (see table 9); the financially cautious John Steele, medical

[105] Hospital for Sick Children, minutes of the board of governors, 7 May 1875, GOSH, 1/6/1; St Bartholomew's Hospital Medical School Session 1877–78, London 1898/9, 17; London Hospital, minutes of the house committee, LH, A/5/40–2.
[106] Anne Witz, Professions and patriarchy, London 1992, 137.
[107] London Hospital, annual report 1899, LH.
[108] Christopher Maggs, The origins of general nursing, London 1983, 131.
[109] Dingwall, Rafferty and Webster, Social history of nursing, 59.

Table 10: Income from loans
(% of total income)

Hospital	1850–5	1870–5	1890–5
German*	11.6	1.9	7.2
Hospital for Sick Children	0.0	1.8	5.2
London	4.8	0.0	0.0
St Bartholomew's**	0.0	14.6	2.5
University College	6.3	2.5	9.4

* Figures for the German Hospital start from 1851, the first year in which detailed accounts were published
** No ledger exists for 1850 to 1855
Source: Annual reports 1850–95; St Bartholomew's, general account books, SBH, Hb/23/3–4

superintendent at Guy's, felt that overall 'nurses earn good round sums for the Hospital'.[110]

All medical schools charged their students tuition fees. The money was divided between the doctors who taught there and, because medical schools did not generally receive financial assistance from the hospitals to which they were attached, the medical school's running expenses. However, where most teaching hospitals had a symbiotic relationship with their medical schools based on mutual service, University College Hospital used tuition fees as a general source of income. Fees were paid straight to the doctors and University College, and both voluntarily redirected their share back to the hospital. In the first three decades after University College Hospital opened, fees formed an important part of its income: between 1850 and 1855 they represented 30.8 per cent of its funding. By the end of the nineteenth century the situation had changed. The level of fees redirected to the hospital had halved and their significance in the structure of income had declined as funding from other sources increased, so that between 1890 and 1895 fees represented 4.1 per cent of income.[111] A change in the financial importance of fees did not alter the governors' attitude to them. They continued to regard fees as important and were concerned to maintain the reputation of the hospital's medical school to keep the number of fee-paying students up.

When all other sources of funding left a deficit, governors borrowed to circumvent financial problems, keep beds open, pay tradesmen's bills and meet the cost of new wards or clinical facilities (see table 10). Borrowing was a short-term and long-term strategy and at certain periods all hospitals sought loans, though some with more frequency than others. Governors were prepared to borrow large amounts to balance the books and meet what was considered 'extraordinary' expenditure (see appendix). If the *Charity Record &*

110 *Charity Record & Philanthropic News* xi (1891), 25.
111 UCH, annual reports 1850–95, UCL.

Philanthropic News could complain that loans were an expensive way of raising money, it also realised that they were often essential in keeping hospitals
running.[112] At the London a policy of loans joined with the sale of stock kept
the hospital open and matched the demands placed on it that the benevolent
resources available within the local community could not afford to meet.
Between 1850 and 1860 the governors borrowed a total of £14,000, most of
which was repaid from the sale of invested property.[113] At University College
Hospital loans were seen as the first resort in any financial crisis. The
endowed hospitals had to have the Charity Commission approve every loan
they took out, but this did not dissuade them from borrowing and even St
Bartholomew's borrowed money, though for improvements rather than debt.

Loans were sought from several sources. In the first few years after an institution's foundation small amounts were borrowed from the treasurer, a policy
adopted by the Hospital for Sick Children until the 1870s to avoid the
impression that it was in debt. Money could also be borrowed internally when
resources were transferred between the building fund and the general fund. In
1883 the Royal Hospital for Diseases of the Chest had to 'borrow' £700 from
its building fund to cover expenditure when donations fell.[114] It was a move
the governors repeated frequently, though such a policy ensured that building
work was delayed. Other hospitals established deposit accounts for this purpose. Internal borrowing, however, was unreliable. As the demands of the
institution grew and new wards were built or sanitary improvements under-
taken it became insufficient, forcing governors to turn to banks and building
societies. When the builders at the German Hospital refused to extend the
governors' credit in 1867, £1,500 immediately had to be borrowed from a
bank.[115] Loans may have been seen as an ideal solution to periodic financial
difficulties, but extensive borrowing created difficulties. The Charity Commission was all too aware of these problems when they refused to sanction
further loans for St Thomas's and Guy's in the 1880s. They informed the governors at Guy's in 1886 that 'while ready and anxious to assist the Governors
in the administration of the Hospital in the present critical condition of its
finances, [the commission] must yet remind them that the repeated recourse
to loans . . . will obviously lead at no distant date to a condition of absolute
insolvency'. The Commission stressed the need to develop other sources of
funding and adopt a better system of financial management to prevent such
situations reoccurring.[116] The governors were appalled, but could do little but
follow the Commission's suggestions. Other hospital governors, without an
external regulation on their borrowing, were aware that there was a limit to
which loans could be sought and at least attempted to repay all loans when

---

112 *Charity Record & Philanthropic News* vi (1886), 103.
113 London Hospital, minutes of the house committee, LH, A/5/27–30.
114 RCH, annual report 1883, LMA.
115 German Hospital, minutes of the hospital committee, 10 Oct. 1867, SBH, GHA 2/4.
116 Guy's to Charity Commission, 1 Dec. 1886, LMA, H9/Gy/A118/20.

money was available to prevent problems from arising. However, considering the widespread level of borrowing it should not be surprising that by the 1890s many hospitals faced financial problems that their deficit financing could not overcome.

Hospital finance was multifaceted and erratic, conditioned by the resources available within the benevolent economy, but at the same time able to draw on a wider number of resources linked to the hospital's function and property. Hospitals as charitable institutions could not rely on charity for all their financial needs. The parameters of hospital funding seemed broad, but the structure of finance was forced to change as the hospital developed and assumed more medical functions.

Commercial philanthropy: the problem of paying patients

Patients were an obvious source of income and it was here that the hospitals' philanthropic credentials came into conflict with their financial needs. Three schemes could be adopted: charges for medicines could be introduced, small fees for out-patient attendance adopted or paying in-patients admitted. Charges for medicines were not as controversial as paying in-patients, which resulted in expensive schemes to provide the high quality of non-medical care linked to privacy that governors associated with private care. Almost every London hospital debated the need to charge patients for some component of their medical care. Discussion was partly stimulated from the 1870s onwards by fears about charitable abuse.[117] Using impressionistic evidence and bold statements that failed to confirm the extent of abuse one way or the other, Victorians were convinced that hospitals' out-patient departments were being used by the middle classes or by an ill-defined group of 'undeserving' patients. Philanthropists (guided by the COS) and doctors extended the argument to see that any free treatment given to those who could afford to pay would inevitably have a pauperising effect. Although the uneasy alliance over abuse between general practitioners and the new elite of hospital consultants frequently broke down, the medical profession repeatedly returned to the problem, encouraging others to take an active interest. Doctors argued that they had a 'duty' to the benevolent public to stamp out abuse and hid behind a rhetoric that shared philanthropists' fears about the habit of dependence. Abuse was quickly cast as a national problem but the focus remained on London.[118]

Some hospital philanthropists felt that it 'would be saying too much' to assert that London's hospitals did not 'relieve a certain percentage' who did not 'deserve' treatment, but in the debate actual numbers did not seem to

---

[117] Lindsay Granshaw, 'St Thomas's Hospital, London, 1850–1900', unpubl. PhD diss. Bryn Mawr 1981, 373–423.
[118] Waddington, ' "Unsuitable cases" ', 26–46.

matter. Despite attempts to quantify abuse by *The Lancet* and hospital reformers, no firm statistics could be produced.[119] Evidence of abuse was seen in anecdotal accounts of out-patient waiting rooms, not in an analysis of the number of patients admitted.[120] Hearsay was enough to confirm fears at a time when abuse was also being seen in other areas of benevolent action. In the debate, rhetoric was more important than reality. Concern was motivated by wider fears about the pauperising effect of indiscriminate philanthropy and this merged with a desire on the part of hospital doctors to regulate the conditions under which they worked. It was this latter point that was at the heart of the debate.[121] Conditions in out-patient departments were seen as appalling and the large number of people attending meant that hospital doctors were not only overworked but also often forced to see patients too quickly.[122] For general practitioners, fearful of becoming 'Medical Tradesmen' and worried about their livelihoods, any limitation of free treatment was desirable in a highly competitive market for medicine. Doctors therefore headed organisations like the Hospital Outpatient Reform Association or the Hospital Reform Association to promote reform.[123] Debate remained fierce and was not abated by an authoritative statement from the King's Fund in 1910, which asserted that there was no sharp financial distinction between those considered deserving and the slightly better-off.[124]

With the extent of abuse impossible for contemporaries to measure, few

[119] For historians levels of abuse are no less easy to determine. Hospitals failed to keep detailed records of out-patients. However, an analysis of in-patient admissions at St Bartholomew's, Guy's, the German Hospital and the London, which were mainly drawn from those waiting in out-patient departments, does suggest that London's hospitals maintained their working-class character with only a small proportion of patients drawn from the middle or professional classes. Granshaw's study of St Thomas's comes to a similar conclusion: St Bartholomew's, statistical tables of medical and surgical registrars, SBH, MR 9/62–84; German Hospital, annual reports 1850–98, SBH; Guy's Hospital, register of admission and discharge, 1854–96, LMA, H9/Gy/B2/1–5, H9/Gy/B3/1–12, H9/Gy/B25/2; London Hospital, register of surgical operations, 1852–62, LH, M/3/74; Granshaw, 'St Thomas's', 62–7. The culture of private medical assistance among the middle class and the stigma of pauperism often associated with charitable care acted as an important disincentive to those who could afford to pay. In addition, with contemporaries claiming that even the poor 'hate going' to out-patient departments where they were 'always harried' and expected to sit for hours in 'close association with dirty people', the departments themselves were sufficiently discouraging: cited in F. B. Smith, *The people's health, 1830–1910*, London 1990, 255.

[120] SC on *Metropolitan Hospitals, First Report*, 172. If the COS could claimed that only 36% of patients admitted to the Royal Free Hospital in 1875 were suitable candidates for treatment, most hospitals by 1897 preferred to claimed that incidents of abuse were 'very small indeed': Charles S. Loch, *Cross purposes in medical reform*, London 1884; *Lancet* i (1897), 1657.

[121] Waddington, ' "Unsuitable cases" ', 26–46.

[122] Samuel Squire Sprigge, *Medicine and the public*, London 1905, 57–9.

[123] *Medical Times & Gazette* ii (1864), 270; *Lancet* i (1870), 497, 500; *Medical Times & Gazette* i (1873), 240–1; *BMJ* ii (1897), 1272–7; *Hospital*, 31 Oct. 1896, 73.

[124] King's Fund, *Enquiry into the management of out-patients departments*, London 1912.

were willing to put forward a contrary view or radical solution that chal-lenged the voluntary nature of the London hospital system. Philanthropists were not prepared to move away from the language of deserving/undeserving poor or advocate any solution that would break down the tripartite structure of medical care: private practice, hospital care and poor law relief. London's hospitals were unwilling to implement far-reaching reforms. They were caught between a half-hearted desire to encourage reform to assure public opinion, the need to attend to the sick poor and a desire to use numbers treated as an advertisement of their public utility. It was impossible for Lon-don's hospitals to ignore the need for reform however. The debate produced a number of possible solutions. Only the inquiry system advocated by the COS and a move to charge patients so they would not be pauperised by hospital care were implemented with any degree of enthusiasm.[125] Inquiry aimed to stamp out abuse; payment worked with the realisation that abuse could not be prevented. The idea that patients should pay something towards the cost of their care had already been accepted in Europe and America where it was argued that contribution schemes strengthened the national character of independence. In England practical schemes took longer to emerge. William Guy, a physician at King's College Hospital and honorary secretary of the Statistical Society, had first recommended an out-patients' payment scheme in 1856 after he had become convinced that many patients could afford to pay something for their treatment.[126] A similar view was adopted by the gov-ernors of the Hospital for Sick Children in 1860, but no plans were made to put the scheme into practice.[127] Other influences linked to the demand for institutional care for the middle classes can be detected. Southwood Smith had endorsed a programme in 1842 to open a hospital for the middle classes in London, but it failed after three years through lack of support. The notion received further backing from the Home Hospital Association, which estab-lished a home hospital in London in 1880. It aimed to offer hospital treat-ment in a homelike atmosphere as an alternative to care in normal lodgings, which were deemed ill-suited for new, more sophisticated forms of medical treatment. The pay principle was implicit and the association endeavoured to promote the contributory system.[128] The extent of the association's influence is uncertain. Governors generally remained cautious, worried about the effect pay beds would have on fundraising and expected intense opposition to any payment scheme. Most pay beds were initially outside the voluntary sector in nursing homes, cottage and private hospitals, but by 1883 thirty-four hospi-tals were charging their patients.[129]

[125] Waddington, ' "Unsuitable cases" ', 39–45.
[126] Cited in Granshaw, 'St Thomas's', 386.
[127] Hospital for Sick Children, minutes of the medical committee, 2 May 1860, GOSH, 1/5/2.
[128] BMJ ii (1878), 806.
[129] Hospital, 22 Mar. 1902, 426; J. L. Clifford-Smith (ed.), Hospital management, London 1883, 52–3.

Table 11: Income from poor-law in-patients
(% of total income)

Hospital	1850–5	1870–5	1890–5
Guy's	0.2	0.4	0.1
London	0.3	0.6	0.4
University College	0.0	0.5	0.1

Source: Annual reports 1850–95; Guy's, financial abstracts, LMA, H9/Gy/D/19/1–2, A/94/1

Informal patient charges, however, already existed at many hospitals. The creation of the new poor law in 1834 established a network of local unions, but with many unable to treat every case of sickness that applied for relief, unions sent some of their patients to local voluntary hospitals for treatment. The result was the creation of an 'internal market' between healthcare sectors. Steele, in an attempt to rationalise the payment system introduced at Guy's, willingly explained in 1882 that 'from time immemorial, it has been the custom for guardians in London, as well as in the country, to send special cases to the hospital for the benefit of the superior medical skill and treatment it affords'.[130] Marland's work on Wakefield and Huddersfield suggests that this was not limited to London, while Amanda Berry has shown that it was a feature of late eighteenth-century hospital care.[131] Most paupers were admitted under subscription rights, but those hospitals that relieved a large number of poor-law patients established a separate system of fees (see table 11). Charges were small. At Guy's poor-law patients were admitted at 1s. per day, while the London charged the Whitechapel Union 1s. 6d. per day per pauper. Despite the relatively high charge (higher than paying patients were later expected to pay), the Whitechapel guardians felt they had acquired a good deal and signed a treatment agreement to ensure the admission of their paupers.[132] The union's decision was not usual. St Pancras Union contributed fifty guineas annually to University College Hospital and in 1866 twenty beds were allocated to the union on a semi-permanent basis. University College Hospital charged 10s. per patient per week in addition to the union's subscription for this privilege.[133] The financial advantage was decidedly in the hospital's favour, which justified high charges by claiming a superior level of care. Co-operation between poor law unions and voluntary hospitals was more extensive than contemporaries acknowledged, but a transfer of the cost

[130] BMJ ii (1882), 805–6.
[131] Marland, Medicine and society, 84–5; Amanda Berry, 'Community sponsorship and the hospital patient in late eighteenth-century England', in Peregrine Horden and Richard Smith (eds), Locus of care: communities, institutions, and the provision of welfare since antiquity, London 1998, 126–50.
[132] Whitechapel Board of Guardians' minutes, 19 May 1857, LMA, St.B.G/Wh/21.
[133] UCH, minutes of the general committee, 25 July 1866, UCL, A1/2/1.

of care between the two institutions remained limited to large general hospitals, located near densely populated areas. Only in the twentieth century were payments from local authorities for a range of services extended.[134]

Payment schemes not connected to the poor law attracted staunch opposition and were seen as the 'modern philanthropy of commerce'.[135] Opposition focused on four main points: payment, it was feared, would encourage subscribers to withdraw their support, discourage patients and deprive hospitals of clinical material and represent a break with the hospitals' charitable nature. The British Medical Association remained critical, believing that payment would damage the economic position of general practitioners, a view shared by many doctors who felt that it created unfair competition.[136] For the COS, any hospital payment scheme would paradoxically limit providence and prevent the development of character by creating the notion that nominal payment gave a right to relief.[137] One speaker at a conference of hospital administrators organised by the SSA in 1882 believed that 'even the bankrupt condition of a hospital is not sufficient to justify its committee in beginning to trade in medical relief'.[138] Criticism and concerns about opposition failed to dissuade several hospitals from admitting paying patients, and other writers stressed the financial background behind their controversial decisions. For one writer in *The Times* in 1882 payment by patients was the best way to generate additional funds for the ailing London hospitals, a view shared by Henry Burdett who was closely involved in the foundation of the Home Hospital Association.[139] The *Charity Record & Philanthropic News* reluctantly came to the same conclusion in 1883. A moral gloss was added to make the journal's suggestion more palatable when it explained that payment would remove the 'semi-pauperism' that hospitals encouraged.[140] As the initial hope that paying patients would bring vital income into the hospital faded with experience, paying patients were made to serve another purpose. Image and utility were crucial in London's highly competitive benevolent economy, for a closed bed created an unfavourable impression and reduced the number of patients that could be treated. A paying bed, however, provided additional income and ensured that beds were kept open, increasing admissions.

Individual hospitals did not rationalise their moves to charge patients, but admitted them out of financial necessity. At the Poplar Hospital a 4d. outpatients' charge was introduced soon after the hospital opened because it

134 Cherry, 'Before the National Health Service', 315.
135 Charles S. Loch, 'Confusion in medical charities', *Nineteenth Century* xxxii (1892), 299.
136 *Lancet* i (1884), 363.
137 Loch, 'Confusion in medical charities', 306.
138 Cited in Clifford-Smith, *Hospital management*, 46.
139 *Times*, 14 June 1882, 7; 15 Jan. 1883, 12.
140 *Charity Record & Philanthropic News* iii (1883), 233.

Table 12: Payment from patients
by hospital type, 1897

Type	No.	In-patients	Out-patients
General	28	£6,337	£1,906
Chest	7	£4,179	–
Children's	14	£2,074	£1,111
Lying-in	6	£335	£619
Women's	7	£1,652	£1,383
Fever	1	£2,384	–
Lock	2	£2,514	£1,444
Dental	2	–	£1,391
Epilepsy	4	£2,511	£894
Fistula	2	£685	£89
Ophthalmic	5	£538	£512
Orthopaedic	3	£1,532	–
Skin	4	£451	£3,667
Stone	1	£181	£2,057
Throat	5	£734	£4,895
Cottage	3	£394	–

Source: *Hospital Saturday Fund Journal*, Sept. 1897, 4

faced mounting debts.[141] St Thomas's adopted a similar course on financial grounds. Whether a hospital decided to charge its patients or not depended on its nature, its financial situation and on what types of patient it treated (see table 12). In the care of consumptives and those suffering from cancer, for example, private-paying institutions greatly outnumbered public ones until 1907.[142] Specialist hospitals were believed to charge most of their patients and a report by the Hospitals Association in 1897 noted that they were 'largely dependent on the payment of patients' for their income. Of the forty-one specialist hospitals in 1895, 73 per cent charged for treatment, though few drew as much income from this source as the Grosvenor Hospital for Women and Children where money from patients represented one third of the total income.[143]

Payment schemes, however, were less widespread in general hospitals, despite rising demand from middle-class patients for institutional medical care. St Thomas's was the first major hospital to admit paying patients. Its decision pushed the issue before the public and involved the hospital in an

[141] Barnes, 'The Docker's Hospital'.
[142] See Michael Worboys, 'The sanatorium treatment for consumptives in Britain', in John V. Pickstone (ed.), *Medical innovations in historical perspective*, New York 1992, 47–71.
[143] *Hospital*, 31 Dec. 1887, 236; *Lancet* i (1897), 1031.

internal struggle between the governors and the less enthusiastic medical staff that lasted from 1878 to 1881. The impetus came from the hospital's financial position. The long-term expenditure involved in its move to Lambeth acted as a continuous drain on the hospital's endowed income and imposed higher running expenses. Rents for landed property and donations did not increase as expected, the former declining with the agricultural depression.[144] Tired of St Thomas's incessant financial problems, the Charity Commission suggested a payment scheme, which after lengthy discussion was adopted. The medical journals approved of the idea but disliked the scheme, and *The Lancet* condemned the governors' dismissive attitude to the medical staff.[145] On 1 March 1881 St Thomas's was opened to paying patients. Over the next nine months a total of 237 patients were admitted, producing a profit of £400, but from 1886 admissions declined and the scheme was not the success the treasurer had envisaged.[146]

Though the governors of the London discussed an out-patient payment scheme in 1880, it was Guy's that initially followed St Thomas's lead.[147] In 1883 it admitted its first paying patient after four years of intense financial problems linked to falling rental income as a result of the agricultural depression. Once more the Charity Commission, reluctant to sanction further loans, had taken the initiative and suggested the admission of paying patients. With few other alternatives available the governors were forced to agree with the Commission's proposals.[148] Unlike St Thomas's there was little internal debate and two schemes were adopted. The governors suggested that patients could be admitted to the wards under two forms of payment: the first admitted them to the general wards at a cost of one guinea per week, the second was a three-guinea fee for admission to a separate paying ward of twelve beds. The three-guinea charge bought nursing care, rudimentary medical care from a resident medical officer and a separate cubicle. All treatment had to be negotiated with the medical staff or with an approved hospital consultant; general practitioners were excluded. Initially thirty-eight beds were allocated rising to fifty in 1886.[149] The medical staff put forward another method of payment whereby a 3d. out-patients' fee was levied on the patient's second visit. A clear statement of inability to pay from a doctor, priest or the COS granted free treatment. It was argued that this would have a less damaging effect on patient admissions and allow doctors to give free emergency treatment while at the same time discouraging unnecessary or trivial cases. In a memorandum in 1897 it was stated that 'the paying patient system was . . .

144 Granshaw, 'St Thomas's', 401–19, 390–3.
145 *Lancet* i (1880), 19.
146 Granshaw, 'St Thomas's', 421.
147 London Hospital, minutes of the house committee, LH, A/5/39–40.
148 Guy's to Charity Commission, 21 Mar. 1884, LMA, H9/Gy/A172/2.
149 Guy's Hospital, minutes of the court of committees, 23 July 1884, LMA, H9/Gy/A3/11; memorandum book of John Steele, LMA, H9/Gy/A164/1.

Table 13: Guy's Hospital: payment from patients
1886–98

Year	Paying ward		Other ward		Out-patients	
	No.	£	No.	£	No.	£
1886	77	£721 10s. 7d.	262	£1,038 18s. 0d.	63,077	£715 5s. 2d.
1887	84	£702 10s. 2d.	311	£1,467 12s. 10d.	56,353	£656 0s. 7d.
1888	81	£889 5s. 0d.	333	£1,245 14s. 0d.	59,175	£670 12s. 0d.
1889	89	£1,093 6s. 9d.	283	£984 14s. 0d.	53,885	£631 7s. 0d.
1890	183	£1,672 14s. 6d.	284	£1,077 2s. 0d.	57,412	£657 9s. 5d.
1891	196	£2,221 6s. 0d.	273	£1,030 3s. 6d.	62,621	£750 16s. 4d.
1892	224	£2,326 13s. 0d.	316	£1,091 19s. 11d.	63,335	£730 16s. 4d.
1893	216	£2,091 7s. 0d.	279	£867 1s. 1d.	64,656	£752 8s. 1d.
1894	208	£2,300 0s. 4d.	641	£1,211 15s. 0d.	68,945	£807 3s. 1d.
1895	216	£2,718 2s. 6d.	301	£1,247 10s. 0d.	76,109	£874 15s. 11d.
1896	301	£2,502 17s. 6d.	321	£1,289 9s. 0d.	78,762	£920 0s. 0d.
1897	277	£2,305 17s. 6d.	298	£955 17s. 6d.	80,265	£941 6s. 1d.
1898	353	£3,120 7s. 0d.	16	£87 3s. 0d.	80,862	£956 6s. 7d.

Source: *Hospital Saturday Fund Journal*, Sept. 1987, 4

originally a temporary measure expedient to raise money', but as income from other sources did not improve it became permanent. The low number of patients admitted in the first few months encouraged the view that the scheme was a failure, but it was not abandoned as the governors and staff anticipated that reforms would make the scheme more attractive.[150] By 1890 improvements in the paying ward ensured that admissions had risen and the initial hopes were justified.

The German Hospital, unlike many other general hospitals, had always admitted paying patients through its separate sanatorium. The aim was to provide treatment for members of the respectable working and middle classes who could not be nursed at home. The institution remained small. Exceptions were made to admit patients who could only speak English, but the sanatorium was generally reserved for German nationals or German-speaking patients. Charges were on a sliding scale, linked to the type of room rather than the treatment required, though from 1857 syphilitic patients were charged one guinea more than other patients to bring admissions in line with costs – and to discourage them.[151] The sanatorium was a service for those who could afford to pay, removing all concerns over hospital abuse. It represented a 'highly important branch' of the hospital, but it received few patients and made little money.[152]

Income from patients could not solve the London hospitals' incessant

---

[150] Guy's Hospital, minutes of the finance committee, LMA, H9/Gy/A24/1; minutes of the medical committee, 22 Mar. 1884, LMA, H9/Gy/A20/1.
[151] German Hospital, minutes of the hospital committee, 24 Sept. 1857, SBH, GHA 2/2.
[152] *Charity*, June 1887, 5.

need for funds in the short or long term. After a slow start at Guy's the income from paying patients did gradually rise (see table 13). According to the *Hospital* in 1890 payment schemes provided 15 per cent of provincial hospitals' income, but in 1893 only 2 per cent of the total income of London's general hospitals and 7.5 per cent for specialist hospitals.[153] The difference reflected the number of general hospitals in London prepared to admit paying patients. At the German Hospital payment from patients remained marginal, contributing 1.9 per cent between 1850 and 1854, and 2.7 per cent between 1890 and 1895.[154] Profits were never substantial and payment was not in proportion to the cost of treatment. At Guy's in 1886/7 eighty-four paying in-patients produced a profit of only £103 10s. 1d.; by 1890/1 this had risen to 187 patients with a profit of £850 4s. 4d.[155] However, there was an immediate effect on the number of cases treated. Out-patient admissions at St Thomas's and Guy's, despite the optimism of the *BMJ*, fell dramatically when payment was introduced and only slowly recovered.[156] The hope of long-term profits had to be balanced against the immediate fall in admissions that threatened the hospital's appearance of utility, and the small amount of income that paying patients generated.

Patient payment schemes, despite continued criticism, did not prove an expensive and potentially damaging dead-end. Financial pressure eventually forced other hospitals to follow Guy's and St Thomas's and introduce patient charges. By the 1920s, patient payments had become a major source of finance, with 60 per cent of hospitals in London having pay beds by 1929.[157] When St Thomas's introduced its scheme, this was still unthinkable with payment being seen by many as an extreme solution.

Changing patterns of hospital finance

Hospital finance, even in 1850, was not in 'that flourishing condition . . . which everyone would wish'.[158] In the pursuit of financial security and from a desire to balance the books, governors gradually and erratically adapted the structure of their hospital's income. A change in the nature of the hospital required an alteration in how it was financed and governors, often preoccupied with financial concerns, responded in the face of change. Hospitals were flexible enough institutions to adapt to new financial demands and conditions, though change was rarely immediate and often the result of crisis man-

153 *Hospital*, 26 Apr. 1890, 47; Henry Burdett, *Hospitals and asylums of the world*, iii, London 1893, 119.

154 German Hospital, annual reports 1850–95, SBH.

155 Guy's Hospital, weekly reports of superintendence, LMA, H9/Gy/A67/7–8.

156 *BMJ* i (1884), 184.

157 Cherry, 'Before the National Health Service', 319–20.

158 *Medical Times & Gazette* xxi (1850), 10.

Table 14: German Hospital: income,
1851–95 (%)

	Source	1851–5	1870–5	1890–5
Balance		8.4	4.1	1.6
Direct	Subscriptions	23.5	13.2	18.0
Philanthropy	Donations	39.9	37.4	34.4
	Legacies	2.1	2.5	6.3
	Collections	8.3	0.2	0.5
Indirect	Sunday Fund	–	1.9	6.1
Philanthropy	Saturday Fund	–	0.4	1.8
Property	Rent	–	–	2.0
	Deposits	–	8.5	–
	Dividends	2.0	13.8	18.6
	Insurance	0.7	–	–
	Sale of property	–	–	–
	Sale of stock	1.6	13.6	0.1
	From waste	–	–	–
	Tax	–	0.1	0.5
	Tithes	–	–	–
Function	Students	–	–	–
	Nurses	–	–	–
	Patients	1.9	2.1	2.7
Loans		11.6	1.9	7.2
'Sundries'		–	0.3	0.3

Source: Annual reports 1850–95, SBH

agement and opportunity. The result was an unco-ordinated process of financial diversification.

This could take several forms. Existing sources of funding might be modified. For example, the London's move to reinvest its government bonds in mortgages was an attempt to increase income that simultaneously modified an existing resource. Income from direct philanthropy was changed in a similar manner as new means of soliciting benevolence were adopted or old ones declined in importance. Financial diversification equally resulted from the development of existing resources so that they changed their relative importance within the structure of income. The governors at the German Hospital achieved this after 1869 by placing a renewed emphasis on investments. New sources of funding also encouraged diversification. The foundation of the Sunday Fund and Saturday Fund in the early 1870s created a new channel for voluntary contributions that benefited London's non-endowed hospitals and increased the money they received from the benevolent economy. Other London hospitals made existing services into a financial asset and attempted

Table 15: St Bartholomew's Hospital: income, 1863–95 (%)

	Source	1863–5	1870–5	1890–5
Balance		7.0	1.1	3.7
Direct	Subscriptions	–	–	–
Philanthropy	Donations	1.5	0.9	0.5
	Legacies	0.2	2.1	2.7
	Collections	–	–	–
Indirect	Sunday Fund	–	–	–
Philanthropy	Saturday Fund	–	–	–
Property	Rent	77.7	56.2	73.2
	Deposits	–	–	–
	Dividends	10.2	7.9	4.2
	Insurance	–	1.8	2.0
	Sale of property	–	12.8	4.5
	Sale of stock	–	–	–
	From waste	0.5	0.3	–
	Tax	0.8	1.3	2.0
	Tithes	0.4	0.1	2.0
Function	Students	0.1	0.1	0.8
	Nurses	–	–	1.8
	Patients	–	–	–
Loans		–	14.6	2.5
'Sundries'		1.6	0.8	0.1

Source: General account books, SBH, Hb/23/3–4

to make new ones self-funding. New financial strategies did not have to be grand to modify the hospital's income structure.

All hospitals, to one degree or another, experienced a process of financial diversification. In the 1850s University College Hospital had nine main sources of income, by the 1890s it had sixteen. At the Royal Hospital for Diseases of the Chest the number rose from seven to ten, and from nine to seventeen at the Hospital for Sick Children. The different approaches to diversification can be seen at the German Hospital (table 14), St Bartholomew's (table 15) and Guy's (table 16). The German Hospital displayed a pattern of diversification that reflected a process of crisis management in the 1860s, followed by a period in which the governors built up their investments to increase 'reliable' income. Financial diversification at St Bartholomew's, on the other hand, was not the product of an anxious pursuit of funds, rather a response to new financial opportunities and demands. At Guy's the situation was different. Here diversification was a lesson in crisis management after the hospital's income had been dramatically affected by the agricultural depression.

Table 16: Guy's Hospital: income, 1853–95 (%)

	Source	1853–5	1870–5	1890–5
Balance		–	–	–
Direct philanthropy	Subscriptions	–	–	–
	Donations	0.4	0.2	23.0
	Legacies	–	2.1	–
	Collections	–	–	–
Indirect philanthropy	Sunday Fund	–	–	1.0
	Saturday Fund	–	–	1.2
Property	Rent	95.6	95.8	58.2
	Deposits	–	–	–
	Dividends	3.8	1.5	4.2
	Insurance	–	–	–
	Sale of property	–	–	0.1
	Sale of stock	–	–	–
	From waste	–	–	–
	Tax	–	–	–
	Tithes	–	–	–
Function	Students	–	–	–
	Nurses	–	–	2.6
	Patients	0.2	0.4	9.7
Loans		–	–	–
'Sundries'		–	–	–

Source: Financial abstracts, LMA, H9/Gy/D/19/1–3; treasurer's reports, LMA, H9/Gy/A/94/1

Each hospital had its own financial approach and response to financial problems. The German Hospital displayed a careful and at times cautious financial policy where diversification was a consequence of an attempt to meet the hospital's running costs and the financial strain of rebuilding. The Hospital for Sick Children and the London had a similar approach to their finances, whereas Guy's and University College Hospital, if not reckless, were not as careful in their administration. The result was the same. Each hospital in London, and to a lesser extent each hospital in England, underwent a process of financial change as it evolved and aged. Governors, in their pursuit of new sources of funding, unconsciously and erratically diluted charity's financial contribution. However, if common sources of income can be found in the internal economy of hospital finance, it might also be possible to identify common factors that encouraged this widespread, if not uniform, process of financial diversification. It is the explanation for these changes that the next chapter addresses.

4

Financial Diversification: An Explanation

Financial diversification was not a random phenomenon. All London hospitals changed the structure, and sometimes the nature of their income. It was a process that accelerated from the 1860s onwards as hospitals increasingly faced a financial crisis that dogged them until the foundation of the National Health Service in 1948. Governors responded by expanding the number of sources from which they drew their income. However, there was more to the process of diversification than a deepening financial crisis.

Contemporaries were pessimistic about the hospitals' economic fortunes, but few analysed the reasons behind the apparent crisis. In a speech in support of the Metropolitan Hospital Sunday Fund in 1887, Baron Ferdinand de Rothschild provided a rare analysis of hospital finance. He identified the agricultural depression, competition within the benevolent economy, the growth of specialist hospitals and a disregard for physical ailments as the main reasons for the misfortunes that faced London's hospitals.[1] Others blamed the 'widespread and just dissatisfaction' with how medical charities were administered, or the lack of co-operation between the medical and philanthropic sides of the hospital.[2] Governors, however, did not acknowledge these influences. Instead they publicly lamented their problems and directed their efforts into fundraising. Any interpretation of financial diversification therefore has to reconcile the pressures exerted on the hospitals' finances with the hospitals' experiences. Rothschild's analysis is a good starting point, but he fails to give the complete picture. A broad analysis is needed. With no clear statements from governors it is difficult to be precise, but a framework that looks at expenditure, rebuilding, the experiences of different institutional types, community resources, competition, the national economy and the damaging effect of criticism does provide a model through which the experiences of individual hospitals can be located and explained.

Ever-increasing expenditure

In his evidence to the Select Committee on Metropolitan Hospitals, Lieutenant-Colonel Emanuel Montefiore, the long-serving secretary of the Charity Organisation Society's medical advisory committee, was careful to

---

1 *Hospital*, 29 Oct. 1887, 73–4.
2 *Charity Record & Philanthropic News* iv (1884), 362; *Charity*, Nov. 1887, 151.

Figure 7: University College Hospital:
income against expenditure, 1851–98

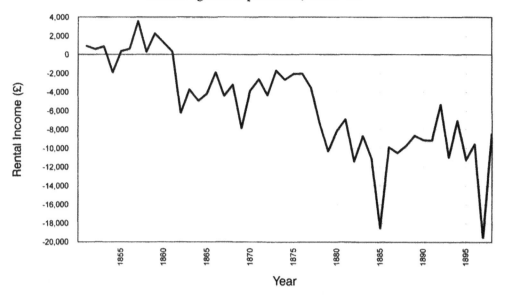

Source: Annual reports 1850–98, UCL

explain that expenditure was the main evil in hospital finance.[3] It exerted an enormous pressure on income, forcing the development of new sources of funding and a reliance on deficit financing. In 1855 the governors of the Royal Hospital for Diseases of the Chest anxiously explained that they had been compelled to 'turn their attention to other modes of supply' because expenditure had exhausted the hospital's traditional sources of income.[4] Few hospitals, however, were in the same position as University College Hospital (see figure 7). Here the governors stumbled from one crisis to the next and subscribers were constantly misled over the seriousness of the hospital's financial position. By 1897 a deficit of over £19,000 forced the governors to close nearly a quarter of the hospital's beds. For the BMJ this was 'convincing proof that the chronic financial difficulties of the hospitals in London [had] reached a serious crisis'.[5] From the 1860s onwards economies were attempted – champagne was removed as an item of medical expenditure – but the hospital's resources were insufficient to meet annual expenditure.[6] As spending increased, debts mounted and bills were left unpaid until additional money could be raised to pay them. The governors practised a policy of brinkmanship, paying only those creditors who pressed hardest. With such a burden of

3 SC on Metropolitan Hospitals, First Report, 15.
4 RCH, annual report 1855, LMA.
5 BMJ ii (1897), 1805.
6 UCH, minutes of the house committee, 23 May 1887, UCL, A1/3/3.

Figure 8: Royal Hospital for Diseases of the Chest:
expenditure, 1850–98

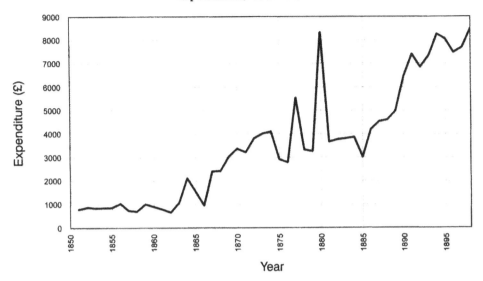

Source: Annual reports 1850–98, LMA

debt they energetically worked to develop new sources of funding and sold invested property to raise additional capital. A few benefactors, like George Moore in 1876, recognised that this could only reduce future income and when they left money to the hospital they stipulated that it had to be invested.[7] However, given University College Hospital's financial position, the governors felt that they had few alternatives and relied on fortuitous legacies to bail them out of their financial difficulties.

University College Hospital was an extreme but not unusual case. The Middlesex shared its propensity for debt and the Norfolk and Norwich Hospital had to launch its first major appeal in 1801 when income failed to cover running costs.[8] It was a crisis that was repeated at other institutions throughout the century. Even the prosperous St Bartholomew's had to sell £3,000 of its investments in 1854 to meet expenditure.[9] Public appeals were a more common approach to an expenditure crisis: the London launched its first public appeal in 1807 to 'rescue it from serious embarrassment' and followed it with a further appeal in 1814. The foundation of a quinquennial appeal in 1878 was an attempt to reduce mounting debts and represented a move away

---

7   UCH, minutes of the general committee, 20 Dec. 1876, UCL, A1/2/4.
8   SC on Metropolitan Hospitals, Second Report, 123; Steven Cherry, 'The role of the provincial hospital: the Norfolk and Norwich Hospital, 1771–1880', Population Studies xxvi (1972), 297.
9   St Bartholomew's, minutes of the board of governors, 7 June 1854, SBH, Ha 1/21.

Figure 9: London Hospital:
expenditure, 1850–98

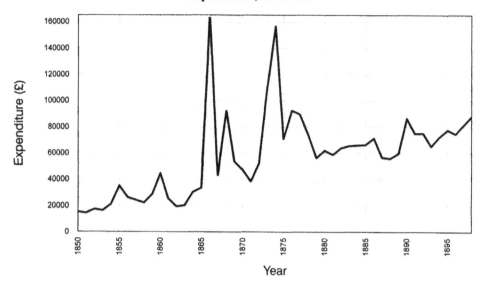

Source: Annual reports 1850–98, LH

from the London's traditional reliance on dividends and subscriptions.[10] Appeals, however, were only a short-term solution that did nothing to reduce total expenditure. Governors found it harder to cut spending than raise money, though all institutions regularly made economies.

From the foundation of the voluntary hospitals in the eighteenth century administrators had been anxious to anticipate any allegation of mismanagement and defend every increase in expenditure to maintain public confidence.[11] In an attempt to justify large items of spending, expenditure was divided into 'ordinary' and 'extraordinary' to alleviate subscribers' concerns. Capital costs and rebuilding schemes were placed under 'extraordinary' expenditure to emphasise the unusual nature of the capital outlay. This could not hide the fact that expenditure increased dramatically (see figures 8 and 9). By 1890 metropolitan hospitals were on average spending £2,000 per day and from 1891 to 1911 annual expenditure rose from approximately £643,000 to £1,360,000.[12] Not even the most prudent of administrators could prevent this dramatic increase. Growth rates varied between institutions: at St Bartholomew's there was a 70 per cent increase in spending between 1860 and 1895; at the Hospital for Sick Children it was 76 per cent, while expendi-

10 London Hospital, annual report 1850, LH.
11 Ann Borsay, ' "Persons of honour and reputation": the voluntary hospital in the age of corruption', *Medical History* xxxv (1991), 286–7.
12 Pinker, *English hospital statistics*, 162.

Table 17: Hospital for Sick Children:
expenditure, 1860, 1895

	1860			1895			Increase (%)
Administration	£0	0s.	0d.	£490	16s.	6d.	100.0
Building improvement	£0	0s.	0d.	£822	0s.	2d.	100.0
Medicine	£217	13s.	2d.	£1,284	12s.	7d.	83.1
Provisions	£1,068	14s.	8d.	£2,397	3s.	2d.	55.4
Salaries	£617	7s.	4d.	£3,016	10s.	9d.	79.5
TOTAL	£1,903	15s.	2d.	£8,071	0s.	2d.	76.4

Source: Annual reports 1860, 1895, GOSH

ture rose less quickly at the Cancer Hospital.[13] The trend, however, was the same across London.

Why did expenditure increase in this manner? The 'excessive amounts spent by hospitals in advertising and collecting, printing stationery and post-age' were persistently attacked, and critics wanted to claim that governors were either extravagant or unable to control funding.[14] The reasons for the universal rise in spending lay elsewhere, however, as shown in tables 17 and 18. Large extravagances were uncommon. The governors of the German Hospital spoke for many hospitals when, after investigating their expenditure in 1856, they found that it was an increase in 'essential items' that was raising costs.[15] George Goschen, the conservative Chancellor, was closer to the truth when he explained in 1887 that 'the expenditure of an hospital was increased by new inventions in medical science, and that the very perfection at which medical science has arrived had increased the expenditure of hospitals'. Under these conditions 'it cost more to cure a man than formerly'.[16] At Guy's expenditure per patient rose from £46 to £81 between 1868 and 1887–9, from £40 to £66 at the Westminster, and from £38 to £115 at the London Fever Hospital. This was against a metropolitan fall in the average length of stay. Antiseptic procedures, new 'surgical appliances and dressing', and changes in nursing were seen as the main reasons for this rise, while at the London Fever Hospital it was connected with the introduction of new antitoxins.[17]

Changes in therapeutic practice with the development of new clinical aids, advances in surgery and moves towards scientific medicine, signified

13 St Bartholomew's, general account books, SBH, Hb 23/3–4; Hospital for Sick Children, annual report 1855, 1895, GOSH; Burdett, Hospitals and asylums, iii. 172.
14 Hansard, 3rd ser. cccxxxviii. 1552.
15 German Hospital, minutes of the hospital committee, 10 Apr. 1856, SBH, GHA 2/2.
16 Charity Record & Philanthropic News vii (1887), 147.
17 Burdett, Hospitals and asylums, iii. 172; Pinker, English hospital statistics, 121.

Table 18: St Bartholomew's Hospital: expenditure, 1855, 1895

	1855			1895			Increase (%)
Administration	£746	5s.	6d.	£3,512	10s.	10d.	78.8
Building improvement	£158	10s.	0d.	£1,095	8s.	0d.	85.6
Medicine	£627	7s.	4d.	£3,275	19s.	9d.	80.9
Provisions	£2,409	10s.	10d.	£3,610	16s.	6d.	33.3
Salaries	£1,098	11s.	8d.	£5,558	9s.	5d.	80.2
TOTAL	£5,040	5s.	8d.	£17,052	4s.	6d.	70.4

Source: General account books, SBH, Hb/23/3–4

new procedures for medical practitioners and more expensive ones for hospitals. New specialisms meant new departments and more equipment.[18] Whereas the introduction of X-ray equipment after 1896 was rapid, acceptance of many of these new procedures was either piecemeal or resisted, as discussed in chapter 6. Old and new existed side-by-side, but the London hospitals (and especially the metropolitan teaching hospitals) were quicker at incorporating new techniques into their medical regime than many of their provincial counterparts. Governors in London, for example, were expected to buy clinical thermometers as a routine item of expenditure by the 1880s. In the decade before, improvements in instrument making with the adoption of nickel-plated and enamelled instruments to replace iron ones (which were prone to rust) forced governors to virtually re-equip their hospitals.[19] The introduction of chloroform had encouraged an 'operating mania' and more

[18] See Stanley J. Reiser, *Medicine and the reign of technology*, Cambridge 1990, for the rise of clinical technology. For the growth of specialism and the change in therapeutic and surgical practice see Rosemary Stevens, *Medical practice in modern England: the impact of specialisation and state medicine*, New Haven 1966; Richard H. Shryock, *The development of modern medicine*, London 1948; Youngson, *Victorian medicine*. Christopher Lawrence, ' "Incommunicable knowledge": science, technology and clinical art in Britain, 1850–1914', *Journal of Contemporary History* xx (1985), 502–20, and W. F. Bynum, *Science and the practice of medicine in the nineteenth century*, Cambridge 1996, offer more thought–provoking analyses. Other studies, like Lindsay Granshaw, 'Knowledge of bodies or bodies of knowledge?: surgeons, anatomists and rectal surgery, 1830–1985', in Christopher Lawrence (ed.), *Medical theory, surgical practice*, London 1992, 232–62, or Anne Hardy, 'Tracheotomy versus intubation: surgical intervention in diphtheria in Europe and the United States, 1825–1930', *BHM* lxvi (1992), 336–59, illustrate the development of particular practices. John H. Warner, *The therapeutic perspective*, Cambridge 1986, and M. J. Vogel and Charles E. Rosenberg, *The therapeutic revolution: essays in the social history of American medicine*, Philadelphia 1979, look at these developments from an American perspective, but offer an insight into the evolution of modern medicine and how changes were perceived and adopted.
[19] UCH, minutes of the finance committee, 10 Feb. 1884, UCL, A1/3/3; Smith, *The people's health*.

invasive procedures that required longer post-operative treatment. Chloro-form also involved the appointment of a new, paid class of practitioner, the anaesthetist. The timing of appointments varied and though the Hospital for Sick Children did not find it necessary to hire one until 1895, most London hospitals saw an anaesthetist as an essential member of their staff by the late 1870s.[20] Changes in the nature and quantity of prescriptions had similar financial implications. If St Bartholomew's could dispense 900 gallons of cod-liver oil, 1,200 ounces of quinine and three hundredweight of ammonia to anxious patients in 1869, the number of prescriptions and drugs used had multiplied by the 1890s contributing to the 81 per cent rise in expenditure on medicines in the period. It was not just a case of more prescription to a greater number of patients. In the treatment of burns, for example, the more expensive lanolin gradually replaced the use of turpentine, vinegar, or more commonly treacle, in dressings.[21] Although staff working at the London were prepared to make do with the old operating theatre and wooden operating table until the 1890s, they pressed the governors to buy spirometers (for measuring lung capacity) and other new equipment for quantifying patients' symptoms from the 1850s onwards.[22]

The 1880s and 1890s saw further developments in hospital medicine that had greater financial implications. It was in this last quarter of the nineteenth century that the diagnostic and therapeutic function of the hospital underwent a revival and a period of rapid change. While some surgeons did use lint dressings or lac plasters before 1870 as a means of reducing infection, the difficult introduction of Lister's antiseptic system encouraged the use of carbolic and more dressings as regular draining and re-bandaging was initially required. St Thomas's interest in antiseptic techniques saw a move from carbolic sprays to the use of sterilised water in 1890; to the purchase of two autoclaves and two larger sterilisers for bulky items. The surgeon Harrison Cripps's enthusiasm for an antiseptic approach led the governors at St Bartholomew's in the early 1890s to buy three sterilisers and provide a separate theatre with a brass and glass operating table for him. They were not prepared, however, to pay for the operating theatre to be rebuilt in marble and alabaster in 1896, forcing Cripps to pay for this himself. Lister's methods failed to kill airborne bacteria and did not stop hospitals from being unhygienic institutions (with both St Bartholomew's and University College Hospital criticised for their sanitary arrangements in the 1890s), but they did

20 UCH, medical and surgical registrars' reports, UCL, MR/3a/8; *Journal of the Royal Statistical Society* (1911), 367–8; Hospital for Sick Children, minutes of the committee of management, 20 Mar. 1895, GOSH, 1/2/21.
21 *The Lancet* ii (1869), 577, 678; St Bartholomew's, general account books, SBH, Hb 23/3–4; Smith, *The people's health*, 258.
22 E. W. Morris, *A history of the London*, London 1926, 201; London Hospital, physicians and surgeons' report book, 28 Nov. 1851, LH, A/17/7.

make them more expensive.[23] If bacteriology had less impact on ward practices, it did have financial implications with hospitals providing and equipping new laboratories. In teaching hospitals the need to educate students in the most modern methods made such developments appear a necessity. One of the first measures in the redevelopment of the London's in the mid-1890s after the appointment of the Sydney Holland as chairman, was the opening of a new clinical laboratory in 1896. A similar laboratory was built at St Thomas's in the following year. At the Royal Hospital for Diseases of the Chest, the analysis of sputum by a pathologist became an important guide for treatment even if cod-liver oil remained the main medicine prescribed.[24]

The mathematically-minded Philip Hensley, senior physician at the Royal Hospital for Diseases of the Chest, expressed a common view among doctors in 1885. Writing in the *Charity Record & Philanthropic News* he commented that he 'had never considered the question of expense in recommending what he thought was right for the patients of the hospital'.[25] The rate of progress should not be exaggerated; new techniques often had a difficult reception. Hospitals remained conservative institutions and doctors' junior position in management ensured that they had little control over spending and were forced to match their medical demands to the governors' assessment of the individual hospital's financial position. This acted as a brake on development rather than an insuperable barrier. Governors lacked the professional knowledge to argue effectively against new equipment when their medical staff insisted that it was a medical necessity. The widespread purchase of microscopes in the 1880s might be seen as symbolic of the interactions between medical science, governors and hospital doctors. They became a common but disputed item of medical expenditure. When the medical staff at the German Hospital claimed that a microscope was 'absolutely necessary for the Institution in order to keep pace with the progress of the knowledge and discoveries of the causes of disease made in late years', the governors were in no position to argue and agreed the expenditure. Doctors in other hospitals made similar claims with varying degrees of success.[26]

---

[23] T. H. Pennington, 'Listerism, its decline and its persistence: the introduction of aseptic surgical techniques in three British teaching hospitals, 1890–9', *Medical History* xxxix (1995), 48–51. At University College Hospital the storage of soiled bedpans in ward lobbies was identified as the main reason for the smell in the wards in 1885, while in 1898 the King's Fund could still find the sanitary arrangements 'objectionable': UCH, finance committee, 1 June 1885, UCL, A1/3/3; Prince of Wales Hospital Fund, report on UCH, June 1898, LMA, A/KE/259/1.

[24] London Hospital, minutes of the house committee, 20 July 1896, LH, A/5/46; RCH, minutes of the finance committee, 28 July 1885, LMA, H33/RCH/A5/1.

[25] *Charity Record & Philanthropic News* v (1885), 197.

[26] German Hospital, minutes of the hospital committee, 11 Sept. 1884, SBH, GHA 2/8. Staff at the Royal Hospital for Diseases of the Chest were less successful. In 1884 the governors initially opposed the purchase of a microscope, considering it unnecessarily expensive at a time when funds were strained: RCH, minutes of the medical council, 3 Jan. 1883, LMA, H33/RCH/A3/1.

The effect of these changes was to drive up medical expenditure. At the London, expenditure on drugs and chemicals rose from £3,315 7s. 2d. in 1889 to £4,995 11s. 4d. in 1897, a rise of 33.6 per cent in nine years. The finance committee was aware of this problem: as part of a thorough review of the London's financial situation initiated by Holland a special 'drugs' auditor was appointed in 1897 to check the contracts and purchasing. The increase was equally striking at the German Hospital where from 1854 to 1898 medical expenditure rose by 331.1 per cent.[27] Doctors demanded new drugs and instruments, and governors had to pay for them. In most London hospitals a compromise was reached and doctors modified their demands and attempted to control spending.

Developments in scientific medicine and therapeutic practices were not the only advancements in patient care that affected expenditure. Wages spiralled, reflecting both the employment of more staff and the need for higher salaries for more skilled workers. By 1895 the Hospital for Sick Children employed a casualty medical officer, medical and surgical registrar, a pathologist, an anaesthetist, a dispenser, clinical clerks, and a number of house surgeons and physicians to assist with the 1,627 in-patients and 74,224 out-patients; it had started with a small honorary staff. A similar trend can be seen at the Royal Hospital for Diseases of the Chest. General hospitals employed essentially the same medical officers but in larger numbers. At the London, for example, only the apothecary, his two assistants, and the two house surgeons and two resident pupils were paid in 1851. By 1898 there were two resident maternity assistants, a medical registrar, a surgical registrar, seven dispensers, four clinical assistants, four resident receiving room officers, ten house surgeons and physicians and numerous clinical clerks and dressers.[28] Although such staff were paid comparatively low salaries (often only between £20 and £100), the need to employ them pushed up the wages bill.

In was nursing, assisted by the move to train nurses with the growth of nursing sisterhoods and the work of the Nightingale School at St Thomas's, that contributed most to the rising expenditure on salaries. Extensive programmes of nursing reform did not initially prove expensive and created a new source of income. However, reforms encouraged the emergence of a new assertive class of matron who demanded a higher nurse–patient ratio and improved facilities. Between 1861 and 1901 the number of nurses nationally rose from 24,821 to 64,214.[29] Similar rises occurred at a local level. When University College Hospital opened in 1834 it had approximately fifteen

[27] London Hospital, annual reports 1890, 1898, LH; minutes of the finance committee, 17 May 1897, LH, A/9/51; German Hospital, annual reports 1854, 1895, SBH.

[28] Hospital for Sick Children, minutes of the committee of management, 20 Oct. 1896, GOSH, 1/2/18; 21 Oct. 1891, GOSH, 1/2/20; annual report 1895, GOSH; RCH, minutes of the finance committee, LMA, H33/RCH/A5/1; London Hospital, annual reports 1850, 1898, LH.

[29] See Abel-Smith, History of the nursing profession; F. B. Smith, Florence Nightingale: reputa-

nurses and a matron, whose low salaries encouraged them to steal from the wards. When the All Saints Nursing Sisterhood took over the nursing in 1862 the number immediately rose to include a head sister, four head nurses, and twelve other nurses. Numbers had increased again by 1892 to ten sisters and sixty-five nurses. It was not just numbers that pushed up the cost of nursing. Trained nurses were more expensive. In the 1830s nurses were paid on average between 6s. and 9s. per week; a trained nurse fifty years later could expect to earn £25–40 after qualification. The transition could be expensive: within a year of employing the All Saints Sisterhood nursing costs had risen from £1,000 to £1,300 at University College Hospital. When St John's House Nursing Sisterhood took over nursing at Charing Cross Hospital in 1866 expenditure doubled overnight.[30] The creation of training schools involved the need to provide additional accommodation to house probationers and extra domestic staff to look after them and the income they generated at best made them self-financing. The transition to a new system of nursing was not always smooth, as the nursing dispute at Guy's outlined in chapter 6 shows. However, the need for trained nurses were increasingly seen as essential if the hospital wanted to offer the most advanced medical care available. Nursing reform consequently contained an inherent trend that favoured higher wages and a rise in expenditure.

An increase in medical and nursing costs is only part of the explanation. An expansion of hospital administration saw more staff being employed to run the hospital and ironically more being spent on advertising and fundraising. Modernisation, with the introduction of telephones, flowers in the wards in the 1870s and better lighting and heating in an effort to create an ordered, pleasant and sanitary environment all increased the day-to-day running costs. Contemporaries identified a further reason for spiralling costs. At a meeting at Mansion House in aid of the London in 1888, the duke of Cambridge solemnly explained that the growth in patient numbers naturally forced expenditure up.[31] Admissions statistics are notoriously inaccurate. Governors needed 'to make a goodly show of work in the eyes of the public, with the object . . . of attracting subscribers', and admissions became a useful tool in their claim for support.[32] However, even allowing for misleading statistics the rise could be dramatic (see table 19). The general increase in patient numbers was experienced across all hospital types. Even at St Bartholomew's, which had no need to attract philanthropy until 1904, admis-

tion and power, London 1982; L. Holcombe, Victorian ladies at work, Newton Abbot 1973, 204–5.

[30] Merrington, University College Hospital, 245, 249, 251–5; Abel-Smith, History of the nursing profession, 6; Maggs, Origins of general nursing, 48; R. J. Minney, The two pillars of Charing Cross: the story of a famous hospital, London 1967, 103–5.

[31] Cited in London Hospital, scrapbook, LH, A/26/31.

[32] Morell Mackenzie, 'The use and abuse of hospitals', Contemporary Review lviii (1890), 507.

Table 19: Admissions to principal London general hospitals, 1809–95

Hospital	In-patients		Out-patients	
	1809	1895	1809	1895
London	1,406	10,599	877	152,411
Middlesex	555	3,404	522	41,707
St Bartholomew's	3,849	6,674	45,410	59,063
St George's	1,450	4,191	1,211	28,392
St Thomas's	2,789	6,150	4,322	112,056
Westminster	627	2,934	687	24,247

Source: Rivett, *The London hospital system*, 140

sions doubled between 1861 and 1881.[33] Expansion can be explained by the developments in medicine and nursing discussed above, which served to alter the public's harsh perception of the hospital. Hospitals built on their new popularity; the result was a rapid increase in admissions as they became viable locations for medical care. Doctors fuelled this increase with their desire for a greater pool of interesting cases for teaching and research, while the growth of the Sunday and Saturday Funds raised the hospitals' profile and gave the impression that contribution implied a right to treatment.[34] In many cases, such as at the London and at St Thomas's, patients had to be turned away. Hospitals rested precariously between their new 'popularity', their need for more patients, and the constraints of finance.

The link between an increase in patient numbers and rising expenditure is not hard to make. Governors struggled to cut spending, but they could not reduce admissions without damaging their image and public support. More patients demanded more beds, services, medicines, bandages and dressings, adding to the hospitals' medical bill. Between 1861 and 1891 the number of beds in Britain's voluntary hospitals doubled, but even this barely matched demand or the rise in the metropolitan population. The financial pressures this increase in patients and beds produced were reflected in the cost of treatment: between 1864 and 1891 the average weekly cost of in-patient care in London rose by 203.3 per cent.[35] Although the London hospitals were always more expensive than their provincial counterparts, a similar increase

[33] St Bartholomew's, statistical tables of medical and surgical registrars, 1861–81, SBH, MR 9/58–86.
[34] Brand, *Doctors and the state*, 193.
[35] Fleetwood Buckle, *Vital and economical statistics of hospitals and infirmaries etc. of England and Wales for the year 1863*, London 1865; Pinker, *English hospital statistics*, 49, 81; SC on Metropolitan Hospitals, Second Report, 799–802.

occurred outside London as a growing number of patients had to be cared for, housed and fed.

The link between spending and patient admissions can be clearly seen in the amounts governors increasingly had to spend on provisions, especially as from 1873 the agricultural depression saw a marked fall in food prices. Food was the largest component in expenditure, representing a quarter of the London hospitals' running costs in 1896. Provisions were not bought on the open market as they could not be stored in the quantities required, so governors negotiated contracts with suppliers. Fluctuations in price were not accounted for and the system often resulted in poor quality food as contractors bought the cheapest goods available to remain within their costing. According to the *Hospital*, which ran a series of articles in 1896 and 1897 on expenditure, patients could be fed on a minimum of 4s. per week.[36] Governors were not inclined to be extravagant, even with the medical staff prescribing specialist diets, but as admissions rose so too did the amount of food required. At the German Hospital the number of in-patients increased by 164.3 per cent between 1854 and 1895 and the cost of provisions by 240.2 per cent. When in 1859 the governors criticised the medical staff for what they believed was their extravagant purchasing of beers and spirits, the doctors in their defence cited increased admissions as the main reason for the high expenditure.[37] Other London hospitals experienced a similar rise that defied efforts to economise.

It was an inescapable consequence of development that as hospitals came to treat more patients and expand their medical remit so their expenditure also rose. To care for the sick increasingly meant new wards, more doctors, more specialist departments, new techniques and better provision. Under these conditions traditional sources of funding came under pressure. The solution was to either close wards and restrict treatment, a move that aroused opposition and went against the hospitals' medical and philanthropic character, or develop additional sources of funding. The result was a more diverse financial strategy, often not by intention but by necessity.

Building mania

One factor that promoted an increase in expenditure needs to be considered separately. Henry Burdett, speaking at a meeting of the British Medical Association (BMA) in 1881, felt that a building mania had enthralled London's hospitals. With a wave of new hospital buildings and improvements in the 1860s and 1870s the physical evidence for this was clear. As a widely recognised expert on hospital charity and administration, Burdett argued that this

[36] *Hospital*, 25 Apr. 1896, 61; 28 Mar. 1896, 436.
[37] German Hospital, annual reports 1854, 1895, SBH; minutes of the board of household management, 11 Apr. 1859, SBH, GHA 8/4.

Figure 10: German Hospital: income against expenditure, 1851–98

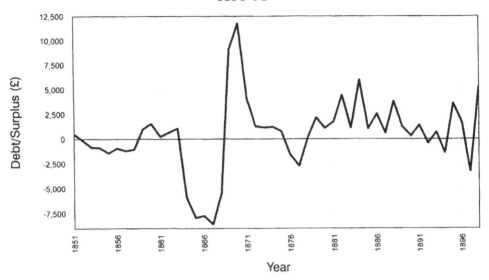

Source: Annual reports 1851–98, SBH

had resulted in a dramatic rise in expenditure, while new wards remained empty.[38] Overcrowding and changes in how hospital patients were treated made new buildings essential. The inadequacies of existing hospitals, highlighted by the *Builder* and by the survey conducted by Bristowe and Holmes for the Privy Council in 1863, contrasted with new ideas on hospital design popularised by Florence Nightingale in her *Notes on hospitals* and later works like Douglas Galton's *Healthy hospitals*. The emphasis Nightingale and others placed on the pavilion plan added an extra dimension to governors' enthusiasm to rebuild, motivating them to construct new edifices and add additional rooms in the interests of a 'well-tempered' and sanitary environment.[39] The governors at the Royal Hospital for Diseases of the Chest decided to build an extra room for the 'examination of sputum' in 1898 on the grounds that this was healthier. St Mark's Hospital for Fistula undertook a more ambitious project three years later. It rebuilt on sanitary grounds, having unsuccessfully attempted to make improvements to the old building. The new hospital, to cope with the number admissions, was twice the size of the old one, but debt forced the governors to sell investments and wards remained

---

38 *BMJ* ii (1881), 646.
39 Florence Nightingale, *Notes on hospitals*, London 1863; Douglas Galton, *Healthy hospitals: observations on some points connected with hospital construction etc.*, Oxford 1893; Taylor, *Hospital and asylum architecture*. Not all areas were motivated by these concerns. In Manchester the Royal Infirmary was rebuilt as part of the civic improvement of the Piccadilly district where it was located: Pickstone, *Medicine and industrial society*, 100.

Figure 11: Royal Hospital for Diseases of the Chest: income against expenditure, 1850–98

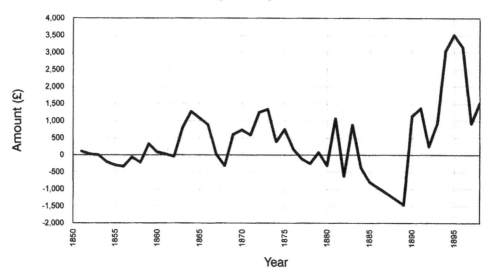

Source: Annual reports 1850–98, LMA

empty, vindicating Burdett's earlier assessment.[40] Even ignoring financial problems the result was not always successful. Despite rebuilding the governors of the Hospital for Sick Children still had to close the hospital periodically because of outbreaks of disease. According to Brian Abel-Smith, 'the new spacious hospitals were expensive to build and expensive to run', a view borne out by the testimony of contemporaries and the financial experiences of London's medical institutions.[41]

Building exerted a considerable pressure on hospital finance. New buildings raised running costs and increased overall expenditure, but the main pressure was felt during construction. Debt peaked in the years when new wards or clinical facilities were built, as shown by the experiences of the German Hospital (see figure 10) and the Royal Hospital for Diseases of the Chest (see figure 11). Loans were invariably sought to meet building costs until enough income could be raised from philanthropy to meet the accumulated debt. This policy was adopted by the Royal Hospital for Diseases of the Chest. In 1889 the governors sold £6,000 in consolidated stock 'for the purpose of paying sundry debts incurred in the building of the new wing of the Hospital'.[42] At the German Hospital a different solution was found when rebuilding left the institution financially embarrassed. At first legacies and invest-

---

[40] RCH, council minute book, 19 Dec. 1898, LMA, H33/RCH/A1/8; Granshaw, St Mark's Hospital, London, 75–6.

[41] Abel-Smith, The hospitals, 154.

[42] Charity Record & Philanthropic News ix (1889), 292.

ments were liquidated, followed by a series of loans and in 1869 a bazaar was organised 'for the purpose of raising the means of liquidating the debt still owing on the New Building'.[43] 1867 marked a turning point and successful appeals enabled the governors to build up the hospital's surplus income and investments. The governors had apparently learnt their lesson. For the rest of the nineteenth century they attempted to avoid over-extending the hospital's finances and built up investments to provide a reliable income that partially freed them from the vagaries of direct philanthropy.

Few administrators were as prudent as the governors of the Hospital for Sick Children who attempted to save their annual profits until they could afford to build. However, this was not always possible, especially when initial estimates were exceeded. Occasionally the governors were forced to borrow to cover their expansion and when they ambitiously bought St John's and Elizabeth Hospital in 1898 they had to borrow £4,000.[44] Most hospitals, however, built when there was a need rather than the funds or when building costs were low, a phenomenon that counters Whitehand's view of an institutional building cycle.[45] At University College Hospital and the London expenditure peaked during years of rebuilding (see figures 7 and 9). It was not, however, until 1888 that the chairman of the London's house committee acknowledged this pressure on the hospital's finances.[46] Similar problems were encountered at all hospitals and resources were modified accordingly. The Brompton faced financial problems after opening a new building in 1882, and the Swansea General and Eye Hospital experienced building-related financial difficulties after 1876. At the Swansea General the governors were forced to court working-class organisations to raise income and they opened a provident dispensary in 1877 to relieve the hospital's strained resources, a move that proved highly profitable.[47] St Thomas's equally had to adopt a new financial strategy after 'the folly of overbuilding'. Its move to Lambeth left it financially embarrassed with only thirteen of the twenty-one wards open. When combined with a fall in income from the hospital's endowments, pressure was exerted in the face of considerable opposition to admit paying patients.[48] Most hospitals did not, however, adopt controversial sources of funding. Instead they relied on their investments to overcome the

---

43 German Hospital, minutes of the hospital committee, 11 Apr. 1867, 10 Oct. 1867, SBH, GHA 2/4; bazaar committee to Weber, 7 Aug. 1868, GHA 14/3.

44 Hospital for Sick Children, minutes of the finance committee, 21 June 1898, GOSH, 1/8/2.

45 J. Whitehand, 'Building cycles and the spatial pattern of urban growth', *Institute of Geographers (Transactions)* lvi (1972), 39–55.

46 Cited in London Hospital, scrapbook, LH, A/26/31.

47 Bishop and others, *Seven ages of the Brompton*, 68; T. G. Davies, *Deeds not words: a history of the Swansea General and Eye Hospital, 1817–1948*, Cardiff 1988, 75–7.

48 Henry Burdett, *Hospitals and the state with an account of the nursing at London hospitals and statistical tables showing the actual and comparative cost of management*, London 1881, 11; Granshaw, 'St Thomas's', 390–421.

financial strain of building. The governors of St Bartholomew's sold £6,000 in consolidated stock between 1870 and 1872 to pay for a new chemical theatre. The decision had been reached because the house committee was aware that the 'ordinary' income for that year was insufficient to pay for the work.[49] The move to sell did not create anxiety partly because it was seen as a temporary measure. When traditional sources of finance could not pay for expansion, new sources of income had to be found so altering the hospitals' financial make-up and encouraging diversification to avoid debt.

Nature of the hospital

The financial experiences of individual hospitals were influenced by the nature of the institution. Each different 'type' of hospital (endowed, general, specialist, ethnic) faced characteristic restraints and advantages in raising or redirecting income. This could either be a benefit, as in the specialist hospitals, assisting governors in their fundraising; or a disadvantage, as in the teaching institutions, by placing an additional burden on expenditure.

The growth in the market for medical education, the development of an anatomico-clinical approach, and the restrictive regulations introduced by the Royal College of Surgeons in the 1820s all encouraged an institutionalisation of medical education during the late eighteenth and early nineteenth century that favoured the hospital.[50] Training and treatment merged in the teaching hospital, creating a new type of institution that became a feature of the Victorian medical environment. Although these elite and protected institutions were integral to the medical establishment, it was widely acknowledged that 'hospitals associated with medical schools' were 'somewhat more expensive than others'.[51] Their internal educational logic required them to admit more patients to give students access to interesting cases and also made it necessary for them to provided a wider variety of treatment techniques. Other hospitals, without an educational function, did not have the same pressures exerted on them. Only by continual improvement could London's teaching hospitals maintain their competitive edge in their efforts to attract students. A higher level of expenditure and a greater pressure on resources was the consequence. University College Hospital epitomises the pressures exerted on teaching hospitals. Founded in 1834 to provide clinical experience for medical undergraduates, contemporaries felt that University College Hospital had a profound influence on medical education, but its educational function produced a continual pressure for expansion that drove the hospital into debt. The governors attempted to keep pace

[49] St Bartholomew's, minutes of the board of governors, SBH, Ha 1/23.
[50] See Susan Lawrence, *Charitable knowledge: hospital pupils and practitioners in eighteenth-century London*, Cambridge 1996.
[51] *Hospital*, 5 Jan. 1889, 214.

with developments in medical science, imposing demands on the hospital's finances that the normal careful management of resources was ill-equipped to meet. For example, an 'electrical room' for galvanic treatment was provided in 1867 to allow the medical staff to teach the diagnostic and curative uses of electricity. The room and the equipment cost £50 at a time when the hospital could not afford to pay its other bills. From 1869 and 1880 drug expenditure alone rose by 146.7 per cent and from 1876 to 1881 £1,922 was spent on surgical equipment.[52] The result of these demands was a permanent financial crisis.

To a certain extent the large general hospitals in London all experienced these pressures as they modified their charitable credentials to provide teaching facilities. The London had always benefited from its medical school, even though from 1853 it was managed and financed independently. Medical students provided key services during their training that the hospital did not have to pay for, but from the 1870s onwards the governors were increasingly aware that the college was facing a pressing financial crisis. To protect the hospital's reputation, the governors agreed in 1876 to assist the college. Initially the agreement covered a set grant of £2,000 that was awarded annually for three years. However, when this temporary agreement was renewed in 1879 the governors and medical staff, after prolonged negotiation, agreed to assume joint responsibility for the college's finances.[53] The governors, in adopting an additional strain on the London's already insufficient resources, acquired a leading managerial role in the college at the invitation of the lecturers. Where the governors had previously had no control over the allocation of the college's resources, they were now able to direct them to their benefit.[54] However, it is doubtful if this was ever sufficient to match the college's financial demands. Those teaching in the college continued to be paid by dividing the student fees between them, but now any shortfall in the college's expenses was met from the annual grant. The hospital also subsidised the college's rebuilding. In 1885 the governors lent the college £15,000 at 3 per cent interest and in doing so had to borrow £4,000 and sell £5,000 of its annuities to meet the hospital's normal running costs.[55] Unlike University College Hospital, the London's move to fund the medical college did not directly promote financial diversification, but it exerted additional financial pressure that made diversification desirable.

The situation was different at specialist hospitals, which fared better than their general counterparts. Though specialist hospitals were widely attacked

---

52 UCH, minutes of the medical committee, 23 Oct. 1867, UCL, UNOF/2/3 (1).

53 London Hospital, minutes of the house committee, 4 Apr. 1876, LH, A/5/37; minutes of the medical council, 31 Mar. 1879, LH, Mc/A/1/3.

54 Other institutions lacked this sharp contrast between the medical college and the hospital, allowing governors more control over the allocation of financial resources.

55 London Hospital, minutes of the house committee, 9 May 1885, 30 Mar. 1886, LH, A/5/42.

by doctors, large sections of the public willingly gave money to them because they evoked sympathy or, in the case of subscriptions from businesses, because they held a material benefit and provided a cheap alternative to insurance. The Royal Hospital for Diseases of the Chest attracted particular support from the printing and textile firms where chest diseases were common.[56] This natural advantage in attracting charity, when merged with their energetic fundraising tactics, ensured that specialist hospitals were able to increase their charitable support by playing on their nature. The Hospital for Sick Children was adept at this. The hospital was particularly fortunate as contemporaries hastened 'to extend the hand of mercy' to sick children.[57] The *Hospital* felt that the Hospital for Sick Children was perhaps 'the most popular of all hospitals in the eyes of the public' and the *Illustrated Times* noted that few people could resist the sympathy it inspired.[58] The governors played on the institution's nature, issuing a regular stream of pamphlets. On these emotional grounds many gave money, but not even the Hospital for Sick Children could rely on sympathy alone. In 1893 Adrian Hope, the hospital's dedicated secretary, complained about the 'serious decrease in subscriptions and donations' and the governors were forced to sell some of the hospital's assets to forestall a deficit.[59] However, the hospital's nature did generate a sufficient flow of charitable resources to ensure that the need to develop a diverse financial base was less acute.

Whereas specialist hospitals could play positively on their nature to attract charitable funding, endowed hospitals did not have to make public appeals. Guy's and St Thomas's did solicit philanthropy from the 1880s onwards as the agricultural depression eroded the mainstay of their financial support, but until the late 1870s all endowed hospitals were largely reliant on their invested funds. Income from charitable sources was often marginal. Endowed hospitals did diversify their finances, but until the late 1870s this was a less anxious development and often a response to opportunity rather than need. After 1876 Guy's and St Thomas's, with their traditional sources of funding greatly reduced, pursued a policy of crisis management that saw them adopting innovative and widely criticised sources of funding. The general opinion, however, was that these institutions were well financed. It should not therefore be surprising that many hospitals sought to mimic them and invest surplus income to build up a pseudo-endowed status to reduce their dependence on unreliable sources of funding.

The hospitals' nature played an important role in influencing the financial strategies adopted by individual hospitals. The income available to an individual hospital was not entirely dependent on its type, but this was an important factor in contributing to the pace of financial diversification. In teaching

---

[56] Wohl, *Endangered lives*, 260, 277.
[57] *Hospital*, 19 Mar. 1887, 420.
[58] Ibid. 5 Aug, 1893, 290; *Illustrated Times*, 24 Apr. 1858, 302.
[59] Cited in Hospital for Sick Children, press cuttings, GOSH, 8/153.

hospitals there was a pressing need to develop new sources of funding; at the endowed hospitals this need was not present until the late 1870s.

Community resources

It was to the local community that governors first directed their appeals and new institutions initially drew most of their support from their surrounding districts. At the Royal Hospital for Diseases of the Chest in the 1850s the majority of subscribers came largely from Clerkenwell, declining middle-class Shoreditch, the City, and Hoxton, which had been built-up during the 1820s and 1830s with homes for clerks and minor professionals. All these areas were near the hospital. Only gradually was its geographical appeal extended, though local businesses and organisations like the *Clerkenwell Chronicle* and the Clerkenwell Conservative Women's Club continued to appear in the list of benefactors. Hospitals serving an immigrant population, like the French Hospital, Queen's Square, or the German Hospital in Dalston, drew support from a different type of community that was concentrated in a number of areas throughout London.[60] Burdett, given his close involvement in reforming the financial position of the Seamen's Hospital in Greenwich, exalted the benefits of local collection schemes. He believed they established exclusive areas of support and limited competition.[61] Where this might work in Greenwich or Birmingham where Burdett had been superintendent of the Queen's Hospital, it was inappropriate for London. *The Lancet* felt that 'it is noteworthy that the London Hospitals are badly off mainly because they are in London'.[62] Provincial hospitals could become the centre of civic pride, but in London the sheer number of charitable institutions ensured that hospitals had to compete for contributions.

Levels of local identification varied with the institution, but no locality 'even if it were very rich' could sustain a hospital, though some were better suited than others.[63] Charity was not the exclusive preserve of the middle classes. Working-class benevolence at a formal and informal level was important to local communities, but with hospitals interested in regular subscriptions and donations they came to rely on money from a small, often wealthy constituency in the community. Where this was wanting they faced consider-

---

60 RCH, minutes of the finance committee, LMA, H33/RCH/A5/1. Although German immigrants were not concentrated in any one locality, they mainly settled in three areas: East London, particularly Whitechapel and Stepney; West London, in Westminster, St Marylebone, Paddington, Kensington and St Pancras; and North London, predominantly in Kentish Town, Camden and Islington where a German Church had existed since 1862: Panikos Panayi, *The enemy in our midst: Germans in Britain during the First World War*, New York 1991, 17–19.
61 *BMJ* i (1877), 405.
62 *Lancet* ii (1898), 1647.
63 Cited in London Hospital, press cuttings, LH, A/26/31.

able problems in motivating local benevolence. Population movements not only deprived hospitals of their original patient clientele, but also distanced them from their traditional networks of local support. In 1890 the governors at the London complained that 'the former inhabitants of East London, who contributed largely to this great institution, have moved to the suburbs'.[64] It was a widespread problem. As the middle classes moved to the suburbs and northern heights, arousing fears of social dislocation, local support for hospitals in central London dwindled.[65] According to Roy Porter, these 'aspirant folks', who were most likely to form the mainstay of the benevolent public, 'were always moving somewhere new, more modish further from the brick-yards, the fog and the riff-raff', and from London's hospitals.[66] Geographical divisions between patients, hospitals and their supporters increased as the metropolis swallowed more land and expanded outwards. London's high degree of localism and system of loosely connected 'villages' further fragmented the benevolent economy. What made matters worse was that some areas had a habit of parsimony. The North London Hospital was continually under financial pressure as it was 'impossible to charm any money out of the tight-buttoned pockets of the people of North London'.[67] Though this was an exaggeration, it serves to show that community resources were important in determining the supply of direct philanthropy and the shape of the hospitals' financial experiences.

Shifts in the community base of patients admitted to London's hospitals highlight these changes in local support. The ability of subscribers to recommend patients through the letter system, although challenged by doctors' increased dominance of admission criteria, was not removed. To some extent where patients came from reflected not only a widening of a hospital's appeal as it established a metropolitan, national or even (in the case of St Bartholomew's) an imperial reputation, but also where subscribers lived. According to a study of metropolitan institutional mortality by Graham Mooney, Andrea Tanner and Bill Luckin, hospitals had a 'triple-tiered catchment area' based on their immediate area, coterminous neighbourhoods and national importance.[68] Over time this distribution changed but the bias remained clearly metropolitan. In 1867, 15.3 per cent of patients at the Royal Hospital for Diseases of the Chest came from the predominately poor Clerkenwell which was near the hospital on City Road. Other local areas within a mile of the institu-

---

[64] Ibid.

[65] See F. M. L. Thompson, *Hampstead: building a borough, 1650–1970*, London 1978, or H. J. Dyos, *Victorian suburbs: a study of the growth of Camberwell*, Leicester 1967.

[66] *Hospital*, 15 Dec. 1888, 175; Richard Dennis, *English industrial cities of the nineteenth century: a social geography*, Cambridge 1984, 52–6; Roy Porter, *London: a social history*, London 1994, 208.

[67] *Hospital*, 6 Nov. 1886, 95.

[68] Graham Mooney, Bill Luckin and Andrea Tanner, 'Patient pathways: solving the problems of institutional mortality in London during the late nineteenth century', *SHM* xii (1999), 227–69.

tion provided 69.1 per cent of the patients. By the 1880s, if the number of patients from Shoreditch and Islington had dramatically increased, admissions from the local community had fallen to 55 per cent. Slum clearance, street improvements and residential decline with the expansion of the City all helped reduce the hospital's community base as professionals, businessmen 'and finally shopkeepers quit from Cheapside and Clerkenwell for suburbs like Primrose Hill and Herne Hill'. In the 1890s a further widening of the catchment area was reflected in the large number of subscribers with addresses in west and north London.[69] At the Hospital for Sick Children patients and subscribers came from across London and the south east by the early 1890s whereas in the 1850s addresses in Grays Inn Road, Southampton Road, Guildford Street, Durry Lane, Cleveland Street and Great Ormond Street itself had dominated.[70] Of course Londoners' willingness to walk and a growing system of transport ensured that not all patients needed to attend their local hospital. 'Bus and tram journeys per Londoner increased fivefold between 1881 and 1891', though many tram routes avoided the central districts where hospitals were located.[71] Patients did move from one out-patient department to another until they received the treatment they expected and were more than prepared to walk to the appropriate specialist hospital. With few hospitals south of the Thames, Guy's served an enormous population, while the Great Northern was the only hospital located in north London with a population of 900,000.[72] Socially and geographically patients moved away from a network of deference, a move that broke down community support for individual hospitals and at the same time made them more metropolitan in nature.

The London's position clearly shows the problems a hospital could face when patients and subscribers moved away. Located in a district 'where the density of the population renders the poor liable to disease of all kinds, and the nature of their employment exposes them constantly to the dangers of serious accident', it was the only 'general Hospital for the whole of the East End'. The German Hospital in Dalston and the Metropolitan Hospital were not considered large enough to be of any serious consequence in meeting the health needs of those living in London's East End. Continuing economic crisis in east London in the 1860s compounded by strikes and the collapse of the Poplar shipbuilding industry in 1866 limited the amount of money available for formal benevolence. Overcrowding, the effect of railway clearance and a series of typhus epidemics from 1861 to 1869 equally strained resources.

69 RCH, annual reports 1868, 1880, LMA; Porter, London, 209; RCH, register of subscribers and donors, 1890–2, LMA, H33/RCH/D1/1.
70 Hospital for Sick Children, register of applicants for admission, 1881–92, GOSH, 9/1/22; register of donors, 1890–7, GOSH, 6/1/4; admissions register, 1852–5, GOSH, 9/1/1–2.
71 Porter, London, 227; Theo Barker and Michael Robbins, A history of London transport, London 1963.
72 Guy's Hospital, patient statistics, 1868, LMA, H9/Gy/A262/1; Charity Organisation Reporter, 28 June 1883, 1883; Lancet i (1890), 515.

Fierce competition between dock companies in the 1880s saw further reductions in the workforce, while regular employment was always hard to find. Although Charles Booth's survey demonstrated that no more than 30 per cent of those living in east London suffered from want, there were few wealthy or middle-class subscribers. The East End was characterised by high population growth fuelled by rural migrants and immigrants and by unemployment and underemployment.[73] The London continued to benefit from local philanthropy, mainly stimulated by the People's Five Shilling Subscription Fund, but the local charitable resources were insufficient to meet the hospital's needs. The London's position was not unique. Speakers at University College Hospital's jubilee dinner in 1884 complained that many of the hospital's wealthy subscribers had moved away from Russell Square, which became a fashionable area for student digs. The worry was that this had reduced the 'quantity' of its local support.[74]

The absence of wealthy subscribers heightened the pressures exerted by the overcrowded nature of the medical market in central London. The charitable resources available within the community were strained by the number of institutions in any one area. A series of maps prepared by Frederick Mouat at the Local Government Board between 1881 and 1883 to support his argument for a state run medical service (see chapter 8), pointed to a high concentration of hospitals in the West End. The Lancet was alarmed by the density and the BMJ asked the charitable public to think hard before they established another hospital there.[75] By 1887 the Hospital could complain that 'hospitals have sprung up without any definite regard to the requirements of the population or growth of individual communities, with the result that there is a tendency for the work of each institution to be overlapped by that of its neighbour'.[76] The area within two miles of Charing Cross was particularly overcrowded in institutional terms. University College Hospital had two general hospitals located within a mile with the Middlesex only six minutes walk away, while ten of the fifteen large general hospitals were within one-and-a-half miles of Charing Cross. All theoretically drew on the same community resources. Contemporaries became increasingly anxious about the distribution of the capital's hospitals and for the BMJ this was the source of the problems facing London's hospitals.[77] There was some discussion in 1894 of the possibility of relocating certain hospitals outside London to relieve this medical congestion and the Prince of Wales Hospital Fund con-

[73] Jones, Outcast London, chs iii–v; Anne Hardy, 'Urban famine or urban crisis?: typhus in the Victorian city', Medical History xxxii (1988), 212; Charles Booth, Life and labour of the people of London, i, London 1889, 37–8; Lara Marks, 'Medical care for pauper mothers and their infants: poor law provision and local demand in East London, 1870–1920', EcHR xliii (1993), 519–21.
[74] Charity Record & Philanthropic News iv (1884), 188.
[75] BMJ ii (1878), 35.
[76] Hospital, 19 Feb. 1887, 343.
[77] BMJ i (1883), 776; Burdett, Hospitals and the state, 5.

tinued to campaign for redistribution. Increasingly, hospital reformers turned their attention to the problems of location and the prospect of state regulation was discussed in a climate where voluntarism seemed unable to provide the necessary co-ordination. Such schemes were repeatedly opposed. Doctors and administrators 'cherished their proximity to wealth, medical resources and private practice' and resisted moving. They feared that patients would be attracted away from teaching hospitals, while voluntarism had its own 'centrifugal tendencies'.[78]

Hospitals therefore jealously guarded their community resources and new institutions initially found it hard to compete. Both the Sunday Fund and the Prince of Wales Hospital Fund were initially attacked because governors feared they would threaten local collections and subscriptions.[79] Hospitals equally resisted more localised schemes, especially the establishment of other institutions in their locality. The German Hospital and the North Western London Hospital advised the duke of Westminster in 1883 that his support for a new hospital in the area would be unwise as there was no clear need.[80] A similar move to found a hospital in Camberwell, despite the urgent need for institutional medical care south of the Thames, was resisted because 200 beds were empty at Guy's and St Thomas's.[81] These were not altruistic attempts to save subscribers' money, but efforts to protect the financial base of the four hospitals concerned.

Poor distribution in economic terms emphasised the difficulties many hospitals faced in collecting local charitable resources. To compensate, governors extended their appeals beyond their immediate locality to the metropolis and were forced to supplement the charitable resources available within the community with different sources of income.

Charity against charity: competition with the benevolent economy

The availability of charitable resources extended beyond the local community to London as a whole. The metropolitan benevolent economy was shaped by London's economy and society and represented a highly sophisticated market. The *Hospital* compared it to a divided and leaderless state and within this 'chaos of benevolence' hospitals had to compete with other voluntary associations.[82] Charity was 'distinguished for its fitfulness and its impulse', and as a writer in *Truth* explained in 1883, it needed only a touching story of disaster to open its purse strings.[83] Foreign ventures were a particular

---

78 *Hospital*, 3 Feb. 1894, 314; Prochaska, *Philanthropy and the hospitals of London*, 9.
79 *Morning Post*, 2 Sept. 1897, 2.
80 German Hospital, minutes of the hospital committee, 26 Apr. 1883, SBH, GHA 2/7.
81 *Times*, 24 June 1895, 11.
82 *Hospital*, 22 Sept. 1888, 397.
83 *Truth*, 19 Apr. 1883, 539.

drain on the emotions and money of subscribers. Governors and journals constantly lamented that charity had been directed away from 'kith and kin' to help the foreigner and convert the heathen while hospital beds remained closed. Appeals did not have to be directed overseas to have an effect. The *Manchester Guardian* commented in 1891 that 'when "General" Booth got his £100,000, careful observers predicted that it would be mainly drawn from the subscription list of other charities' and 'what is true of this fund is true of all other new charitable undertakings'.[84] Hospitals in comparison launched regular appeals and contributors were easily distracted by other, more immediate problems that were sensationalised by special appeals and newspaper funds. Even the governors of Hospital for Sick Children, normally highly successful in motivating charity, complained in 1890 about the difficulty in attracting funds in such a competitive environment.[85] The *Charity Record & Philanthropic News* saw this as a crucial problem for hospital finance and Lord Derby warned subscribers to 'help the novelty if you will and think it right, but do not help it at the cost of the old and well-tried institutions'.[86]

Competition was not limited to the different objects of charity. 'There was a keen and continuous competition between hospitals' and the total number of medical charities in London was 'larger than the public can be induced to support'.[87] When Guy's announced its first public appeal in 1886, the *BMJ* hoped that it would not divert benevolence away from those institutions that depended on charity.[88] The view was too optimistic. One hospital's appeal was often another's hardship, and the *Hospital* asked administrators who had had a successful appeal to refrain from capitalising on their success and let the less fortunate 'scramble for bread'.[89] When appeals occurred simultaneously the result was to reduce their general effectiveness. The chairman of the London complained that the hospital's 1888 appeal had not been as 'entirely satisfactory as they had expected – due, of course, to the increased number of hospitals that were compelled to appeal for funds'.[90]

Particular acrimony was directed at specialist hospitals. They were rounded on as 'a nuisance to the public' and attacked by the medical profession who saw them as damaging to general practice.[91] Doctors' professional self-interest merged with governors' anxieties. By the 1870s the pace at which specialist hospitals were being founded had slowed and initial antagonism was gradually modified as many specialist hospitals had become leading institutions and general hospitals had started to establish their own specialist wards. However, throughout much of the period they were castigated as over-

---

[84] Cited in London Hospital, press cuttings, LH, A/26/8.
[85] *SC on Metropolitan Hospitals, Second Report*, 472.
[86] *Charity Record & Philanthropic News* ii (1881), 72; *Hospital*, 10 Jan. 1891, 228.
[87] *SC on Metropolitan Hospitals, First Report*, 16; *Lancet* i (1858), 48.
[88] *BMJ* ii (1886), 1230.
[89] *Hospital*, 14 June 1890, 160.
[90] Cited in London Hospital, press cuttings, LH, A/26/5.
[91] *Lancet* ii (1857), 650; Peterson, *The medical profession in mid Victorian London*, 272–80.

stocking and overcrowding the existing medical market. Contemporaries felt that the specialist hospitals' aggressive fundraising deflected charity to unnecessary causes. According to Sir Andrew Clark, president of the Royal College of Physicians, these institutions 'divert the funds in a direction in which they ought not to be employed, and rob the great hospitals of the support which they ought to receive'.[92] Specialist hospitals were shown to be the bloodsuckers of philanthropy and the 'robbers of the poor', but even these institutions faced competition. When St Martin's Hospital for Fistula opened in 1868, the older St Mark's immediately felt the economic consequences and beds were closed.[93] However, specialist hospitals were generally in a healthy financial position. In 1875 £106,385 went to thirty-six specialist hospitals with 113 beds; in the same year eight general hospitals with 2,268 beds received £110,199. By 1887 the total deficit of the teaching hospitals exceeded £32,000, while the specialist hospitals had a surplus of £90,000.[94] For concerned contemporaries this was a clear misapplication of resources. Part of the antagonism came from a sense of injustice. Specialist hospitals were invariably better at attracting philanthropy than their general counterparts. With general hospitals providing their own specialist departments from the 1850s onwards competition was felt to be intensified. Specialist hospitals' general unpopularity as fraudulent institutions combined with deep-seated concerns about hospital finance to make them unwelcome competitors for already limited resources.

The fickle nature of philanthropy and the intense competition within London's benevolent economy worried hospital administrators, especially as charitable resources fluctuated. In 1888 donations in London were an estimated £840,000; in 1890 they were £769,000.[95] Given charity's highly volatile nature, competition was a problem. It served to reduce the philanthropic income available to individual institutions on an annual basis, straining resources and encouraging at best a search for more reliable sources of income and at worse an anxious pursuit of funds.

Benevolence in the national economy

Britain's economic performance played an important role in controlling the flow of income to the London benevolent economy. A depression in industry or agriculture restricted the amount of income available to charity, while periods of relative and perceived affluence encouraged the charitable public to give more and ensured that investments and land had a higher return. Fluctuations in the London economy made governors anxious rather than

92 *Hansard*, 3rd ser. cccxxxviii. 1551.
93 Granshaw, *St Mark's*, 59, 70–1.
94 *BMJ* i (1877), 405; *Hansard*, 3rd ser. cccxxxviii. 1551.
95 *Lancet* i (1890), 97.

Figure 12: Guy's Hospital: income against expenditure, 1853–98

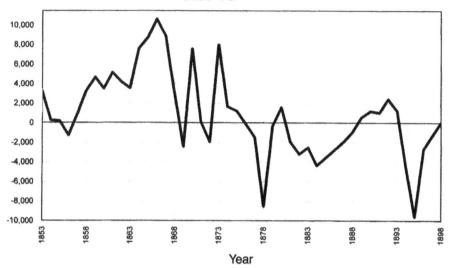

Source: Abstracts of accounts, LMA, H9/Gy/D191/1–3

optimistic and often increased pressure on traditional resources. Under these conditions new sources of funding became desirable.

In 1895 the *BMJ* blamed the hospitals' financial troubles on the depression in industry.[96] Depressions 'struck the well-to-do to a great extent', affecting 'the income of those who have been amongst the most prominent supporters of charities' and reduced charitable income as subscribers economised by giving less.[97] The journal predicted that 1895 would be an anxious year for hospitals.[98] It was not, however, an atypical year. Hospitals were 'exposed to the periodic recurrence of seasons of depression' and, according to Lord Aberdare, under such circumstances 'the difficulty of obtaining money is exceptional'.[99] Governors were all too aware of these problems. The governors of University College Hospital felt in 1887 that the hospital had suffered from the effects of the agricultural and industrial depression, which added to its 'life of struggling'.[100] In 1875 the governors of the German Hospital recognised that the uneasy feeling in the City would limit the flow of philanthropy. In response they withdrew £1,000 from their deposit account to cover the expected fall in income.[101] Fluctuations in the nation's economic

---

96 *BMJ* i (1895), 31.
97 *Charity Record & Philanthropic News* vii (1887), 147.
98 *BMJ* i (1895), 31.
99 *Lancet* i (1877), 888; *Hospital*, 11 Dec. 1886, 174.
100 *Charity Record & Philanthropic News* vii (1887), 147.
101 German Hospital, minutes of the hospital committee, 8 July 1875, SBH, GHA 2/6.

performance were not always damaging however. Prosperous years could see an increase in philanthropy. In 1895 the Sunday Fund was able to distribute a record amount because profits from the 'South African Boom' were partially redirected into the fund. Such events were uncommon and it was more the problems faced by the national economy that worried governors.

Endowed hospitals were particularly susceptible to economic fluctuations. Direct philanthropy was not an accurate barometer of Britain's economic performance, but land prices and dividends, on which endowed hospitals relied for the main part of their funding, were. This relationship was marked if governors had invested unwisely. At St Thomas's and Guy's a reliance on agricultural property produced a severe financial crisis from the late 1870s onwards (see figure 12). Agricultural prices had been falling since 1872 but it was not until 1879 that this began to deepen into depression. England's gross annual land value fell by 23.7 per cent between 1879 and 1893, with the capital value falling by 50 per cent.[102] The value of the estates Guy's held in Essex fell by 59 per cent between 1889 and 1891; those in Herefordshire by 28 per cent. In such a climate the governors could not dispose of the hospital's rural property, income fell and the level of debt rose. Falling land values was not the entire reason for the financial problems that faced Guy's and St Thomas's. They were primarily affected by the declining ability of their tenants to pay rent (see table 20). Initially the governors at Guy's attempted to ignore the problem as they felt that the situation was temporary and that recovery would be quick. However, after 1879 everything was attempted to stabilise income. Rentals were greatly reduced, 'arrears blotted out, remissions given, large sums expended on buildings', but in 'spite of it all', the hospital's tenants were 'still unable to pay in full'.[103] Compromises were made at an individual level in the hope that by writing off part of a tenant's debt the rest might be repaid, but this policy was unsuccessful, leaving accumulating arrears.

The Lancet was one of the few journals to recognise that Guy's and St Thomas's had 'fallen upon evil days entirely on account of [the] agricultural depression'.[104] Those outside the hospitals' administration, however, blamed financial mismanagement. At a meeting of the Sunday Fund in 1888 Dr Jabez Hogg claimed that Guy's had embarked on too ambitious a programme of speculation that had left the hospital financially embarrassed.[105] The BMJ added that the financial position was a 'curious comment on late expenditure on the treasurer's house and the chapel'.[106] Bad luck was added to an already deteriorating position at Guy's. Damage to the sluice on the Lincolnshire property involved an 'unexpected' expenditure of £8,500, absorbing the £7,500 raised among governors and staff that Edmund Lushington, the treas-

---

102 Royal Commission on Agricultural Depression, PP 1897 xv. 22–3.
103 Ibid. 9.
104 Lancet i (1896), 1651.
105 Guy's Hospital, letter book of treasurer, 1888, LMA, H9/Gy/A104/14.
106 BMJ ii (1880), 855.

Table 20: Guy's Hospital: income from landed property, 1875–91

Year	Rural property		Urban property	
	gross	net	gross	net
1875	£41,840	£30,919	£7,549	£6,533
1876	£41,679	£31,179	£7,977	£7,188
1877	£41,993	£31,396	£8,313	£7,567
1878	£40,367	£30,486	£7,888	£7,186
1879	£42,005	£33,421	£7,844	£7,177
1880	£41,379	£33,809	£8,109	£7,657
1881	£40,842	£25,983	£8,071	£7,512
1882	£38,399	£24,439	£8,111	£7,320
1883	£37,885	£26,281	£7,924	£7,150
1884	£35,186	£18,646	£7,993	£7,277
1885	£33,592	£20,612	£7,800	£7,193
1886	£31,938	£20,736	£7,622	£7,050
1887	£29,631	£19,504	£7,560	£6,852
1888	£31,210	£19,905	£7,639	£6,865
1889	£28,797	£18,652	£7,728	£7,154
1890	£28,191	£17,495	£7,634	£7,016
1891	£27,550	£17,222	£7,678	£7,035

Source: John Steele, 'Agricultural depression and its effects on a leading London hospital', *Royal Statistical Journal* (1892), 12

urer, had hoped to use to meet the hospital's debts.[107] With few resources to draw on, beds were closed at both hospitals and loans were negotiated. The financial situation became increasingly intolerable. With no tradition of appealing to the benevolent public, and in the face of the Charity Commission's refusal to sanction further borrowing, both hospitals attempted to solve the situation by admitting paying patients.[108] The resultant income was insufficient to solve the hospitals' financial problems and in 1886 Guy's launched its first public appeal to raise further funds. St Thomas's was quick to follow. Guy's and St Thomas's had been reduced by financial circumstances to seek charity and in recognition the Sunday Fund included Guy's in its grants in 1887. Both hospitals now joined the non-endowed hospitals in competition for charitable resources at a time when they were diversifying their income away from direct philanthropy.

No other hospital was affected as dramatically by changes in the country's

[107] *Graphic*, 14 May 1887, 514.
[108] See Guy's to Charity Commission, 21 Mar. 1884, LMA, H9/Gy/A172/2; Granshaw, 'St Thomas's', 401–19, 390–3.

economic performance as Guy's and St Thomas's, which were forced by external economic factors into an anxious pursuit of alternative sources of funding. If the experiences at Guy's were severe, they do highlight how hospital income was closely linked to factors outside London's benevolent economy as well as the strains acting on it. Every metropolitan hospital encountered these pressures to a greater or lesser extent and this encouraged the pursuit of new sources of funding as traditional sources of income could not be relied on.

The damning effect of criticism

Governors could not depend on the smooth flow of philanthropy to fund their institutions. The charitable resources available within the community and the benevolent economy were restricted and liable to fluctuate; the country's economic performance added an additional dimension. However, these were not the only problems. Governors faced a further difficulty as support could be alienated by criticism and scandal. According to The Lancet in 1881, there was growing disapproval of how the London hospitals were managed. The COS, the Social Science Association, the BMA and the Hospitals Association were in the forefront of this movement, though other bodies interested in hospital reform also added their damning views. Given this critical environment, the benevolent, 'who were never too numerous' had ample 'reasons for buttoning up their pockets and withholding or reducing their subscriptions'.[109] The result was an alienation of support that was quickly translated into economic terms, increasing the pressure on the hospitals' already meagre resources.

Attacks on the hospital system reduced the subscribing public's confidence in the London hospitals, but certain campaigns had a noticeable effect. One example is the financial consequences of a debate over vivisection into which the London hospitals were unwittingly drawn. John Passmore Edwards, pacifist and a philanthropist particularly interested in education and museums, claimed that the hospitals' finances were being damaged by the practice of vivisection. Although the BMJ dismissed the idea, the antivivisection lobby had an impact.[110] It is doubtful how many subscribers adopted Baroness Burdett Coutts's call in 1876 for a charitable boycott of those hospitals that employed vivisectionists, but the Star certainly felt that contributions would increase if the practice ceased.[111] By 1897 the government had only issued eighty-six vivisection licences and there is little evidence to support the antivivisectionists' accusations that animal experiments were being

109 Lancet ii (1881), 800.
110 BMJ ii (1895), 1398.
111 Richard D. French, Antivivisection and medical science in Victorian society, Princeton 1975, 271; Star, 9 Oct. 1896, 1.

funded by charitable contributions.[112] However, this did not stop antivivisectionists from criticising hospitals with medical schools. In 1898 the London Hospital came under attack from the National Anti-Vivisection Society for its £2,000 subsidy to the medical college. The society sent a letter to all the hospital's subscribers implying that the subsidy would be used to fund vivisection, pointing to the work carried out there by Leonard Hill and Harold Barnard on cats and dogs.[113] The governors were concerned enough to counter these accusations. Burford Rawlings, secretary to the National Hospital for the Paralysed and Epileptics, noted that antivivisectionists did 'their utmost to prevent subscriptions' to hospitals that they believed practised vivisection.[114]

Criticism was generally limited to individual hospitals. The press was quick to notice any scandal, blowing every minor incident out of proportion. Criticism damaged the hospital's standing with the public and governors did their best to avoid any scandal or sign of difficulty that would adversely affect their income. This was not always possible. At Guy's the nursing dispute in 1880 damaged the hospital's public image and provoked an intense debate about the need for hospital reform, but the hospital's endowed income prevented public acrimony from being translated into economic hardship. The London and the German Hospital were not so fortunate when they were exposed to public censure in the 1890s.

Evidence given to the Select Committee on Metropolitan Hospitals and reports in the press concerning the London's nursing arrangements in 1890 provoked a crisis in the hospital that drastically affected the amount of charity received for that year. Some concern had been expressed when Eva Lückes was appointed matron in 1879 to reform the system of nursing. From a privileged background, the stubborn and determined Lückes had trained at the Westminster, worked as a night nurse at the London and been a matron at Pendlebury Children's Hospital. Some of the governors and members of the medical staff felt that she was 'too young and pretty' to be effective.[115] However, as a close friend of Florence Nightingale she set about her work quickly and with zeal. She dismissed the old nurses, and set about improving conditions, establishing a new two-year system of training and insisting on separate bedrooms and regular and longer holidays. Both the staff and the governors, after some uncertainty, supported her actions, probably because Lückes did not attempt to challenge their authority and limited her work to improving the standard of nursing. It was not until 1890 that differences and opposition became apparent. Witnesses presenting evidence to the Select Committee

---

[112] *Hospital*, 15 May 1897, 117–19.
[113] *Morning Leader*, 21 June 1898, 7.
[114] *Hospital*, 30 Nov. 1895, 154.
[115] Gore, *Lord Knutsford*, 53.

on Metropolitan Hospitals accused Lückes and the London of 'sweating' its nurses and exposing them to poor living conditions.[116]

A disgruntled minority around Mrs Yatman, whose daughter Ellen had been a probationary nurse at the London, and Ethel Bedford Fenwick (former matron at St Bartholomew's, nursing reformer and wife of Dr Bedford Fenwick, physician in charge of the nurses) savagely criticised Lückes's work. In their attack they were joined by the Reverend Henry T. Valentine. An embittered chaplain who had been dismissed from the London in 1889 for ritualism, Valentine had promised to 'leave no stone unturned to do the Hospital injury'.[117] In claiming that nurses were sweated, Lückes's opponents were playing on images much used by the liberal press and social commentators in their discussions of working conditions in the East End. The 1888 House of Lords select committee had defined the evils of the sweating system as long hours, low pay and poor working conditions.[118] Nursing at the London appeared to fit this stereotype with Ellen Yatman and several other nurses claiming that they were underfed and overworked for a pittance, a view corroborated by Dr Bedford Fenwick. However, the nurses' situation at the London was no worse than the conditions faced by nurses in other hospitals. Nursing by the late 1880s had taken on the 'classic contours of a women's occupation, overcrowding, stagnating wages, uncontrolled entry and varying standards of training' with work characterised by hasty gulped-down meals, constant tiredness and rigid discipline.[119] In the attack on Lückes wider issues were at stake. It can be seen as part of a campaign to improve nursing conditions at all London hospitals with nursing reformers keen to promote registration using the Select Committee to further their cause by attacking Lückes. The opinionated Ethel Bedford Fenwick held opposing views to Lückes. An active campaigner for women's suffrage, she was a forceful advocate of the professionalisation of nursing and registration and had split the Nurses Section of the Hospitals Association in 1887 when she formed the more extremist British Nurses Association to campaign for the state registration of nurses.[120] Lückes's opposition to registration and her faith in training were well-known and contributed to the attacks on the London. Letters from former nurses testifying against Lückes had not been submitted spontaneously and it is probable that Ethel Bedford Fenwick was involved in soliciting them.[121]

Whatever the motivations behind the accusations, criticism had a damag-

116 *Citizen*, 5 Dec. 1891, 7.
117 A. E. Clark-Kennedy, *London pride: the story of a voluntary hospital*, London 1979, 142.
118 James Schmiechen, *Sweated industries and sweated labour: the London clothing trade, 1860–1914*, London 1984, 134–5.
119 Martha Vicinus, *Independent women: work and community for single women*, London 1985, 102–9.
120 See W. Hector, *The life of Mrs Bedford Fenwick*, London 1973; Dingwall, Rafferty and Webster, *Social history of nursing*, 78–9.
121 Anne Marie Rafferty, *The politics of nursing knowledge*, London 1996, 51–2.

ing financial effect. Despite all but at small minority at the London express-
ing 'unabated confidence in the administration of the Hospital', the
governors were concerned that the hospital was 'being most unwarrantly
damaged . . . in the confidence of the public'.[122] They were alarmed because
the hospital was under considerable financial pressure and needed public support. Certain sections of the press were scathing and even the *East London
Advertiser*, normally a warm supporter, was hostile. The *Pall Mall Gazette*
launched a virulent campaign and the *Hospital* felt that the editor had 'done
his best to ruin the London'.[123] Personal animosity animated much of the dispute, but the effect was not lost on the subscribers. Income fell by £10,000
and the hospital was forced to sell part of its invested stock to meet the deficit.[124] Although the charges were eventually proved false and the Lord's committee returned a generally favourable verdict on the hospital, the London
suffered financially.[125] Efforts were made to restore public confidence, but
income from direct philanthropy took several years to return to its pre-1890
level and in the meantime the governors had to borrow more money.

At the German Hospital an internal crisis two years later had similar economic consequences. Accusations surrounding the chaplain's Lutheran proselytism and attempts by the nurses to persuade Jewish patients to convert
sparked a controversy that offended both Jewish and Catholic subscribers.
The hospital had been founded on liberal principles, but Baron von
Schröeder's statement as chairman at the governors' annual meeting in 1894
contradicted this sentiment. In response to a question from the rector of the
Roman Catholic Church of St Boniface, Schröeder declared that the hospital
was 'decidedly a Protestant institution'. He was merely reaffirming a principle
adopted in 1891.[126] However, by 1894 the local Catholic and Jewish community had begun to find the situation intolerable. Complaints had been made
earlier in the year that Catholic patients had been forced to attend services in
the Lutheran Church next to the hospital and that Mr H Gülich, the hospital's superintendent, had prevented a Catholic patient from receiving the last
rites. Both events contradicted 'Rule XXVI', which clearly stated that all
patients had the right to their own minister. Between January and May 1894
accusations of proselytism were brandished in the press. A number of governors resigned over the issue and Dr [?] Ludwig, a physician at the hospital,
resigned on the grounds that his position under such a regime was 'inconsi-
stent with my dignity' and because the governors found his attacks on the

---

[122] London Hospital, minutes of the court of governors, 2 Mar. 1892, LH, A/2/14.
[123] *Hospital*, 5 Aug. 1893, 290.
[124] *Hospital Gazette*, 5 Mar. 1892, 119; *Morning Post*, 26 Dec. 1891, 4.
[125] SC *on Metropolitan Hospitals, Third Report*, pp. xvi–xx.
[126] German Hospital, minutes of the special general court, 8 May 1894, SBH, GHA 6/2;
minutes of the annual general court, 26 Jan. 1894, GHA 5/2; minutes of the hospital committee, 8 Mar. 1894, Dec. 1891, GHA 2/9.

hospital's poor treatment of Jews unacceptable.[127] The local Jewish community supported Ludwig's accusations and Davidson, chairman of the visitation committee of the United Synagogue, considered breaking the Synagogue's connection with the German and sending its sick to the Metropolitan Hospital. A special meeting was called to 'help save the German Hospital for the German Colony in London and prevent its becoming the property of a sect'.[128] Whereas Schröeder tried to claim that he was basing his statement on the respective number of Protestant, Jewish and Catholic patients treated, others attacked the hospital's recent Protestant bias. They were clear that the German Hospital had been established as a national rather than a Protestant institution. Amid accusations of a suppression of free speech and concerns about the counting of votes, a motion was passed that confirmed the German's non-sectarian nature by a majority of thirty-eight. In addition, it was asserted that Schröeder's original statement was not in 'accordance with the opinion of the majority of the Subscribers'.[129] The dispute ended, but not without damaging the hospital's subscriptions. The *Charity Record & Philanthropic News* noted that such proselytising meant 'goodbye to . . . generous and sympathetic support'.[130] Donations fell from £3,253 16s. 8d. in 1892 to £2,695 14s. 5d. in 1893, recovering only slightly in 1894 once the dispute had ended. The governors fought shy of mentioning the dispute in the 1894 annual report as they were afraid that support might be damaged still further.[131]

Contemporaries were aware of these problems, and hospital scandals remained a constant theme in the press. The consequences were rarely disastrous, but they were often serious enough to provoke alarm and forced governors to rely more heavily on non-charitable sources of funding. As the *Hospital* wrote in 1893, hospitals needed 'less criticism and more cash'.[132]

Conclusion

The problems facing hospital finance were varied. It is perhaps because hospitals did not rely on any one source of income, but developed a diverse financial base that they managed to survive expansion and the transition away from a philanthropic base. The need to develop new sources of funding was always present. Financial diversification was in part inspired by the restricted nature and uncertainties of direct philanthropy, and linked to the hospitals'

127 Ibid. 19 Apr. 1894, SBH, GHA 2/9.
128 German Hospital, minutes of the annual general court, 8 May 1894, SBH, GHA 5/2; 'A word in season to the governors and friends of the German Hospital', 1894, SBH, GHA 18/3.
129 German Hospital, minutes of the special general court, 8 May 1894, SBH, GHA 6/2.
130 *Charity Record & Philanthropic News* xiv (1894), 201.
131 German Hospital, annual reports 1892–4, SBH.
132 *Hospital*, 3 June 1893, 153.

experiences as medical institutions, their location, nature and expenditure. However, perhaps it should be recognised that invariably it was the opportunity to move away from traditional sources of funding that sealed the hospitals' financial strategy. Without the opportunity to charge probationary nurses, redirect clinical fees, even sell land or make public appeals, the hospital had to struggle on with its traditional resources until a solution was found. Such an important transformation in the hospitals' financial character and a dilution of charity's significance in the structure of income, raises questions about how financial diversification influenced the hospitals' administration.

PART II

PHILANTHROPY AND CONTROL

5

Charity and Control: Voluntarism and the Management of the London Hospitals

A subscribers' democracy?

The diversification of income and a dilution of charitable resources in the financial structure of London's hospitals did not occur in a vacuum. At the same time as the hospitals' funding was changing, the administrative environment also altered. It would be convenient to link the two: to argue that a change in finance encouraged a dilution of the philanthropist's power. Does such a view match the evidence?

Brian Abel-Smith has argued that nineteenth-century hospital administration represented an idiosyncratic mix of institutional variations.[1] Differences did exist. Each hospital developed its own administration to match its institutional needs, but it would be true to say that hospitals conformed to a certain managerial norm, that hospitals in Wakefield, Bristol or Chichester had a similar administrative structure to their counterparts in London.[2] Just as similarities existed between hospitals, they also existed between charitable agencies. According to Morris, by the 1830s voluntary societies had emerged as a flexible and adaptable 'cultural norm', sharing a number of organisational features.[3] Hospitals fitted within this pattern and shared common characteristics with other benevolent societies. Charitable organisations were governed by a 'subscriber democracy', where 'one subscriber, one vote was the general rule'. They internalised the idea of an urban democracy where membership was limited to those who contributed.[4] The hospital's voluntary nature was reflected in its management, but the 'subscriber democracy' was modified in favour of a hierarchical administrative system. Authority continued to be vested in the subscribers, with presidents and vice-presidents remaining largely ornamental. However, though subscribers retained the theoretical right to influence the hospital, in practice managerial responsibility was awarded only to those who had given a certain amount. Ten guineas represented the minimum for a position on the hospital's management with some institutions setting a higher premium: at the Hospital for Sick Children, for example, fifty guineas were required. These subscribers became the

---

1 Abel-Smith, *The hospitals*, 34.
2 Marland, *Medicine and society*, 98–9.
3 Morris, *Class, sect and party*, 184.
4 Ibid.

hospitals' governors. Management based on such subscriber representation would have created enormous logistical problems when thousands were encouraged to contribute. By limiting the number of governors through a monetary qualification, a smaller administrative unit was created. Doubts existed about whether this was the most rational basis for management, but it was widely accepted as the best system that could be devised.

The endowed hospitals, by virtue of their older foundations and economic base, were run on slightly different principles, substituting nomination for subscription. St Bartholomew's, St Thomas's and Guy's had no large body of subscribers as they relied (at least until the late 1870s) on endowments for their financial security. With few philanthropists involved directly in the hospitals' funding an alternative basis of management had been created. The small number of benefactors and the high contribution required for a governorship ensured that the administration was a self-perpetuating oligarchy, selecting its own candidates for inclusion.[5] At Guy's, where the number of governors was limited to sixty, this system gave the hospital a strong Evangelical character. Nomination produced few active governors however. Under these circumstances the main administrative duties passed to a treasurer, as each hospital's only permanent lay official. Treasurers were appointed at other hospitals, but they did not adopt the same prominent role. The governors at St Bartholomew's and Guy's, without an active financial interest in the hospital, seemed content to let the treasurer run the institution. From the 1850s onwards the medical press was concerned that such a system encouraged autocracy. Until the appointment of Sydney Waterlow at St Bartholomew's in 1874 and Edmund Lushington at Guy's in 1876 it was not so much autocracy that characterised management but inactivity. Endowed hospitals had a poor record of reform and much of this can be attributed to their governors' disinclination to become actively involved.

The notion that financial commitment was naturally linked to managerial responsibility was a powerful concept in the administration of benevolent societies. However, at St Bartholomew's and University College Hospital an external non-elected authority claimed an influence in each hospital's affairs. Whereas St Thomas's had succeeded in shaking off the City of London's influence by 1782, at St Bartholomew's the City retained the right to appoint aldermen and the Lord Mayor as governors.[6] Aldermen (with the exception Waterlow) did not take much interest in the hospital and were a minority group, but the City remained keen to exercise its privilege and took St Bartholomew's to court in 1863 when it felt that its rights had not been upheld. The City won the case, taking the moral high ground that it had a right to appoint governors as in the past it had made substantial contributions.[7] At

[5] At St Bartholomew's governorships cost £100 in 1864: minutes of the board of governors, 24 Feb. 1864, SBH, Ha 1/22.
[6] Granshaw, 'St Thomas's', 57; Medvei and Thornton, *Saint Bartholomew's*, 23.
[7] *Medical Times & Gazette* ii (1863), 472.

University College Hospital it was University College that exerted a right to participate in the hospital's management, basing its claim on the college's role in founding the institution. To protect University College's interests and to ensure that the hospital continued to provide clinical training, the college secretary was appointed as an ex-officio officer on the management committee. This was enough for University College and the secretary was disinclined to participate in the hospital's affairs. In both cases the rhetoric of financial support was used to justify involvement.

All hospitals organised their governors into a general court that sat periodically to discuss the institution's business. The frequency of these meetings varied between hospitals: most met on an annual basis at the start of the 'Season' when governors were guaranteed to be in London, though at the Hospital for Sick Children and St Bartholomew's the court assembled every three months. The responsibilities of the general court, as outlined by the Charity Commission in 1840, remained unchanged throughout the nineteenth century. Courts convened to appoint 'the presidents, treasurers, and all other officers and ministers . . . and to do every other act of good government'.[8] Important decisions, especially those linked to finance and appointments, required a special meeting. General courts could provide the opportunity for intense conflict, as seen at the German Hospital in 1894 over the hospital's religious character, but mainly they remained quiet and orderly, a chance to review the year's work. The unwieldy nature of these bodies required an administrative streamlining. Managerial responsibility was transferred to an annually elected committee, a move that *Charity* felt promoted the most efficient form of management.[9] Others feared that this would encourage subservience to the hospitals' permanent officials; instead administration passed to a small clique. The general court remained a hospital's ultimate executive authority, but management had effectively devolved to its elected representatives.

Management committees met weekly, or every two weeks, and discussed every administrative detail. The names of these bodies changed at each institution: at Guy's it was called the court of committees, at the German Hospital the hospital committee, while the London was administered by the house committee. The functions of these committees remained the same however. All major decisions had to be referred back to the general court, but as the management committees consisted of the leading governors, and the courts generally gathered annually and were poorly attended, it was these committees that shaped the hospitals' development. Some critics felt that this produced a closed shop and made a farce of elections, echoing similar criticisms made of local government.[10] The same men were returned year after year, but rather than creating a closed shop it ensured a certain degree of continuity.

8 *Thirty-Second Report of the Charity Commission*, 9.
9 *Charity*, Apr. 1887, 217.
10 *Times*, 26 Dec. 1889, 9; Garrard, *Leadership and power*, 79.

Not all took up their posts with equal enthusiasm: whereas Sir Francis Gold-smid was the tireless chair of University College Hospital despite his active involvement in the cause of Jewish emancipation, Robert Hawthorn after his appointment as a governor in 1850 never attended a meeting.[11] To promote continuity at the German Hospital the hospital committee was chosen from the eighteen most active members of the previous year's committee. Six new governors were elected to the committee annually to prevent stagnation. In 1854 this was reduced to three.[12] Committees were invariably poorly attended and small quorums were specified in the hospitals' rules to compensate. At the Hospital for Sick Children, the committee of management had a membership of twenty and a quorum of seven, and even then meetings had to be periodically cancelled due to poor attendance.[13] It was a common problem. In hospitals 'the work of very many is performed habitually by the attendance of the same four or five'.[14] From among this small group a chairman was elected who became the hospital's spokesman and guiding influence in the administration. Chairmen did not acquire the same degree of influence that the treasurers of endowed hospitals possessed; their authority was moderated by the larger number of governors who were willing to become actively involved. However, chairmen did wield considerable influence by virtue of their long-standing attachment to the institution and their willingness to attend every meeting.

Not all issues were discussed by the entire committee. Matters requiring detailed investigation were delegated to subcommittees of governors. At St Bartholomew's and University College Hospital management via sub-committee became the main vehicle for administrative change; at other hospitals they were established periodically to discuss a wide range of issues. At the German Hospital a subcommittee was appointed in 1851 to look into the purchase of a portrait of the duke of Cambridge, the hospital's president; at the London subcommittees were convened to discuss, for example, the employment of a new chaplain in 1889, or building plans in the following year.[15] These subcommittees could become semi-permanent features of the administration. The annual dinner and the organisational activity needed to make it a success saw the formation of dinner committees, elected annually for short periods. Where building occurred over several years, as at the Hospital for Sick Children, building committees met until the work was completed. The flexible nature of such committees ensured that they were adapted to organise a number of fundraising activities.

---

[11] UCH, minutes of the general committee, 22 July 1850, UCL, A1/2/1.
[12] German Hospital, minutes of the annual general court, 26 Jan. 1854, SBH, GHA 5/1.
[13] Hospital for Sick Children, staff rules, GOSH, 5/1/3a.
[14] *Times*, 11 Dec. 1850, 4.
[15] German Hospital, minutes of the hospital committee, 28 Aug. 1851, SBH, GHA 2/2; London Hospital, subcommittee minutes, LH, A/9/122; minutes of the court of governors, 1 Apr. 1890, LH, A/2/14.

Management committees did not supervise the hospitals' day-to-day administration. In industry owners delegated the immediate management of the workshop or factory to trustworthy employees, ensuring a minimal bureaucratic framework. According to Lesley Hannah, it was only after 1914 that industry moved away from its family basis and started to develop the factory office as more than an adjunct to the workshop.[16] In hospitals a similar process of delegation occurred, but here governors exercised a higher degree of control through regular visits to the wards and a system of reports. Medical responsibility on a daily basis was delegated at a ward level to the matron and at a wider level to the doctors who were expected to submit regular reports. At Guy's this duty was passed to a paid medical superintendent who looked after the management of the wards. The medical staff had initially opposed the move until they were threatened with a salaried status.[17] Other non-medical administrative duties were allocated to other male employees. Paid collectors working on commission gathered subscriptions and where large estates were held a land agent was employed. Such officers were appointed because it was felt to be 'unreasonable to expect a gentleman either in business or out of business, to devote sufficient time' to the hospital's daily management.[18]

Of these paid officials, it was the secretary or steward that had the largest administrative burden. According to the *Charity Record & Philanthropic News* a secretary had to be 'a man of business, a good accountant and bookkeeper, a diplomat, special pleader, architect and builder, a house steward, tinker, clerk of the works, and occasionally office boy and porter'.[19] No treasurer or chairman, even when residing in the hospital, could be expected to carry out these duties. Considerable responsibility was therefore placed on the secretary or steward. At University College Hospital with the chairman living in Westbourne Terrace and the dean in Harley Street this left Newton Nixon as the secretary the *de facto* head of the hospital for much of the day. Such men generally had a colonial or civil service background and were indefatigable in their efforts. Adrian Hope, secretary of the Hospital for Sick Children from 1885 to 1904, fits this model. He worked in the Bank of England before serving as secretary to the governor of Ceylon and clerk to the council of the island. After a year in Paris in 1884 he returned to England and worked voluntarily as an assistant auditor for London's workhouses until he took up his post at the Hospital for Sick Children. The hospital's success was largely due to his tireless work and fundraising. Before his appointment to University College Hospital Nixon had worked at the London School Board.[20] Constant attendance ensured that these posts were salaried, though anomalies con-

16 Leslie Hannah, *The rise of the corporate economy*, London 1983, 71–2.
17 Cameron, *Mr Guy's Hospital*, 197–8.
18 Granshaw, 'St Thomas's', 49–51.
19 *Charity Record & Philanthropic News* xii (1892), 214.
20 *Charity*, Feb. 1889, 553; SC on *Metropolitan Hospitals, Second Report*, 253–64.

tinued to exist with the secretary of the Royal Northern Hospital paid on commission until 1894. On average secretaries earned between £100 and £400 *per annum*, a rate of pay that compared favourably with local government officers' salaries in 1914 where 88 per cent were paid below £260. Within the hospital these men remained the highest paid officials, with chaplains only earning between £100 and £300.[21] However, from the 1880s onwards administrators increasingly complained about their poor level of pay and high level of responsibility. Governors gradually responded by raising salaries, appointing additional clerks and creating new posts by dividing the secretaries' duties, thus demonstrating an increased professionalisation of hospital management. Hospitals nevertheless continued to be run by governors and not by paid administrators even in 1900. An attitude that favoured a professional and bureaucratic administration was slow to emerge. Hospitals remained bastions of amateurism where other organisations were moving towards a professional management structure and professional administrators were taking a key role in social-reform organisations.[22]

Administrative change

The transition from a philanthropic imperative to a medical environment with the addition of new wards, new treatments, out-patient departments and telephones was marked by a shift in the hospitals' administrative structure.[23] The institutional environment under which hospitals had initially grown was ill-suited to the process of medicalisation. The result was administrative expansion in an environment where the 'ostentatious worship of the voluntary system' persisted.[24] Rather than altering the hospitals' charitable foundation, governors adapted and extended the administration because an alternative to voluntarism was unthinkable in a society where philanthropy and amateurism were revered. Existing committees were modified; additional functions were grafted onto old committees, and through a process of organisational subdivision new committees were created.[25] St Bartholomew's stood

---

[21] Eric C. O. Jewsbury, *The Royal Northern Hospital, 1856–1956*, London 1956, 73; P. J. Waller, *Town, city and nation: England, 1850–1914*, Oxford 1991, 286; Abel-Smith, *The hospital*, 33–4.

[22] Harris, 'Political thought and the welfare state', 122.

[23] The Hospital for Sick Children was particularly slow in discussing the need for a telephone. The committee of management only raised the issue in 1898, while the house and finance committee at University College Hospital had one connected in 1883: Hospital for Sick Children, minutes of the committee of management, 13 July 1898, GOSH, 1/2/21; UCH, minutes of the house committee, 2 Nov. 1883, UCL, A1/3/3. These technological changes were in advance of many businesses as in general office technology remained crude until after 1914: Hannah, *Rise of the corporate economy*, 77.

[24] *Times*, 2 Aug. 1892, 11.

[25] These changes were reflected in a transformation of the nature of record keeping. Narra-

apart from these developments, limited by its royal charter and constrained by the institution's conservatism. The house committee's work did increase from the 1870s onwards and a series of subcommittees was appointed to discuss specific administrative and medical changes, but no new committee was formed until 1892. At other hospitals, to prevent an unmanageable structure from emerging, an administrative subdivision occurred as management became too complex for one committee to encompass.

General hospitals founded in the institutional expansion of the eighteenth century and the teaching hospitals of the early nineteenth century were the first to augment their administration in the period after 1850. The new specialist hospitals followed. Development was often linked to an increase in the institution's size and an expansion in its functions, and most committees were added after periods of building. However, while doctors were often at the centre of these developments the best they were able to obtain was a junior partnership in the hospital's formal administration. In response to change, lay finance committees were created to control increasing expenditure; house committees were set up to regulate 'house keeping and drug expenditure, furniture and repairs etc., the hiring and discharge of servants and nurses' and to 'take the responsibility [for] the internal management of the institution'.[26] Estate committees were founded to supervise the hospitals' property, and medical committees were established by doctors in their bid to exercise some degree of authority over the medical environment. These new committees invariably met monthly and submitted regular reports outlining their suggestions to the management committees. Agreement was often a foregone conclusion as the new committees were subsets of existing ones. As a result management committees were freed from many of their duties, and though they retained responsibility for all the decisions taken, they were involved in less administrative detail.

Administrative expansion is best illustrated by the experiences of the Royal Hospital for Diseases of the Chest. The admission of in-patients in 1850 strained the established managerial structure and in 1853 the management committee appointed a subcommittee to investigate. No immediate changes were made, but in 1857 the management committee abandoned its quarterly meetings at the London Tavern, Bishopsgate, and met monthly in the hospital. The decision to extend the hospital in 1862 prompted further change. A building committee was appointed and a finance committee was established to raise money for the venture. The opening of the new hospital saw further development: in 1864 Robert Smart, the secretary, was awarded £10 for his extra work and in 1866 an honorary secretary was appointed to assist him. To manage the new domestic arrangements a temporary house committee was formed and after a probationary period of three months it was

---

tive accounts began to disappear from the annual reports and new systems of records were established: Craig, 'A survey of hospital records', 164.

26 RCH, minutes of the house committee, LMA, H33/RCH/A4/2.

made permanent.[27] By 1881 the Royal Chest's management had increased sufficiently for the secretary to be awarded another £150 pay rise, and in 1885 an election committee was established to discuss staff appointments, followed by a drug committee in 1886. The result was a dramatic increase in the hospital's running expenses and in 1886 the Sunday Fund felt disinclined to award the hospital a full grant.[28] Similar developments can be seen at other hospitals. The Hospital for Sick Children was managed solely by the management committee until 1857/8 when finance, dinner and drug committees were added. By 1878 the hospital was governed by eight committees and a chapel committee was established in 1891.[29]

Administrative expansion was not limited to the specialist hospitals, but in the case of general hospitals increased size was less of a factor in development. New committees were founded at these hospitals in response to specific concerns. The London Hospital, anxious about its financial position in 1864, founded a finance committee and when the governors decided to award an annual grant to the medical college in 1876 a joint college board was formed.[30] The retirement of a long-serving treasurer or chairman often provided a chance to re-evaluate how the hospital was run. At Guy's the administration was investigated in 1896 when Lushington retired. The difficulty of finding a new treasurer saw a change in the hospital's government. The treasurer's post was made non-resident and a new administrative structure was adopted. A school and staff committee was established to deal with the medical arrangements and a house committee was set up to concentrate on domestic affairs. Concern over the hospital's poor financial position saw the foundation of a finance committee to co-ordinate fundraising and the Act of Incorporation was modified in 1898 to increase the governors' control over the hospital's landed property.[31] The immediate effect was an increase in activity and the governors became less inclined to let the treasurer make all the decisions. Comparable administrative changes were made at the London in 1897 when the tireless Sydney Holland was appointed chairman.[32]

A static administrative structure could not support a change in the nature of the hospital. Medicalisation, building and financial anxiety required bureaucratisation and administrative expansion. Gradually duties were devolved from the main management committee to smaller bodies to cope

[27] RCH, governors' minute book, 3 Sept. 1857, 6 July 1862, 7 Sept. 1864, 31 Aug. 1866, LMA, H33/RCH/A1/2.

[28] Ibid. 6 July 1886, LMA, H33/RCH/A1/6.

[29] Hospital for Sick Children, minutes of the committee of management, 13 Nov. 1857, 29 June 1858, GOSH, 1/2/6.

[30] London Hospital, minutes of the house committee, Dec. 1864, LH, A/5/32; 4 Apr. 1876, LH, A/5/37.

[31] Guy's Hospital, minutes of the general court, 3 June, 30 July 1896, LMA, H9/Gy/A1/4; minutes of the staff and school committees, LMA, H9/Gy/A23/1; minutes of the house committee, LMA, H9/Gy/A25/1; minutes of the finance committee, LMA, H9/Gy/A24/1.

[32] Clark-Kennedy, The London, ii. 127–36.

with the increase in the hospitals' functions and work. Simultaneously specialist paid staff were appointed to deal with the day-to-day management. The result was an increase in administrative complexity and the development of a more organised and efficient approach to hospital management. The emphasis, however, remained on voluntarism.

'Interested control': the Sunday Fund and hospital management

Governors resisted external pressure for reform. However, the Metropolitan Hospital Sunday Fund used the governors' own rhetoric of financial commitment and managerial responsibility in its work to reform hospital management. *The Lancet* maintained that the fund was bound to 'exercise a most powerful influence on all points connected with hospital management' as 'advice to charitable institutions comes with most force when it is accompanied by assistance'.[33] It was an opinion that acted as the mainstay of the journal's support. Hospital reformers initially predicted that its activities would solve the more obvious problems in hospital management and allied themselves with the movement to further their aims. Sydney Waterlow was quick to confirm the fund's potential. He explained that by 'holding the power of the purse in the name of the public we have an influence over them [medical charities] which it would be difficult to exercise in any other way'.[34] At the grass roots level similar ideas were discussed. In 1880 the Hammersmith branch stressed the need to extend the fund's investigative and reforming potential, especially over the geographical distribution of hospitals, and these interests were repeated elsewhere.[35] Policy was never as clear cut as this, but there was an awareness that it represented a positive instrument for intervention. From the start the COS saw the fund in these terms and attempted to influence its policy. In fact, both organisations had similar intentions. The COS strove to reform and organise charity; the Sunday Fund wanted to reform hospitals and organise collections. However, the COS's brand of organisation was resisted after Waterlow persuaded the fund that the COS's ideas were irrelevant to the movement. In the face of opposition the COS's enthusiasm waned and it diverted its attention to the foundation of a central hospitals board.

The Sunday Fund initially justified reformers' hopes. Management was vested in a council, consisting of fifty clerical and fifty lay members who elected a distribution committee to conduct the main work of the fund. It replaced the individual's choice of philanthropic outlet with careful investigation. The rules governing the committee's work stipulated that only hospitals that produced printed reports with an audited balance sheet for three

33 *Lancet* i (1875), 247; ii (1874), 22.
34 Cited in Owen, *English philanthropy*, 486.
35 *BMJ* ii (1880), 892.

years were entitled to consideration. The endowed hospitals, with which many of the initial organisers were associated, were therefore excluded as they made no attempt to publicise their financial circumstances outside the hospital.[36] Grants were based on two calculations: the cost of in-patients per bed, and the cost of out-patients per head. These were determined by matching expenditure against the number of patients treated. Those institutions found to be too expensively managed were either penalised or excluded to encourage reform. In the distribution of collections the fund departed from the established 'cultural norm' for a benevolent society. Authority continued to come from a well-publicised annual general meeting that elected a committee of management, but the mass subscribing public was denied the right to dictate how their contributions were used. It was perceived that the subscribers' right to influence the hospitals' administration had not solved the hospitals' problems. The fund therefore removed the subscribers from their potentially influential position and substituted itself as the agent of reform. The distribution committee sought to replace the active citizen's arbitrary choice of destination for his philanthropy with a centralised system based on the careful investigation of each hospital's benefit to the community. Those giving to the fund had to place their faith in the fact that it would distribute the grants wisely.

Awards were well-publicised and because they were from a body that claimed to distribute money on the grounds of utility, hospitals were exposed to comparison and public scrutiny, thereby encouraging reform. A small grant or a fall in the award was viewed with considerable anxiety, as this created an impression of poor management. The refusal of a grant 'left a mark'.[37] The Metropolitan Free Hospital felt so strongly about its low grant in 1874 that the hospital's authorities protested violently and complained of corruption, but made no effort to reform its own management. Those concerned with the position of the specialist hospitals attempted to use the Metropolitan Free's grievances to hijack the fund and impose their own views on distribution, involving the fund in an acrimonious public debate that threatened collections.[38] Other hospitals responded in a positive manner, showing the movement's potential as an instrument for reform. When the Royal Hospital for Diseases of the Chest was awarded £82 in 1875, £50 less than in 1874, the governors held an investigation and conducted a programme of strict reform. Strenuous efforts were made to reduce advertising costs and pursue lower tenders, and two beds were added to lower the average cost per

---

[36] Guy's applied in 1887 as the hospital's financial circumstances forced it to conform to the fund's notions. St Thomas's did not approach the fund until 1896 but was prevented from participating as the governors would not agree to the fund's uniform system of accounts or public audit: *Hospital*, 1 Aug. 1896, 397.

[37] Smalley, *Waterlow*, 183.

[38] *Times*, 16 Sept. 1874, 8; 17 Dec. 1874, 8; *BMJ* ii (1875), 372.

bed. Grants rose accordingly.[39] This was exactly what the fund and its supporters hoped to accomplish.

The Sunday Fund ultimately disappointed hospital reformers however. Increasingly it became exclusively 'a collecting body', assuming a less interventionist stance, and the mantle of reform passed to other organisations. Some progress was made in encouraging the adoption of a uniform system of accounting. This was crucial to the fund's work in allowing an effective comparison of institutions that had previously misguided the public with idiosyncratic balance sheets.[40] Hospitals, however, were slow to adopt the fund's suggestions. St Thomas's, for example, disqualified itself from the fund's support by refusing to adopt its uniform system of accounts.[41] An inability to secure reform was not just seen over accounting procedures. Even the pressing issue of hospital abuse, where an increase in admissions was misconceived as a growth in the number exploiting charity, was not dealt with effectively.[42] Although the issue had first been discussed in the 1850s, it was not until 1897, after five years of investigation, that the fund finally encouraged governors to appoint inquiry officers to investigate patients' social backgrounds to reduce abuse.[43] *The Lancet* was disenchanted by 1897 and concluded that Waterlow 'has become increasingly reluctant to see the growing abuse of hospitals, which to everyone else is so apparent, and to use the great power of the council of the Hospital Sunday Fund for its friendly correction'.[44] Waterlow's unenthusiastic attitude was symptomatic of developments within the movement.

Two currents can be detected in the Sunday Fund's change in attitude. The philanthropic public, assaulted by a multitude of charitable appeals, lacked the resources necessary to meet the London hospitals' spiralling expenditure. The fund was all too aware of this dilemma. Initially it had to balance the need to solve the hospitals' economic problems with the desire for reform. By the 1880s an apparent financial crisis in the London hospitals blinkered the fund to the need for reform and consequently it became absorbed in the problems of hospital funding. This combined with a selfish desire to maximise its own income as a justification for its existence. Intervention also carried its own dangers. A preoccupation with hospitals' internal management held the potential of alienating vested interests. It was a position the fund hoped to avoid to ensure its continued popularity. This was highlighted in 1885 when the grant awarded to University College Hospital was attacked. Critics felt that the grant was ill-advised as the hospital employed the Anglican All Saint's Nursing Sisterhood to organise its nurs-

39 RCH, council minute book, 14 Dec. 1875, LMA, H33/RCH/A1/4.
40 *Times*, 18 Dec. 1890, 10.
41 *Hospital*, 1 Aug. 1896, 397.
42 Waddington, ' "Unsuitable cases" ', 26–46.
43 BMJ ii (1897), 1821.
44 *Lancet* i (1897), 672.

ing. Concern was purely sectarian as the nursing at University College Hospital was highly efficient.[45] The fund's general purposes committee investigated and concluded that 'matters relating to the internal administration of hospitals are beyond the jurisdiction of the Hospital Sunday Fund'.[46] This was a complete rejection of the movement's reformist intentions.

The transition from a reforming body to a funding body occurred at no definable point, but from the 1880s the Sunday Fund expected increasingly less from the hospitals it supported. The model, however, was not abandoned but revitalised in the Prince of Wales Hospital Fund, which (as shown in chapter 7) reoriented the nature of active philanthropy.

A governing class?

The dominance of voluntarism in the hospitals' management and the slow pace of professionalisation ensured that by 1900 it was still philanthropists who dominated the hospitals' administration. This raises important questions about the social composition of these managing bodies. The social origins of philanthropists, according to Frank Prochaska, are 'usually difficult to determine'.[47] For all this, historians have tentatively agreed that most subscribers were middle-class, a view confirmed by Hilary Marland's detailed analysis of the subscription lists of medical charities in Wakefield and Huddersfield.[48] In London the structure of the economy strengthened this trend and metropolitan hospitals drew a large proportion of their support from the expanding middle classes. However, according to the Hospital's pessimistic assessment in 1891, only 17 per cent of the population contributed to a hospital.[49] Even fewer gave their time and it was from these philanthropists that the hospitals' governors were drawn. Who were they? Governors can be divided into three groups: those who gave sufficient money to become governors but took no role in the hospitals' management, those who infrequently attended meetings, and those who formed the mainstay of the administration. It is this last group that needs analysis, as it was these men who governed the hospital.

It might be expected that London's hospitals provided an ideal arena for female participation and administrative involvement. Women increased their role in charitable associations during the nineteenth century, building on their formal and informal participation during the seventeenth and eighteenth centuries. As philanthropists they travelled into the city 'in search of adventure and self-discovery', with many fitting charitable work between

---

[45] BMJ ii (1885), 266; S. W. F. Holloway, 'All Saints Sisterhood at University College Hospital, 1862–99', Medical History ii (1959), 146–56.
[46] Times, 2 Dec. 1885, 7.
[47] Prochaska, Women and philanthropy, 41.
[48] Marland, Medicine and society, 117–22.
[49] Hospital, 28 Feb. 1891, 320.

social engagements. Others, like Octavia Hill, showed that women 'have developed an unexpected capacity for organisation' and had 'an enthusiasm for difficult, disagreeable and unpromising work'.[50] In their philanthropic work women displayed considerable organisational skills. They were able to penetrate the homes of the poor, work with male professionals to secure and pass legislation, and raise considerable funds for charitable societies. By the late nineteenth century Louisa Hubbard estimated that at least half-a-million women were engaged in philanthropic work.[51] Through this work they were able to control important resources for the urban poor like housing or access to medical care and this gave them considerable authority. This authority and involvement was not, however, extended to London's hospitals where women continued to play a marginal administrative role. Hospital philanthropy and the structure of London's benevolent economy were at odds in this respect. Arguments that women were suited to hospital management because of their domestic skills were ignored.[52] In the London hospitals male and female philanthropic worlds remained substantially different, mirroring what Leonore Davidoff and Catherine Hall have seen in Birmingham and Jordan has found in Belfast.[53] It was not until 1887 that women were allowed to attend the Sunday Fund's meetings and Sir Edmund Currie's motion in 1893 to admit women to the house committee of the London Hospital was firmly rejected.[54] Women remained largely excluded from hospital management.

There were areas where women were not marginalised. They were highly active in the never-ending task of fundraising and the pastoral task of visiting patients and after-care through Samaritan funds. The division between a male-dominated administration and female participation in (and sometimes dominance of) fundraising might be explained by the voluntary hospitals' medical nature and roots in the eighteenth century. Victorian doctors, anxious about women's attempts to enter the medical profession, subscribed to and helped construct social and biological views of women that showed them at the mercy of their reproductive organs, ideas that only helped confirm 'hegemonic definitions of femininity'.[55] Hospitals partly embodied this medi-

---

50 See Prochaska, *Women and philanthropy*; Mary Clare Martin, 'Women and philanthropy in Walthamstow and Leyton', *London Journal* xix (1994), 119–50; Judith R. Walkowitz, *City of dreadful delight: narratives of sexual danger in late Victorian London*, London 1992, 52.
51 Cited in Patricia Hollis, *Ladies elect: women in English local government, 1865–1914*, Oxford 1987, 11.
52 *Hospital*, 25 Oct. 1890, 61.
53 Leonore Davidoff and Catherine Hall, *Family fortunes: men and women of the English middle class, 1780–1850*, London 1987; A. Jordan, *Who cared?: charity in Victorian and Edwardian Belfast*, Belfast 1994, 199–206.
54 *Hospital*, 17 Dec. 1887, 200; London Hospital, minutes of the house committee, 14 Feb. 1893, LH, A/5/45.
55 Lynda Nead, *Myths of sexuality: representations of women in Victorian Britain*, Oxford 1988, 142–3.

cal view of the female body, while women tended to play a greater role in newer forms of charity. According to Martha Vicinus women did not initially lay claim to 'arenas already controlled by men . . . rather they captured unclaimed areas and pushed out from there'.[56] In finance those running London's hospitals were willing to share the burden, but hospital administration was close enough to business to be seen as a male sphere for which women were unsuited and from which they had to be excluded. Governors certainly believed that fundraising provided a 'respectable' outlet for women's energies that did not involve them in the business of running the hospital. For many women, however, even a limited fundraising role provided an escape from boredom and a chance to play an active role outside the home.[57] This is seen in women's prominent position in organising bazaars. University College Hospital's 1886 bazaar was almost entirely organised by the governors' wives, with Lady Goldsmid, the wife of the hospital's chairman, holding a similarly important role within the bazaar committee.[58] Of the seven women on the German Hospital's ladies committee in 1847, only two were not connected by marriage to the main governing body.[59] As matrons and lady superintendents women achieved some influence over the hospitals' domestic and nursing arrangements, but the administrative environment remained predominantly male.

'Hospital committees', the *Charity Record & Philanthropic News* felt, 'are composed of gentlemen who have a special regard for the charities with which they are associated, who give freely both their money, and what is often of more value, their time.'[60] These two aspects, 'money' and 'time', were crucial in determining the social origins of the managing elite. The financial qualification for a governor, and the expectation that an active governor would be the first to help the hospital in times of hardship, ensured a certain social homogeneity. Only the affluent could afford to make such a financial commitment. The second criteria, the element of 'time', further defined the governors' social class. In 1838 Lord Stanhope noted that only men of leisure could conveniently hold posts and his opinion reflected a social reality.[61] To hold an active position governors had to devote time to the hospitals' affairs and attend monthly meetings. Membership of more than one committee or an active role as a house visitor required weekly visits, while treasurers and chairmen attended almost daily. The provision of a treasurer's house (as at Guy's and St Bartholomew's) did remove the tedium of travelling to the hospital but it also meant that treasurers were expected to be on hand at all times. Where the middle classes were the predominant contributors, only the

---

56 Martin, 'Women and philanthropy', 125; Vicinus, *Independent women*, 15.
57 Prochaska, 'Charity bazaars', 84.
58 UCH, minutes of the bazaar and ball committee, UCL, A1/5/1.
59 German Hospital, minutes of the bazaar committee, 23 Sept. 1847, SBH, GHA 14/1.
60 *Charity Record & Philanthropic News* xvii (1897), 75.
61 Harrison, 'Philanthropy and the Victorians', 359.

Table 21: Social composition of governors, West Bromwich and Dudley, 1867–1900 (%)

	Upper/ Upper middle	Middle class	Professional/ Commerce	Lower middle class	Middle class (unspecified)	Working class	Ur
Hospital	27	18	43	3	2	7	

Source: Trainor, *Black Country elites*, 400–1

leisured and the wealthy could afford to dedicate this much time. Richard Trainor's analysis of the leadership of philanthropic societies in West Bromwich and Dudley (see table 21) and John Garrard's work on Bolton, Rochdale and Salford confirms this view.[62] Active governors were therefore invariably men of wealth, repute and social standing, and often important philanthropists who did not just limit their activities to medical charity.

The *Hospital* observed in 1892 that the most 'active' governors were men largely engaged in 'business' and Jordan notes that business connections were also characteristic of charity in Victorian Belfast. The domination of hospital management by 'business' interests (see table 22) was similar to the way in which they provided the structural basis for local government.[63] London's leading banking and financial companies provided the main background for governors, with those with business interests or connections representing 49.7 per cent of active governors. These men either owned or managed prominent, successful and wealthy banks or companies, particularly brewing, printing and publishing concerns. To the governors involved in the city must be added those who came from largely professional backgrounds and of this group doctors formed the largest section. Governors with independent means, and the clergy were also prominent, while those with aristocratic backgrounds generally played only a marginal role. Support from the nobility, members of the royal family and major landowners was mainly titular and suggested 'the acceptance of responsibility to the community' rather than active involvement. These groups were not as significant as the 'landed-classes' Roy Porter has identified in the eighteenth-century infirmaries.[64] There were of course exceptions. Hospital administration generally reflected society's inequalities of wealth and power, and mirrored the oligarchic mana-

62 Trainor, *Black country elites*; Garrard, *Leadership and power*, 13–37.
63 *Hospital*, 2 Jan. 1892, 161; Jordan, *Who cared?*, 201; Daunton, 'Payment and participation', 201.
64 Richard Roberts, 'Leasehold estates and municipal enterprise: landowner, local government and the development of Bournemouth', in Cannadine, *Patricians, power and politics*, 196; Porter, 'The gift relationship', 49–78.

Table 22: Social composition of active governors, 1850–98

	German Hospital	Guy's	Hospital for Sick Children	London	Royal Hospital for Diseases of the Chest	University College	TOTAL (%)
Aristocracy	0	2	2	0	2	0	3.7
Banking	1	7	4	3	1	2	11.0
Brewing	0	0	0	8	0	0	5.5
Clergy	1	0	2	3	4	0	6.1
Finance	5	9	5	4	10	4	22.2
Independent	2	2	1	2	1	6	8.6
Manufacturing	1	1	1	2	6	0	6.8
Military	0	0	1	2	0	0	1.8
MP	0	2	0	0	1	0	1.8
Publishing	1	2	3	0	1	0	4.3
Professional	2	0	10	2	6	3	14.1
Unknown	6	7	5	1	4	0	14.1
Working class	0	0	0	0	0	0	0.0

Source: Guy's, LMA, H9/Gy/A/96–9; annual reports 1850–98; Dictionary of national biography; Post office directory, 1850–99

gerial structure of other voluntary associations that were also dominated by these groups.[65] Within this framework each hospital had its own particular character, partly shaped by its location and nature. At St George's the governors in the 1880s 'were largely the denizens of Belgravia or Mayfair', while it was 'not uncommon to have two or three dukes, five or six noble lords, sitting at the Board room table'. This was largely due to the hospital's location at Hyde Park Corner.[66] The German Hospital was managed by German immigrants; the London by those with brewing connections, reflecting a major area of employment in Whitechapel. In Cardiff the infirmary received a large amount of its support from the dock interests.[67] No two hospitals were managed by the same occupational groups, a factor that reflected their metropolitan location and the high degree of localism in London, but they were managed by men of similar commercial and business experience and wealth.

Not all hospitals entirely fit this pattern. At the Royal Hospital for Diseases of the Chest, for example, fewer governors came from the upper-middle classes. John Austin, the hospital's difficult secretary, strenuously argued that the hospital was 'supported mainly by local subscribers, employers and working men'.[68] Although there were no 'working men' on the committees, the hospital's governing body did have a more middle-class status, linked to businesses trading on City Road. This difference can perhaps be accounted for by the hospital's character, its importance to areas of employment susceptible to diseases of the chest, and by the fact that long-established chest hospitals like the Brompton attracted the higher social groups interested in chest diseases.

The smallness of the philanthropic world ensured that close links developed between governors and between charitable organisations. Family connections provided an important tie. Hospitals did not become the personal fiefs of leading families, but the involvement of one family member often encouraged others to participate. Lushington came from a legal and political background, but his dedication to Guy's was due to his father's connection to the hospital from 1819 until his death in 1873.[69] At University College Hospital the Goldsmid family was important in the hospital's foundation and early management: Sir Isaac Goldsmid had been chairman from 1833 to 1855 and was succeeded by his son, Francis Goldsmid, who held the post until 1867.[70] Business connections emphasised these links. The East End's major brewing families were active in the London's management. With many governors involved in finance or in the Bank of England as directors, association

---

65 Roger J. Morris, 'Clubs, societies and associations', in Thompson, *Cambridge social history of Britain*, iii. 413.

66 George Turner, *Unorthodox reminiscences*, London 1931, 76.

67 Neil Evans, 'Urbanisation, elite attitudes and philanthropy: Cardiff, 1850–1914', *International Review of Social History* xxvii (1982), 297.

68 RCH, council minute book, 27 June 1889, LMA, H33/RCH/A1/7.

69 Moore, *Zeal for responsibility*, 54.

70 UCH, annual report 1909, UCL.

through work was reflected in participation in hospital management. At the Royal Hospital for Diseases of the Chest the involvement of Edward Sheppard and James Esdaile, both timber merchants, took this to an extreme. Their common business interests and the proximity of their timber yards encouraged their mutual interest in the hospital. Social connections emphasised the smallness of the philanthropic world. Many of the founders of the Hospital for Sick Children were known to each other personally.[71] Guy's practice of nomination ensured that governors came from a small social and evangelical group, with links strengthened between such governors as Philip Cazenove, Henry Hucks Gibbs and Money Wigram by their common membership of the Society of Nobody's Friends. In effect, charity had a small managerial elite.

Working-class governors were not entirely excluded. In specialist hospitals and those located in the East End it was possible for working-class representatives to be elected where there was a small middle-class population and strong labour or trade union interests. Workers' contributions formed a significant component in the income of the Poplar Hospital, but their contribution to the hospital's management was relatively small even after the committee of management appointed working-class representatives in 1891. Working-class governors rarely made up 10 per cent of the governing body.[72] In most hospitals, however, at least until the late Victorian period, the poor 'were excluded from involvement in the government'.[73] Medical charity, and charity in general, seemed hostile to working-class participation in its management.

It was the Saturday Fund that took up the campaign for working-class governors. The fund aimed to raise the level of working-class support for London's hospitals and as a *quid pro quo* it demanded subscribers' privileges and the appointment of working-class representatives. The fund was merely playing on the traditional right of contributors to influence management and pushed for representation to increase its own support. Ironically, however, the fund's own administration contained few working-class representatives.[74] In this it resembled the Bible societies which remained fundamentally middle-class but reflected the character of the local community. The Saturday Fund was not entirely a part of the growth of working-class cultural and leisure associations that developed from the mid nineteenth century onwards, though it acknowledged that the working class had an important role to play in charity.[75] In its aims it partly reflected the mutual aid societies by offering its supporters the possibility of a return on their contribution in times of sickness through admission to a hospital. However, the fund wanted

71 Kosky, *Mutual friends*, 14, 117–28.
72 Barnes, 'The Dockers' Hospital'.
73 Marland, *Medicine and society*, 145.
74 Burdett, *Hospital Sunday and Hospital Saturday*, 24.
75 Yeo, *Religion and voluntary organisations*, 185–235.

to tap the assets of the working classes and was an organisation for them rather than of them.[76] The dominance of its middle-class leadership ensured that it adopted the vocabulary of limited working-class representation for the respectable and thrifty, while it refused to extend this beyond these groups.

If Robert Frewer, the fund's secretary, tried to project the image that hospitals welcomed the movement, in reality many governors were reluctant to agree to its conditions. Large sections of the 'hospital world' were actively hostile to the Saturday Fund, especially as it was feared that it would herald an influx of working-class representatives.[77] This anxiety proved unfounded however. Governors were willing to give the Saturday Fund letters (though the exact number was often argued over), but they felt that the fund's representatives were merely trustees of the money and not subscribers, and therefore not entitled to be involved in the hospitals' management. While large sections of the medical press attacked the fund, many governors resisted its incursions.[78] When the fund passed a resolution in January 1882 to 'appoint a governor to a hospital receiving not less than £50', eleven of the general hospitals, led by Colonel Haygarth of St George's, protested. In response the fund withheld the annual grant to University College Hospital, St George's and the West London Hospital. The fund's firm stance was eroded by the unpopularity of its action and the grants were finally paid in February.[79] Some, however, did give way. In 1879 the Hospital for Sick Children agreed to appoint a representative of the Saturday Fund as a governor, but stated that he would only have access to the general court and not the management committees. Thirteen years later the Royal Hospital for Diseases of the Chest gave in to similar pressure and agreed to appoint Mr R. Costleman, an employee of the London and North Western Railway Board, as an annual governor. The fund claimed this as a victory: it had been trying to have a representative elected since 1887.[80] Although the fund had secured a point of principle, the governors at both hospitals ensured that it had no undue influence. In contrast the German Hospital and the London succumbed to the fund's economic blackmail.[81] Other Saturday funds outside London did have more success at electing their representatives onto 'figurehead' management committees, but in London the fund's influence at an administrative level remained stunted.[82]

[76] See Morris, 'Clubs, societies and associations', 416–19, for the growth of working-class associations.

[77] Charity Record & Philanthropic News ii (1882), 36; Hospital, 4 Jan. 1897, 229; Medical Times & Gazette i (1874), 320.

[78] Charity Record & Philanthropic News ii (1882), 120.

[79] Lancet i (1882), 154.

[80] Hospital for Sick Children, minutes of the committee of management, 18 Dec. 1879, GOSH, 1/2/16; RCH, council minute book, 19 Oct. 1892, LMA, H33/RCH/A1/7; 8 Feb. 1887, LMA, H33/RCH/A1/6.

[81] German Hospital, minutes of the hospital committee, 15 Dec. 1881, SBH, GHA 2/7; London Hospital, minutes of the house committee, 10 Jan. 1882, LH, A/5/40.

[82] Steven Cherry, 'Accountability, entitlement and control issues and voluntary hospital funding, c. 1860–1939', SHM ix (1996), 215–33.

The Saturday Fund was not the only body pressuring London's hospitals to appoint working-class governors. Members of Toynbee Hall, particularly Walter Pye, advocated working-class representation as part of the settlement movement's aim to promote community integration. Others writers concerned with the apparent breakdown in social harmony propounded similar views. However, the practical efforts made by workers' associations to secure representation were more effective.[83] At the City of London Hospital for Diseases of the Chest several bids were made in the 1890s to appoint working-class governors. The first attempt in 1890 by an organised effort of local workmen was firmly resisted.[84] Progress was made in 1893. A Mr Bartlett, the appointed representative of several local collection schemes, approached the hospital with the suggestion that six of his nominees should replace six existing governors. He claimed that these organisations had a right to participate to ensure that their contributions were used wisely. Stephen Olding, the hospital's chairman, saw this as 'revolutionary' and was shocked by Bartlett's effrontery. The *Charity Record & Philanthropic News* recognised the support that local workmen gave to the hospital, but could not justify Bartlett's action and warned of a 'mercenary spirit'. To limit the damage, Olding proposed a compromise and agreed to elect three working-class governors.[85]

The reluctant moves made by City of London Hospital for Diseases of the Chest were symptomatic of a wider change in attitude. From the 1890s onwards a more favourable stance was adopted. Journals gradually became sympathetic to the idea of working-class governors and by the 1920s the view that all contributors should be represented had been reluctantly accepted in part because of the growing economic pressure working-class contributory schemes were able to exert. Hospitals as the 'tied house of a section of the community' were gradually seen as inappropriate.[86] In London a change in rhetoric was not matched by an increase in working-class appointments. During the nineteenth century governors remained a wealthy and exclusive group, and even by 1900 their social composition had not been greatly altered.

Assessing hospital management

The voluntary system the London hospitals embraced was seen as the best possible form of administration, free from state interference and capable of promoting a friendly and homely atmosphere. Hospital reformers, the COS, the Hospitals Association and the Social Science Association did not question the merit of voluntarism, but they readily found fault with its existing

83 *BMJ* i (1886), 837.
84 *Hospital*, 15 Mar. 1890, 382.
85 *Charity Record & Philanthropic News* xiii (1893), 148.
86 Cited in Cherry, 'Accountability', 223.

administration. For the *Hospital* in 1894, 'it is strange that principles of common sense and business prudence as yet gained so little ground among English charitable institutions, managed and supported as they are by businessmen who would shudder at the thought of ordering their private affairs on the lines of incessant debt and difficulty'. For the *Pall Mall Gazette*, hospitals were governed

> by small knots of well-meaning old gentlemen who . . . taken as a class, are profoundly ignorant of the details of the administration over which they preside, and who do nothing except to take an occasional walk through the wards under the safe conduct of the paid officials, whom they seldom or never venture to contradict.[87]

The medical press was inclined to agree. For *The Lancet* 'the whole system of Hospital Government is as bad, as injurious, and as defective as is possible to be conceived'.[88] With doctors at best given a limited role in hospital administration, the medical press remained critical of a style of management that appeared exclusive and dominated by lay concerns. Doctors and hospital reformers were clearly prejudiced. They willingly attacked what they saw as the deficiencies of hospital management whether problems were widespread or not because this served their wider aims. Complaints were generalised and individual hospitals became the subject of violent attacks by the press. These often had dramatic financial consequences for the institution concerned as revealed by the experiences of the London Hospital when its system of nursing was attacked in 1890 and by the furore that surrounded accusations of a Protestant bias at the German Hospital. Endowed hospitals were particular targets for criticism. The closed nature of the administration at St Bartholomew's alarmed contemporaries. In 1869 *The Lancet*, in support of the doctors' calls for an ophthalmic department, felt that the governing body was a 'close[d] corporation'. However, it understood that any 'charge' would 'doubtless be opposed, because rich aldermanic governors will not be disposed to yield the opportunity of toadying wealth and social position'.[89] The medical press followed *The Lancet's* lead and counter-arguments by conservative sections of the press were ineffective. To defend itself the hospital held a public meeting presided over by the prince of Wales after his recent appointment as the hospital's president. William Foster White, the treasurer, made vague promises of improvement and the prince called for the more active involvement of the governors. Limited medical changes were made, but the hospital's administration remained unaltered.[90] Similar superficial reforms were made elsewhere when other institutions were attacked.

Governors were not the arrogant and ignorant men, bent on abusing their

---

87 *Hospital*, 7 June 1894, 303; 2 Jan. 1892, 161.
88 *Lancet* ii (1853), 252.
89 Ibid. ii (1869), 615.
90 St Bartholomew's, minutes of the board of governors, 22 Nov. 1869, SBH, Ha 1/23.

privileges, that the *Medical Times & Gazette* claimed.[91] Examples of dishonest or corrupt governors and administrators are unusual by the nineteenth century. The fraudulent activities of Thomas Coles, the treasurer at Bethlem Hospital who escaped to France in 1835 bringing to light the embezzlement of £10,000 by the receiver and accountant, was an event other voluntary hospitals worked hard to avoid.[92] Bethlem's difficulties were long-standing and seldom reflected in the management of other hospitals, which were more cautious about how their funds were managed. By the mid Victorian period London's hospitals literally could not afford such incidents. If the secretary of the Royal Hospital for Diseases of the Chest could be censured in 1889 for not acting in the best interests of the charity, there was never any question of his honesty.[93] Often the worst that governors and administrators could be accused of was of ensuring that friends and relations secured hospital posts or contracts, but even this was increasingly guarded against. The public nature of hospital governorships, appeals and meetings, the high bonds required from administrators before they took up their posts, and the move to employ independent auditors limited the opportunities for dishonesty even on a small scale.

Hospital administration was far from perfect however. At a meeting to launch the London Hospital's 1883 appeal it was reluctantly admitted that the hospital was not always run well but that the governors 'do the best they can'.[94] The *BMJ* had come to the same opinion over thirty years earlier. It believed that hospital governors managed the ordinary functions well, but their duty ended there and 'if any philanthropic individual suggests some plan for the benefit of the patients out of the ordinary course, he is put down as a visionary, and all but too often treated as a nuisance'.[95] It was assumed that governors were too preoccupied with their own concerns to be 'acquainted with the affairs of the hospital'.[96] Whereas many governors remained uninterested, a small number of men did devote a considerable amount of their time to the hospital. Under such a system, which was open to accusations of corruption, administrative continuity was assured. Issues were dealt with as they arose and there was little forethought or planning. A certain institutional inertia existed as governors were inclined to conservatism and were reluctant to offend subscribers. An interest in reform would be expressed, often to placate the Sunday Fund or the public, but governors were disinclined to commit themselves. Medical developments tended to be the

---

[91] *Medical Times & Gazette* i (1874), 210.

[92] Bethlem Hospital, minutes of the court of governors, 26 June, 4 Dec. 1835, Bethlem Royal Hospital Archives.

[93] RCH, council minute book, 29 May 1889, LMA, H33/RCH/A1/6.

[94] Cited in London Hospital, minutes of public meeting in aid of the London, 13 Apr. 1883, LH, A/10/8.

[95] *BMJ* i (1857), 302–3.

[96] *City Press*, 6 Nov. 1869.

exception, especially in teaching hospitals where governors were keen to be at the forefront of medical advance and were pressurised into adopting new procedures by their medical staff and students. Extensive programmes of reform were delayed and governors strenuously resisted external pressure and criticism: their first reaction was to defend the hospital rather than change it. Reform, however, could not be avoided. Governors kept a careful note of developments in other institutions to prevent themselves from being isolated and when reform was linked to financial considerations they were quicker to modify their opposition. The result was an administration that reacted to situations and responded in the face of change to keep the hospital running.

The governors' financial management was a constant object of attack. Given the London hospitals' permanent financial anxiety from the 1860s onwards this is not surprising. Endowed hospitals were censured for their perceived extravagance, and voluntary hospitals were criticised for their fundraising activities and insolvency. *The Lancet* felt that finance committees were ineffectual and ill-equipped to manage the hospitals' economic affairs.[97] At University College Hospital only fifteen minutes were allocated at meetings in the 1860s to discuss the accounts despite the hospital's precarious financial position.[98] The Charity Commission was appalled at St Bartholomew's accounting procedures, but it was a criticism that could be widely applied.[99] Critics believed that the governors' control of the hospitals' resources was inefficient, but they offered few alternatives other than the uniform system of accounts advocated by Henry Burdett and the Sunday Fund. It was easier to criticise the governors' financial management than question the role charity played in hospital funding.

Finance and fundraising dominated the work of the hospitals' management committees. Governors claimed complete authority over financial concerns: passing votes of thanks for all charitable contributions, negotiating loans, selling stock and land, and approving investments or mortgages. Public appeals were carefully planned and fundraising was discussed in detail. Governors controlled every aspect of the hospital's finance and no money could be spent without their approval. Doctors made suggestions for expenditure and were asked for their opinion on the advisability of certain items of expenditure, but they were rarely consulted over financial decisions. The reasons behind these decisions were not discussed and fundraising rather than expenditure aroused the most interest. The types of resources available and the reasons why new sources of funding were pursued have already been dealt with, as have the financial concerns and preferred system of funding of individual hospitals. The resulting picture is a mixed one. Some institutions like the German Hospital and the Hospital for Sick Children marshalled their resources with care, investing surplus income. Others like University College

97 *Lancet* i (1883), 794.
98 UCH, minutes of the general committee, 3 Nov. 1858, UCL, A1/2/2.
99 St Bartholomew's, Charity Commission to governors, 10 Feb. 1877, SBH, FD 7/5/2.

Hospital and Guy's had a more frivolous attitude, while the London responded as best it could to the pressures it experienced. The financial management of a hospital was rarely linked to any predetermined strategy however. Governors controlled spending, but there was no obvious favouritism in its allocation. Expenditure was not treated at a ward or even department level, and no effort was made to use the hospitals' accounts as a management tool to direct spending or to control expenditure. Instead finance was seen in the context of the institution's overall spending, a view that encouraged a preoccupation with the problems of finance and debt.

A study of the London hospitals' finances suggests that governors spent money when it was available, unless they were dealing with building, and pursued economies when it was not. Equally governors invested any surplus they had and then drew on it in times of need. Hospitals remained governed by their resources and this was the main influence on their management. Perhaps the only strategy that can be detected is the need to keep the hospital open and to match, as best as possible, income to expenditure. This created an over-riding need for more funds. Hospitals' finances were not badly managed, but they were run in a way that created a permanent anxiety for funds and resulted in periodic crises that required heroic feats of fundraising. Governors tried to administer resources as best they could, but it was not always possible to control the pressures that were exerted on the hospital. Given the nature of voluntarism, with its amateur ethic and distrust of professionalism and bureaucracy, perhaps this was the best that could be hoped for. Reform occurred gradually and governors responded to problems as they emerged. If the hospital was not a dynamic institution, it was at least flexible, adapting within the constraints of voluntarism and providing the institutional structure needed to dispense increasingly sophisticated medical relief.

Challenges within the hospital?

The transformation of the hospital into a medical institution did not alter the voluntary rationale behind its management. Hospitals remained voluntary organisations administered by a small philanthropic elite. Few suggested a comprehensive alternative to the voluntary provision of healthcare, even though more patients were treated by poor-law infirmaries. This would suggest a static model. However, though voluntarism remained the administrative rationale, philanthropists' claims to authority were challenged. A diversification of income did not affect the philanthropists' supremacy, but the rise of a medical profession which claimed authority through knowledge rather than through contributions did.

6

Striving for Influence:
Lay versus Medical Control

The voluntary ethic permeated every aspect of the London hospitals' services and management. Governors established their administrative credentials through their voluntary financial commitment, and in all but the most junior posts doctors donated their time and skills free of charge.[1] However, the medical profession's service was not as 'altruistic' as governors and the subscribing public wanted to believe or the profession's rhetoric seemed to stress. Hospitals were only part of a system of institutional posts available to medical practitioners, but whereas an appointment at a provident dispensary or prison might bring much needed income for some, a post at a London hospital conferred an elite status that frequently led to 'large and lucrative practices'.[2] One correspondent in the Medical Times & Gazette even suggested that doctors should pay anything up to £300 per annum for posts because of their commercial significance.[3] The value of working at a London hospital was recognised at a time when appointments were only gradually opened to competition and medical concerns were not initially prominent in the selection of candidates. The 1834 Select Committee on Medical Education revealed a widespread system of nepotism.[4] Hospital doctors and governors favoured relatives and their students, excluding promising candidates sometimes in favour of men who lacked skill but had connections. At St George's Hospital it was the surgeon Sir Benjamin Brodie who ' "ruled the roost" ', with his nominee always being elected. At King's College Hospital a readiness to sign the Thirty-Nine Articles was often more important than medical knowledge.[5] Gradually the system changed with the development of the hospital's teaching functions and the decline of the apprenticeship system, which removed students' link to individual members of staff. However, a

---

[1] All house officers were paid a small honorarium that reflected their junior status in the medical hierarchy. At St Bartholomew's they received £25 with senior house officers paid £80 after 1898. Comparable amounts were paid at other hospitals. More senior resident medical officers had a higher salary of between £50 and £100, a figure comparable to the estimated earnings of doctors a year after qualification: St Bartholomew's Hospital Medical School session, 1898/99, 40–1; Report on Candidates for the Medical Department, PP 1878–9 xliv. 259–305.
[2] Digby, Making a medical living, 224–49; Times, 30 Jan. 1869, 4.
[3] Medical Times & Gazette i (1864), 401.
[4] Select Committee on Medical Education, PP 1834 xiii. 98.
[5] Turner, Unorthodox reminiscences, 77.

limited number of hospital appointments, with only ten vacancies for the post of surgeon at St Bartholomew's between 1861 and 1890, ensured that competition remained intense.[6] Under these conditions it might be expected that doctors were prepared to put up with much. Struggling students and the recently qualified worked long hours in overcrowded and insanitary out-patient departments for a small honorarium and the possibility of a 'lucrative' permanent post. Thomas Wormald was like many seeking senior hospital posts in his willingness to wait twenty-three years as assistant surgeon at St Bartholomew's with no beds of his own until he was appointed surgeon. Anne Digby suggests that outside London doctors' grievances over their working conditions, their calls for remuneration, and their desires for medical 'auto-nomy' were over-ridden by the perceived benefits of being attached to a hospital.[7] However, in London the issue of medical authority became increas-ingly important.

The voluntary relationship between governors, doctors and patients should not obscure the administrative changes that were taking place. Increasingly the interests of the governors and those of the medical profes-sion diverged, creating tension within the hospitals' management. Medical practitioners in London did not mirror the more assertive class of practitioner that Mary Fissell has identified in eighteenth-century Bristol.[8] The nature of Bristol society was more conducive to an extension of medical authority. Here doctors could be part of the provincial social elite where a less marked social distinction existed between them and the hospital's governors. In Lon-don the governors' social importance and wealth clearly separated them from their medical staff who remained essentially part of the new professional mid-dle classes. The reason might also lie in Fissell's definition of authority, as she places less emphasis on the doctors' leverage on policy. When the medical profession's influence in hospital administration is considered it appears that even by the 1890s doctors working in the London hospitals remained in a subordinate position. However, as Jeanne Peterson has argued, from the mid Victorian period doctors started to enter into a managerial partnership with the hospitals' lay administrators.[9] This raises important questions about how this transition was possible when the medical profession had to compete with the governors' charitable authority.

Sociology, medical historians and professionalisation

The extension of medical authority has been seen as an aspect of the profes-sionalisation of medicine. Professionalisation has sparked a prolonged socio-

6 Peterson, *Medical profession*, 141–71, 162.
7 Digby, *Making a medical living*, 125.
8 Mary E. Fissell, *Patients, power and the poor in eighteenth-century Bristol*, Cambridge 1991.
9 Peterson, *Medical profession*, 187–8.

logical controversy over what constitutes a 'profession' and how 'professionalisation' is achieved with medicine often portrayed as the paradigm.[10] The 1950s saw moves to define professional status and a series of models were put forward that created a checklist for progress towards professionalisation. In the 1970s and 1980s a new trend emerged. Emphasis shifted from studying the development of a series of traits, towards looking at professionalisation as a mode of control and power. According to T. F. Johnson:

> not only do 'trait' approaches tend to incorporate the professionals' own definition of themselves in seemingly neutral categories, but the categories tend to be derived from the analysis of a very few professional bodies and include features of professional organisation and practice which found full expression only in Anglo-American culture at a particular time in the historical development of these professions.[11]

Johnson saw professionalisation in structural terms, treating it as an institutional means of controlling occupational activities. Other sociologists have adopted this view in what Witz describes as a neo-Weberian analysis.[12] According to these interpretations power is internalised within the profession to create a system of occupational closure. For Eliot Freidson, it is the 'special knowledge of the profession' that justifies its relation to society and degree of autonomy, with all professional groups claiming an exclusive body of knowledge.[13] He went on to argue that knowledge can be equated with power and used to gain the right to control the working environment.[14] For Rueschemeyer professions use this knowledge to strike a bargain with society in which they offer integrity and self-control in return for freedom from supervision.[15] However, their exercise of 'some degree of supervisory and policymaking authority' is restricted by the 'management's resource allocation decisions'.[16] Where does this leave the medical profession in the nineteenth century? Is it possible to fit the doctors working in the Victorian London hospitals into a model of an autonomous profession in control of its workplace?

Medicine was one of the old liberal professions, but unlike law and the

---

10 See M. S. Larson, *The rise of professionalism*, London 1978; J. Jackson (ed.), *Professions and professionalism*, Cambridge 1970; Witz, *Professions and patriarchy*.

11 Johnson, *Professions and power*, 26.

12 See Frank Parkin, *Marxism and class theory: a bourgeois critic*, London 1979; Noel Parry and José Parry, *The rise of the medical profession: a study of collective social mobility*, London 1976; Gerald Larkin, *Occupational monopoly and modern medicine*, London 1983; Witz, *Professions and patriarchy*, 41.

13 Robert Dingwall and Philip Lewis (eds), *The sociology of the professions: lawyers, doctors and others*, London 1983, 50.

14 Freidson, *Professional powers*, and *Professional dominance: the social structure of medical care*, New York 1970.

15 D. Rueschemeyer, 'Professional autonomy and the social control of expertise', in Dingwall and Lewis, *Sociology of the professions*, 41.

16 Freidson, *Professional powers*, 154.

Church it was associated with trade and remained the lesser of the three, a stepping-stone to more prestigious careers for later generations. Doctors only slowly acquired a professional status and were quickly matched by the new emergent professions such as architecture or accountancy. Although medicine was part of Britain's rising professional society, opinions differ over the extent and timing of its professionalisation.[17] Holmes sees the years 1680 to 1730 as decisive, but this ascribes an undue importance to eighteenth-century practitioners. Most other historians have turned their attention to the period after 1750. Toby Gelfand and Ivan Waddington have adopted Jewson's sociological analysis in suggesting that professionalisation was located in the move from a 'client-dominated' practice in the eighteenth century, to a 'doctor-dominated' practice in the nineteenth.[18] Digby, however, argues that an economic dimension modified the doctor–patient relationship so that 'there is an even balance between the financial standing of the patient and the clinical expertise of the doctor'.[19] Others have adopted a more defined period of professionalisation. For Holloway 1830 to 1858 was the crucial period; by contrast, Peterson places the transformation between the 1858 Medical Act and the 1886 Medical Amendment Act.[20] A more recent view is that of Irvine Loudon who argues that by 1850 'the main structure of the present medical profession had been created'.[21] If the time scales conflict, it seems certain that by the 1850s the medical profession had started to emerge as a concerted, albeit dual, professional group split between the hospital elite and an emerging class of general practitioner.

Following Foucault's *Birth of the clinic* analysis has seen the hospital as the locus for a new relationship between the doctor and the patient in which a new biomedical model of medicine emerged.[22] Foucault's approach has been portrayed as anti-medical: the hospital becomes a repressive institution through which the doctor exerts his authority. According to a Foucaultian analysis, doctors increasingly based medicine on pathological lesions that were only accessible through medical knowledge, transferring the definition of disease from the patient to the doctor, allowing the latter to dominate. A

---

[17] See Alexander M. Carr Saunders and Paul A. Wilson, *The professions*, Oxford 1933, for a classic account, and also T. Gourvish, 'The rise of the professions', in T. Gourvish and A. O'Day (eds), *Later Victorian Britain*, Basingstoke 1988, 12–25, and Harold Perkin, *The rise of professional society: England since 1880*, Princeton 1989.

[18] Toby Gelfand, 'Decline of the ordinary practitioner and the rise of the modern medical profession', in S. Staum and D. E. Larson (eds), *Doctors, patients and society: power and authority in medical care*, Ontario 1981; Waddington, *The medical profession in the industrial revolution*.

[19] Digby, *Making a medical living*, 6.

[20] S. W. F. Holloway, 'Medical education in England, 1830–1858: a sociological analysis', *History* xlix (1964), 299–324; Peterson, *Medical profession*.

[21] Loudon, *Medical care*, 3.

[22] Michel Foucault, *The birth of the clinic: an archaeology of medical perceptions*, trans. A. M. Sheridan, London 1972.

collection of essays edited by Colin Jones and Roy Porter has provided a detailed investigation of Foucault's ideas. However, while the contributors have meticulously analysed Foucault's approach and the power of medicine, discussion remains located within the hospitals' medical environment.[23] Where doctors had power over their patients, could they also use the same body of knowledge in their relationship with the governors?

Scientific medicine – scientific image

Victorian medicine was undergoing a period of change and advance, but it was not an 'age of miracles'.[24] Leeches, bleeding and amputation provided the mainstays of an unregistered medical profession in 1850, where to undergo surgery was 'sure to skirt the borders of death' and prescriptions often embraced it.[25] By the 1890s the situation had improved. Medicine had moved away from the therapeutic chaos of the mid-nineteenth century, but the public and doctors alike were still aware of its shortcomings. Although a more unified body of practitioners had emerged (partly through legislation), a number of medical innovations had created a series of paradigm shifts that left the medical profession often uncertain and divided, split between established practices and new advances.[26] Any survey of medical history reveals a pattern of clinical, surgical and theoretical advance. For Shorth the period of change 'opened shortly after Jenner's description of smallpox vaccination and drew to a close with the introduction of diphtheria antitoxin by Behring and Kitasato'.[27] In the interim, numerous bacteriological discoveries were made, though the cure for many diseases was still awaited. What contemporaries defined as 'orthodox' practitioners began to refine their therapeutic practices. They adopted the heresies of the homeopathic dosages they had once condemned and moved away from 'heroic' therapy to develop the more effective aspects of their old pharmacopoeia.[28] The introduction of anaesthetics in 1846 and the gradual adoption of antisepsis after Lister's work in 1867 changed the practice and perceptions of surgery, making it more effective, invasive and expensive for hospitals. A new approach to disease underpinned these changes and Rudolf Virchow's ideas of cellular pathology marked a final

---

23 See Colin Jones and Roy Porter (eds), *Reassessing Foucault: power, medicine and the body*, London 1994.
24 Guy R. Williams, *Age of miracles: medicine and society in the nineteenth century*, London 1981.
25 Youngson, *Scientific revolution*, 30.
26 Thomas Kuhn, *The structure of scientific revolution*, Chicago 1970, stresses the importance of paradigm shifts in the development of modern science.
27 S. E. D. Shortt, 'Physicians, science and status: issues in the professionalisation of Anglo-American medicine in the nineteenth century', *Medical History* xxvii (1983), 53.
28 Roger Cooter (ed.), *Studies in the history of alternative medicine*, Basingstoke 1988; Philip A. Nicholls, *Homeopathy and the medical profession*, London 1988.

abandonment of humoralism.[29] Illness was beginning to be understood not in terms of the patient's social situation and morality but in relation to scientific formulations based on contagion. However, medicine was also used to confirm accepted social values, especially those over gender, suggesting a less progressive side to medical advance.[30] A balanced view of Victorian medicine shows that the doctor's main function remained the alleviation of sickness; only through the encouragement medical science gave to the public health movement could he deal with its underlying causes.[31]

New practices were not employed uniformly. Even with a dramatic rise in medical expenditure the rate of change should not be exaggerated. The medical profession's innate conservatism and the London hospitals' institutional inertia hampered the adoption of new techniques. A gap remained between science and practice. Therapeutics changed less dramatically than clinical theory so that customary practices still remained important by the start of the twentieth century. Different institutions reacted differently to change. Whereas the old operating theatre at Guy's, which had served the hospital since 1726, was only replaced in 1867, the governors of the German Hospital were keen to be in the forefront of clinical advance. The same enthusiasm for progress was shown at the London, where a clinical laboratory was opened in 1896 and the tetanus antitoxin was in widespread use in 1894 before its clinical value had been proven.[32] New techniques, however, often had a difficult reception and general hospitals were slow to establish specialist departments. Anaesthetics, antiseptic methods and the use of tracheotomies in the treatment of diphtheria, for example, were not immediately embraced and many small operations by the start of the twentieth century were still conducted without an anaesthetic. At St Bartholomew's in the 1880s a mixed antiseptic–aseptic regime existed side by side with antipathetic attitudes towards antiseptic methods.[33] At other hospitals a similar dichotomy in medical practices could be found with a generational split between old and new staff. Hospital funding created further problems. With no control over

---

[29] See David Hamilton, 'The nineteenth-century surgical revolution: antisepsis or better nutrition?', *BHM* lvi (1982), 30–40, who counters the view that antisepsis was as beneficial as many believe.

[30] See Barbara Harrison, 'Women and health', in June Purvis (ed.), *Women's history: Britain, 1850–1945*, London 1995, 157–92; V. Bullough and M. Vogt, 'Women, menstruation and nineteenth-century medicine', *BHM* viii (1973), 66–82; K. Figlio, 'Chlorasis and chronic disease in nineteenth-century Britain: the social construction of somatic illness in a capitalist society', *Social History* iii (1978), 167–97.

[31] John M. Eyler, *Victorian social medicine: the ideas and methods of William Farr*, Baltimore 1979, 198; Wohl, *Endangered lives*.

[32] Guy's Hospital, minutes of the court of committees, LMA, H9/Gy/A3/9; London Hospital, minutes of the house committee, 7 Jan. 1895, 20 July 1896, LH, A/5/46.

[33] A. Winter, 'Mesmerism and the introduction of inhalation anaesthesia', *SHM* iv (1991), 1–27; Hardy, 'Tracheotomy versus intubation', 536–59; Lindsay Granshaw, ' "Upon this principle I have based a practice": the development of antisepsis in Britain', in Pickstone, *Medical innovation*, 17–46; Pennington, 'Listerism, its decline and its persistence', 50–2.

finance doctors were in a weak position when it came to suggesting a rise in medical expenditure. Money was not always forthcoming for doctors to establish the services they wanted or buy the equipment they felt they needed. Henry Lucas, chairman of University College Hospital's management committee, noted that governors and staff tried to 'conform to the wishes of the other', but financial circumstances often caused problems. Medical progress and finance were not always reconcilable.

Medicine was seen by many contemporaries as a menial and subservient activity, but increasingly medical progress gave doctors a vocabulary that stressed the scientific value of medicine. Although there were dissenting voices, large sections of the medical profession explicitly linked progress in science with advances in medicine.[34] If few patients judged practitioners on their scientific knowledge, the rhetoric of science did become an important part of doctors' claim to authority, lending 'support to medicine's assertion that physiology and pathology were subjects increasingly beyond the laymen's comprehension'. Science was the Victorian 'intellectual ratifier of a new world order', a new middle-class ethic that gave social legitimacy to the emergent medical profession. It also carried 'strong messages about the hierarchical organisation of medicine', separating it from empiricism and defining what could be seen as 'legitimate' knowledge.[35] According to Digby, the credibility of the medical profession was 'enhanced by the scientific successes of laboratory medicine and the achievements of hospital surgery'.[36] However, many practitioners gave science a limited role in clinical practice, preferring to retain an emphasis on the value of character.[37] Important differences therefore existed between the profession's public rhetoric and clinical practice that were not always apparent to a lay audience. How hospital governors interpreted these changes is uncertain. Shorth argues that the rhetoric of science was used by doctors 'to gain autonomy from lay control within the hospital system', but where rhetoric stressed the authoritative role of knowledge, most governors were not easily convinced that this necessitated doctors playing an extensive role in hospital management.[38]

[34] See Bynum, *Science and the practice of medicine*, for a wider discussion.

[35] Shortt, 'Physicians, science, and status', 67–8, 61. See also Mark Weatherall, 'Making medicine scientific', *SHM* ix (1996), 175–94, while Colin A. Russell, *Science and social change, 1770–1900*, London 1983, discusses science's impact on popular culture.

[36] Digby, *Making a medical living*, 100.

[37] Lawrence, ' "Incommunicable knowledge" ', 503–20, while the disparity between science and practice is illustrated by John H. Warner, 'Therapeutic explanation and the Edinburgh bloodletting controversy: two perspectives on the medical meaning of science in the mid nineteenth century', *Medical History* xxiv (1980), 241–58.

[38] Shortt, 'Physicians, science, and status', 63.

Contemporaries and medical authority

Antivivisectionists and the Humanitarian League warned about the possibility of medical autocracy; others argued that doctors should devote all their time to the treatment of the sick.[39] Only a few stressed the need for increased medical involvement in hospital management. Doctors and the medical press naturally stood in the vanguard of these demands, working on the belief that hospitals 'determine for the main part the character of the profession'.[40] It was therefore important to extend authority in the very institutions that both educated new entrants and provided the basis for clinical expertise and professional standing.

Thomas Wakley, founder of the radical *Lancet*, complained constantly about the general absence of medical representation and the 'most extraordinary share in direction of merely medical details' governors held without medical knowledge.[41] As late as 1897 *The Lancet* noted that 'the services rendered by hospital physicians and surgeons in their professional capacity surely entitle them to seats on the board of management'.[42] *The Lancet's* opinions helped stir professional grievances and persuade other professional groups and journals to take up the call for representation, though the conservative Royal College of Physicians and Royal College of Surgeons remained half-hearted. In 1881 the metropolitan counties branch of the BMA passed a resolution that 'the necessary arrangements as regards treatment should be under the control of the medical staff'. The *BMJ* added its support and though it remained worried that hospitals robbed general practitioners of business, it regularly campaigned for the medical profession to have 'a large share in the management of hospitals'.[43] The *Medical Times & Gazette* equally felt that a medical officer should be in charge of the hospitals' day-to-day administration on the grounds that his medical knowledge made him a more capable official than any governor.[44] Each journal had its programme for reform, but all shared a common belief that doctors' professional body of knowledge gave them the right to be actively involved. Doctors working in the London hospitals existed in a professional climate that espoused medical representation, legitimised their demands and made representation a professional grievance.

Individual doctors expressed their sympathy for medical representation, but few were as public in their support as Charles West, founder and senior physician of the Hospital for Sick Children. In 1877 West published *On hos-*

---

[39] French, *Antivivisection*, 349–72; David Weinbren, 'Against all cruelty: the Humanitarian League, 1891–1919', *History Workshop* xxxviii (1994), 98–100.
[40] *Royal Commission on the Medical Acts*, PP 1882 xix. 20.
[41] *Lancet* ii (1856), 203.
[42] Ibid. i (1897), 1289.
[43] *BMJ* i (1881), 312; i (1882), 313.
[44] *Medical Times & Gazette* i (1879), 148–9.

pital organisation, which outlined his ideas on hospital management.[45] The book was written in response to his disagreements with the governors of the Hospital for Sick Children and consequently focused on the administration of children's hospitals. West was not easy to work with. Fifteen years before he had resigned his teaching posts at St Bartholomew's claiming overwork. His resignation concealed arguments the year before over changes in the hospital's midwifery arrangements. At the time he had felt that his professional standing had been compromised and that he had been 'forbidden to exercise my own judgement in the management of cases submitted to my care'.[46] West was always worried about the extent and nature of his authority; concerns that underlay his difficulties at St Bartholomew's and the Hospital for Sick Children. In 1876 arguments arose at the Hospital for Sick Children between the obstinate West and the governors over the extent of medical influence and the role of religion in the hospital. The difference led to West's resignation.[47] *On hospital organisation* was a polemic, but it encapsulated many of the medical profession's concerns over their role in hospital management. The book focused on a careful plan for the administration of children's hospitals, but the first fifteen pages outlined West's ideas on medical representation. Basing his ideas on the problems he had experienced at the Hospital for Sick Children, he asserted that harmony was the source of efficiency. To achieve this West felt the administration had to be divided between a medical committee and the governors. Medical representatives would be limited to doctors holding honorary posts to prevent the governors from being outnumbered, but even in the discussion of non-medical issues West was clear that the medical staff should be represented on the basis of their scientific knowledge.[48] The *Medical Examiner* believed that these ideas would create a 'stir in the professional world', but they received a favourable reception because they mirrored professional concerns.[49]

Calls for medical representation, however, also came from outside the medical profession. Dr George Lichtenberg, surgeon to the German Hospital, argued in 1891 that many of the German Hospital's subscribers supported medical representation, and one writer to *The Times* was clear in 1878 that the public were already withholding their subscriptions until doctors were given a greater role in hospital management.[50] Lichtenberg was campaigning for medical representation at the German Hospital, while the assessment in *The Times* was farfetched. Both, however, pointed to a non-medical interest

45 Charles West, *On hospital organisation, with special reference to the organisation of hospitals for children*, London 1877.
46 St Bartholomew's, minutes of the medical officers and lecturers, 24 Mar. 1860, 20 July 1861, SBH, MS 12/1.
47 Hospital for Sick Children, minutes of the committee of management, 9 Feb. 1876, GOSH, 1/2/14; *Pall Mall Gazette*, 6 June 1877.
48 West, *On hospital organisation*, 7–15.
49 *Medical Examiner*, 21 June 1877.
50 *Charity Record & Philanthropic News* xi (1891), 60; *Times*, 23 Jan. 1878, 11.

in medical representation, reflecting society's increasing acceptance of professional service. Without such support doctors' claims would have appeared
less acceptable. Many non-medical journals, albeit reluctantly, came out in
support of the idea. One anonymous writer in the *Quarterly Review* in 1893
argued that 'hospitals exist for patients, and who but the doctor can say what
the patient requires?'[51] If the author's enthusiasm rivalled that of the medical
profession, other contemporaries were more qualified in their support. The
Hospital adopted a moderate stance. It called for the establishment of medical
committees to represent doctors' interests, an opinion that reflected many
governors' attitudes.[52] At a conference on hospital administration in 1883,
speakers expressed their muted favour for the system adopted at St Thomas's
where the medical staff had a representative on the house committee.[53]
Others put forward more systematic plans as part of a general reform of London's hospitals. Frederick Mouat was a key figure in these discussions. A close
associate of Henry Saxon Snell, leading hospital architect and a pioneer
member of the Sanitary Institute, Mouat had been involved in the development of a medical school in India. On his return from India he had joined the
Local Government Board where he had become interested in hospital design
and the need to organise London's hospital services. As part of a detailed plan
to reorganise the structure of metropolitan healthcare rushed out for the
1883 Social Science Association conference on hospitals, Mouat suggested
that all hospital committees should have a medical element. He argued that
medical superintendents should run hospitals on a daily basis and that doctors unconnected with the institution should be on its management because
of their unbiased 'technical and special knowledge'.[54] Mouat's calls for a state
service were widely criticised as an affront to hospitals' voluntary tradition,
but the medical press was heartened by his recommendations for more medical influence.

The medical and lay discussion of hospital management agreed that
increased medical representation was desirable. Doctors, however, were
excluded from one area of management. The *Hospital* warned that 'were it
not that the financial necessities render lay co-operation indispensable' doctors would want full control.[55] In the demands for increased medical representation no attempt was made to encroach on the governors' financial
control. Doctors, in asserting their professional knowledge, recognised that
hospital finance was the governors' own professional sphere. No indication is
given of whether this was a recognition of the hospitals' continued reliance

---

[51] Anon., 'The modern hospital', *Quarterly Review* clxxvii (1893), 471.
[52] *Hospital*, 1 Mar. 1890, 350.
[53] Clifford Smith, *Hospital management*, 10–21.
[54] Frederick Mouat and Henry Saxon Snell, *Hospital construction and management*, London
1883, 10–11.
[55] *Hospital*, 1 Mar. 1890, 350.

on voluntarism, but it does support a view that separate spheres existed in hospital management that were respected in the hospitals' internal politics.

Medical influence and conflict

A survey conducted by *The Lancet* in 1874 revealed that fifteen of the twenty-two hospitals in London with over fifty beds had a doctor in their management.[56] However, a distinction must be made between hospital types, and between formal and informal authority.

Endowed hospitals had a conservative approach to their administration. There, according to the *BMJ*, the medical staff had 'no voice in the management' and were 'under the absolute control of a set of men who . . . are entirely without knowledge of hospital affairs',[57] and who were reluctant to allow their doctors any administrative role. The situation was not the result of the nature of their funding, which in theory should have freed the governors from subscriber pressure to administer the hospital on philanthropic lines. It was a product of the age of these institutions. The endowed hospitals were dominated by their history and tradition, factors that encouraged institutional inertia and hostility to change. At Guy's, as noted below, the position did change in 1880, but at St Bartholomew's the doctors remained excluded from a formal managerial position. It was not until 1843 that a medical committee was established and even moderate suggestions for a joint subcommittee on medical appointments in 1887 proved unacceptable.[58] Superficially the hospital's rules offered the medical staff the chance to stand as governors, but this was not matched with the possibility of being included on any of the managing committees. *The Lancet* criticised the medical staff for their timidity and doctors working at St Bartholomew's felt oppressed by the system.[59] Only in 1904 were medical representatives appointed on the governing body largely on the initiative of Sir Anthony Bowlby after friction over the need to rebuild the hospital had forced a compromise.[60]

Doctors in the newer voluntary hospitals were in a better situation. From 1863 the medical staff at University College Hospital were allowed to send three representatives to the management committee. These representatives were not given voting rights, but from the 1860s onwards the medical staff were increasingly invited to discuss any measures that affected the hospital's medical administration. Similar arrangements existed at St Mary's and the

---

56 *Lancet* i (1874), 420.
57 *BMJ* i (1887), 70.
58 St Bartholomew's, minutes of the board of governors, 24 Jan. 1887, SBH, Ha 1/26.
59 *Lancet* ii (1869), 643.
60 Bowlby to Sir Trevor Lawrence, Contemporary Medical Archive Centre, Wellcome Institute, GC/181/B.4.

Great Northern Hospital.[61] A distinction clearly existed between the endowed hospitals and the eighteenth- and early nineteenth-century hospitals.

Specialist hospitals were in a different position. The BMJ felt that in them doctors exercised a 'quasi-private and semi-autocratic government' where they were both 'practical ruler and official superintendent'.[62] Specialist hospitals did have a high degree of medical involvement in their administration, but the BMJ's assessment was an exaggeration. When the Hospital for Sick Children opened in 1852 the extent of formal medical influence was at first limited and it required a series of changes in 1854, 1877 and 1894 to extend the medical staff's formal participation. From 1855 West and his colleagues were represented in their own medical committee, while the three senior doctors had positions on the management committee. By 1877 medical representatives sat on the drug, management, house and building committees. In 1894, to solve the problem of jurisdiction over appointments, a joint committee was established.[63] Doctors at the Royal Hospital for Diseases of the Chest had to wait until 1867 before a medical council was appointed, but unlike the Hospital for Sick Children a doctor had always sat on the main committee. By the 1880s the hospital's administration was effectively split between the medical council and the management committee and the medical staff were represented at every level of the administration. The need for medical representation was confirmed by the hospitals' specialist nature which made the business experience that gave governors the right to control general hospitals a poor substitute for medical knowledge. Institutionally, specialist hospitals required a greater degree of medical participation. The governors' position was also initially tempered by the fact that the founding inspiration for many of these institutions was invariably a medical one.[64] In specialist hospitals, governors were often in no position to argue, except over expenditure.

The absence of a formal managerial position did not preclude all medical influence. Doctors exercised a certain autonomy over their own working environment, controlling the allocation of beds and the standard of medical education within the parameters laid down by the General Medical Council and the licensing bodies. They also had an informal influence on the hospitals' administration through advice and recommendations that produced a constant flow of information between the hospitals' medical and nonmedical departments. Bruce Clarke, assistant surgeon at St Bartholomew's and actively involved in the management of the medical school there, told the Select Committee on Metropolitan Hospitals that in most hospitals doc-

[61] UCH, minutes of the general committee, 28 Mar. 1863, UCL, A1/2/2; SC on Metropolitan Hospitals, First Report, q. 2138–9.

[62] BMJ ii (1877), 654.

[63] Hospital for Sick Children, minutes of the medical committee, 28 Feb. 1877, GOSH, 1/5/7; minutes of the joint committee, GOSH, 1/7/1.

[64] Granshaw,' "Fame and fortune by means of bricks and mortar" ', 199–200.

tors were often heeded, but not officially.[65] Influence at an informal level, with a voluntary inclusion of the medical staff by the governors in the decision-making process, could be considerable. At the German Hospital this was certainly the case. The governors here opposed the formal inclusion of doctors in the administration, believing that the existing system worked well.[66] Organised into a medical committee (which met erratically in the 1870s and 1880s) the doctors communicated their ideas to the governors through personal representation and letters to shape the hospital's development. In turn, the governors consulted them on matters from the admission of syphilitic patients to the supply of gas.[67] A similar situation existed at other hospitals. At St Bartholomew's and Guy's the medical staff had to rely on their informal authority to exert any influence. Doctors at St Bartholomew's communicated directly with the treasurer and at Guy's their views were interpreted by the medical superintendent, or through direct communication with the treasurer. Until the foundation of a joint management committee for the medical school in 1876, the doctors at the London were in a similar position.[68] Between 1836 and 1867 they used the physicians and surgeons' report book to bring matters to the governors' attention, followed by a system of letters.[69] This suggests a clear distinction between the medical and lay administration. In formal terms, the medical staff had no power over their working environment. All decisions had to be ratified by the governors, but in all matters relating to the London's medical administration the doctors were consulted, though their views were not always accepted. Grievances were discussed on a face-to-face basis. The governors reprimanded any member of staff who did not meet their idea of adequate attendance, but when one surgeon complained in 1853 about the problems cancer patients faced in being admitted, he was given a special dispensation to admit such patients. The decision required a further change in the London's admissions procedure that left the medical staff in a stronger position. This did not mean that the governors were not prepared to refuse petitions from the medical staff without discussion. When a request was made for an ophthalmic ward in 1860 the doctors were firmly told that the London had enough problems allocating beds for accident cases and that such a ward was out of the question.[70] The governors' strident attitude had softened by the mid 1860s onwards. They became more willing to accede to the doctors' requests if a suitable case were made and money were available. Control rested with the governors, but at

65 SC on Metropolitan Hospitals, First Report, 134.

66 BMJ i (1890), 375.

67 German Hospital, minutes of the medical committee, SBH, GHM 1/1; minutes of the hospital committee, SBH, GHA 2/1–10.

68 London Hospital, minutes of the medical council, 10 Apr. 1876, LH, Mc/A/1/3.

69 London Hospital, physicians and surgeons' report book, 1836–67, LH, A/17/7.

70 London Hospital, minutes of the house committee, 13 Dec. 1853, LH, A/5/27; 27 Nov. 1860, LH, A/5/30.

the London and at other metropolitan hospitals the administrative structure concealed a flow of information and influence from the doctors.

Medical authority was at its height both at an informal and at a formal level when a decision needed a medical opinion. Governors, ill-equipped to make an effective judgement on medically related issues, were forced to consult their medical staff. According to Roy Macleod a similar situation existed in parliament where the technical ignorance of the Commons on scientific issues required an increasing level of expert opinion. For Macleod this strengthened the expert's influence.[71] In London's hospitals such issues were intimately connected to the nature of the institution. At the Hospital for Sick Children in 1895 the medical committee was asked to investigate the duties of the registrar and house surgeon, consider the nursing arrangements, appoint two clinical assistants and provide the London School Board with medical certificates for children under the hospital's care.[72] Not all doctors were consulted to this extent, but even at St Bartholomew's the hospital's effective administration often required a medical opinion and Sydney Waterlow as treasurer admitted in 1890 that the governors were 'guided, and I think I may say they are always anxious to be guided, by what they can learn through me is the view of the medical council'.[73] When the general committee at University College Hospital wanted to establish special skin and urinary wards for clinical teaching in 1859, they sought the medical committee's advice.[74] Doctors were prepared to use their professional knowledge under these situations. When a matter was presented to them that they disagreed with they retreated behind the claim that a change could not be supported without 'due regard to the welfare of the patient[s]'.[75] The justification for action or inactivity based on medical knowledge was sometimes hard to separate from the doctors' professional interests.

Doctors in the London hospitals increasingly seemed dissatisfied with this level of informal influence. Peterson suggests that there was a transformation in the 'relations of governors and medical men' where the lay administrators accepted the doctors' 'right to power based on their special knowledge'.[76] Change was rarely inevitable or followed a smooth course however. Hilary Marland in her study of medical charity in Wakefield and Huddersfield feels that 'although the lay officers do seem to have been the dominant force in decision-making, the two groups co-operated well at committee and general meetings, presenting a uniform front on such important issues as admission policies, organisation and funding'. For her the absence of conflict typifies

---

[71] Roy MacLeod, 'Introduction', in Roy MacLeod (ed.), *Government and expertise: specialists, administrators and professions, 1860–1919*, Cambridge 1988, 13.
[72] Hospital for Sick Children, medical committee papers, 6 Mar., 9 Jan. 1895, GOSH, 1/5/52.
[73] *SC on Metropolitan Hospitals, First Report*, 162.
[74] UCH, minutes of the medical committee, 19 May 1859, UCL, UNOF/2/3 (i).
[75] London Hospital, minutes of the medical council, 22 June 1870, LH, Mc/A/1/2.
[76] Peterson, *Medical profession*, 187.

the relationship between lay and medical officers, a view shared by Brian Abel-Smith.[77] More realistically Morris has identified the hospital as an arena of conflict.[78] Hospitals offered manifold opportunities for tension as the hospitals' philanthropic nature increasingly jarred with its new medical functions. The medical profession's steady rise in 'power and influence and respect', noted by William Gladstone in 1890, seemed to obscure the friction that periodically developed.[79] Other observers were not so sanguine and readily identified conflict as part of the reason for the hospitals' financial problems.[80] Scandals adversely affected hospital income, but conflict had a more marked impact on internal management, becoming the main vehicle through which doctors increased their formal institutional authority. Where tension did not erupt into an open dispute, the medical staff's influence often remained stunted, as at St Bartholomew's.

The fault did not always rest with the governors. *Guy's Hospital Gazette* admitted that 'it is, no doubt, often difficult for laymen to appreciate the aims and needs of the medical workers'. Such statements did little to reduce tension with doctors not always sympathetic to other concerns. They could be obstinate, inflexible and arrogant, considering 'their work as a matter of highest importance to the hospital, and in its nature not to be understood by the committee, and, therefore, not to be found fault with'.[81] At the German Hospital, Dr Ludwig Edward Straube was summarily dismissed in 1854. When pressed over the reason, the governors reluctantly explained that during Straube's time as surgeon he had been 'guilty of immoral and disgraceful conduct'. On one occasion it was believed that he had acted improperly towards 'the chastity of Mrs Geuderer' whilst 'visiting her as a Medical Man' at a time when her husband was 'lying' in a dying state, 'if not already dead' in the hospital. Straube, however, believed he had been the subject of 'machinations against me'. He accused the governors of lacking 'all common sense and fairness' and asserted that he had merely been examining Geuderer.[82] *The Lancet* introduced a cautionary note in 1859, explaining that lay governors might not always grasp the importance of medical science, 'but then the modesty that befits science . . . suggests that we may not always be right'.[83] It was a view that was not always heeded. Doctors disliked any external interference and resisted attempts to impose new routines on them. Even the governors' practice of visiting wards, which they saw as an important part of their philanthropic responsibility, aroused opposition because it was seen as disruptive.

77 Marland, *Medicine and society*, 330–1; Abel-Smith, *The hospitals*, 32–45.
78 Roger J. Morris, 'Organisation and aims of the principal secular voluntary organisations of the Leeds middle class, 1830–51', unpubl. DPhil. diss. Oxford 1970, 182.
79 *Charity*, Apr. 1890, 274.
80 Ibid. Nov. 1887, 151.
81 *Hospital*, 1 Nov. 1890, 72; 15 Mar. 1890, 381.
82 German Hospital, minutes of the hospital committee, 29 Dec. 1853, 28 Feb. 1854, SBH, GHA 2/2.
83 *Lancet* i (1859), 634.

'Visiting' was a means to ensure that the hospital environment was regulated and that complaints were investigated, but for the medical staff it suggested that they were being monitored.[84]

Conflict between governors and doctors took many forms, erupting at different points in an institution's history when the medical staff felt their collective interests threatened. From the 1850s onwards doctors increasingly intervened in the admissions process, extending their influence from the casualty departments and internal allocation of beds. Governors seemed willing to let the letter system fall into decline and were aware that 'it would be a dangerous thing for a lay person to say that a case should be rejected which the doctor said should come in'.[85] Problems, however, were encountered over the discharge of patients because governors sought to keep the number of cases high to attract charitable contributions. Whereas the *Hospital* recognised that only a medical practitioner was 'practically competent to say when discharge is safe and right', many governors attempted to impose restrictions on the time patients spent in hospital.[86] One writer in the *Contemporary Review* believed that it was difficult for any doctor to extend a patient's stay beyond three months.[87] This was not always the case and here medical interests clashed with financial concerns. At the London the medical staff had control over the renewal of admission rights, but in 1859 the governors complained that this created an intolerable pressure on the hospital's resources. In response the doctors argued that only through full control could proper treatment be provided.[88] When doctors asserted their professional knowledge over a patient governors often reluctantly agreed to extend treatment. However, they ensured that all extensions still had to have their approval, creating tension with the medical staff who believed that all aspects of patient care should be under their authority. Conflict was shaped by the medical profession's evolving sense of identity and its changing concerns, emerging in areas where medical authority was questioned, or an existing role in administration seemed threatened.

Most hospitals in London had a troubled evolution. The history of the Royal Hospital for Diseases of the Chest was particularly punctuated by friction between its lay administrators and medical staff. In 1867 three doctors resigned claiming an autocratic system of management after one of their colleagues was accused of advertising quack medicines; in 1883 the governors faced a further challenge to their authority. Concerned about attendance, they had attempted to enforce the doctors' visiting times after it was revealed

---

[84] W. B. Howie, 'Complaints and complaints procedures in the eighteenth- and early nineteenth-century provincial hospitals in England', *Medical History* xxv (1981), 345–62.

[85] *SC on Metropolitan Hospitals, First Report*, 521.

[86] *Hospital*, 23 Apr. 1887, 61.

[87] R. Brundell Carter, 'The London medical schools', *Contemporary Review* xxxiv (1878/9), 591.

[88] London Hospital, minutes of the house committee, 4 Jan. 1859, LH, A/5/30.

that Dr Thomas Gilbart Smith and Dr William Murrell had failed to provide locums when they were absent. This was combined with new regulations over prescriptions after accusations had been made that one of the doctors was experimenting on the patients. The medical staff immediately went on the defensive. The flamboyant Gilbart Smith was particularly disgusted that accusations had been made against him, although his recent appointment to the staff of the London Hospital must have taken him away from his duties at the Royal Hospital for Diseases of the Chest. The doctors claimed an 'uncalled interference with those whose practice and experience should qualify them to be the best judges of what is proper in medical treatment', but admitted the need for a voluntary enforcement of more rigorous attendance.[89] They explained that any limitation of prescriptions could only damage the patients and that the proposal would create divisions between in-patient and out-patient care that would 'be twisted to the injury of the Hospital'. The doctors also rather weakly threatened to withdraw from the running of the hospital. The crisis was only resolved with a compromise that left both sides professing victory. The governors acknowledged some of the doctors' grievances and attempted to meet them, while the doctors' attendance improved. Increasingly the governors seemed willing to consult their medical staff and in the discussion over the hospital's new rules throughout 1885 many of the doctors' suggestions were adopted. Medical representatives were appointed *ex-officio* members of the hospital's committees when the new rules were enforced in March 1886 and all appointments were referred to the medical council.[90]

The doctors' stubbornness placed them in a favourable position when a new crisis developed in 1889. Disagreements had emerged between John Austin, the secretary, and the medical staff. Austin explained that since his appointment he had watched 'carefully the increasing tendency to make the Institution less a Hospital for Consumption, for the treatment of poor patients recommended by Subscribers, than a school for the education of Doctors'. He had reason to be suspicious. The hospital had a strong educational link with St Bartholomew's where Philip Hensley, the senior physician, lectured in forensic medicine and James Calvert was a demonstrator, while David Finlay taught forensic medicine and public health at the Middlesex. Whether they used the Royal Chest for their teaching is uncertain however. Austin went on to make other accusations. He claimed that the doctors had refused to admit in-patients recommended by subscribers in favour of ' "emergency cases" '. Here the doctors' clinical judgement was called into question, especially as Austin argued that few of these patients would be discharged alive. Examples of experimentation were cited with Austin claiming that one 'poor child' had only been admitted to give the

89 *Lancet* ii (1867), 400–1; RCH, minutes of the medical council, 28 Dec. 1883, LMA, H33/RCH/A3/1.
90 Ibid. 19 Feb., 10 Mar. 1884, 1 Mar. 1886, LMA, H33/RCH/A3/1.

house physician the 'opportunity of performing his first tracheotomy operation'. Other experiments were alluded to and the death of a patient was used
as evidence of malpractice. After reminding the governors that he was in
regular contact with the local clergy and employers, Austin threatened that if
'the impression got abroad that the Hospital existed for the Doctors rather
than the Patients' it would be damaging.[91]

The medical staff realised the seriousness of the accusations and argued
that they reflected 'in the gravest manner upon [their] professional conduct'.
More importantly the doctors suggested that the allegations alone would
compromise the hospital unless an immediate investigation was made. To
press home their point they resigned. In response the governors called an
emergency meeting. Austin tried to moderate his earlier statements but
Hensley and Finlay, as the medical council's representatives, took a firm line.
As a member of the governing body Hensley explained that if Austin's statements were not 'discountenanced' the medical staff would be placed in an
intolerable position. Hensley called for an expression of confidence aware
that by discussing the issue at a council meeting it would be brought to the
attention of the public and of subscribers. The situation must have been serious for the mathematically-minded Hensley to speak out so firmly as a speech
defect made him shy and contemptuous of publicity. When the treasurer, the
banker Pascoe Glyn, tried to steer a middle course by suggesting that the
number of emergency cases might be reduced, Hensley pressed the threat of
resignation. The governors, already facing an unruly audience at the emergency meeting, were aware that they could only be damaged by such allegations and the mass resignation of their medical staff. Faced with losing the
secretary or all ten of their doctors, they sided with the doctors. They
expressed full 'confidence' in them, accused the secretary of being ignorant,
and reaffirmed their faith in the skill and clinical judgement of the medical
staff. This did not, however, stop them from appointing a committee to look
into the alleged incidences of experimentation to appease the public. It was
Austin not the doctors who was accused of jeopardising the hospital and he
was asked to resign. Austin, with little support outside the hospital, reluctantly agreed, though he remained adamant that it was the doctors who were
at fault.[92] Hensley's position on the council had forced the issue, moving it
from discussion in a subcommittee to debate in a more public forum.

Conflicts at the Royal Hospital for Diseases of the Chest and at other hospitals, though embarrassing for the governors, generally remained essentially
internal disputes. This was not always the case. Although the nursing dispute
at Guy's, which lasted from December 1879 to September 1880, was not
atypical in some respects being mirrored by a similar conflict at the General

---

[91] RCH, council minute book, 27 June 1889, LMA, H33/RCH/A1/7.
[92] Ibid. 8 July 1889, LMA, H33/RCH/A1/7; *Hospital*, 12 Oct. 1889, 31.

Lying-in Hospital, it did have a striking impact on the public.[93] It exemplifies the process by which the medical profession was able to assume a greater role in hospital management.

Medical influence and conflict:
Guy's and the nursing dispute, 1879–80

When Guy's launched its first public appeal in 1886, Frederick William Pavy testified as one the senior physicians 'that the greatest unanimity now existed between the medical and nursing staff . . . [and] that at the present time the nursing staff was everything that could be desired'. Ironically, seven years earlier the system of nursing had incited a virtual state of 'civil war'.[94] Most historians have seen the dispute as a chapter in the history of nursing, not part of the history of the medical profession.[95] Peterson, however, shares the Victorian interpretation: the dispute was more than just a typical struggle between doctors and nurses. She argues that the 'fundamental issue was the authority of the medical officers', but for her this only emerged from the 'summer of 1880'.[96] Her analysis hides the fact that from the start the main issue was not nursing, but the question of authority within the hospital and the role of the medical profession in hospital administration.

The dispute erupted over the appointment of Margaret Burt as matron by Edmund Lushington in December 1879 after the old matron had retired after thirty-four years of service. Lushington had spent twenty-seven years in the Bengal civil service and had been secretary to the finance department there before he was appointed treasurer at Guy's in 1876. Though not a stranger to the hospital given that his father had been a highly active governor between 1819 and 1873, his time in Bengal led some to treat him as an outsider and interloper. The liberal, high-minded Lushington had a difficult reputation to live up to.[97] A laborious speaker, he had a civil service mentality that overlay an anxious concern to improve the patients' material conditions. From the start he had absorbed himself in the hospital's management in an attempt to instil 'the principles of good management and economy' that he felt were absent at Guy's. He worked with tact and an apparent sympathy for the doctors' interests who in return co-operated. After three years of intense activity Lushington turned his attention to the deplorable system of nursing. Intermittent reforms had been attempted before 1879 and had been partly motivated by the medical staff's desire to promote more efficient patient care.

93 For the dispute at the General Lying-in Hospital see minutes of the committee of inquiry, 1880, LMA, H1/GLI/A29/1–21, and weekly board minutes, LMA, H1/GLI/A2/5.
94 *Lancet* ii (1880), 507–8.
95 Moore, *Zeal for responsibility*, 53–97.
96 Peterson, *Medical profession*, 180.
97 Cameron, *Mr Guy's Hospital*, 231; Moore, *Zeal for responsibility*, 54.

However, they had not proved effective. Reliable trained women were difficult to find and progress was hampered by the governors' fitful approach to management. Lushington believed that the basic problem stemmed from the lack of a 'competent female in authority'. In Burt, a trainee of St John's House, he hoped to find this 'competent female'. St John's House was committed to promoting training and improving working conditions for nurses. It was in the vanguard of nursing reform and in 1872 alone had turned down requests from eleven hospitals to take over their nursing. Burt herself had nine years' experience, including a successful spell as the reforming lady-superintendent at the Leicester Infirmary.[98] Lushington was not disappointed. Burt had clear views about the existing nurses: she saw them as untrained, prone to drunkenness and spending their free evenings in pubs and music halls, and failing in their duty to keep patients clean and cared for. To combat this, working conditions were improved, staff dismissed and efforts made to create a unified body centralised under Burt's authority. Other reforms sought to 'secure a thorough training of probationers of whatever social rank, to diminish the menial work of the trained nurses, which had been a serious hindrance to their proper duties in former times'.[99]

Lushington's enthusiasm was not shared by the medical staff, who were prejudiced against the new matron. They saw her as a threat, a view based not on personal acquaintance since only eight of the twenty doctors met her during the dispute, but on her training and work at Leicester.[100] Their antagonism was symptomatic of the medical profession's hostility to nursing reform. Whether new nursing arrangements were instituted by trainees from the Nightingale School or by nursing sisterhoods, doctors generally put up a spirited defence. At the centre of many of these disputes were the nursing sisterhoods, and in particular St John's House.[101]

Doctors were not 'unsympathetic to attempts to improve the practical skills of lower-class nurses so they could administer treatments or monitor the patients' condition more effectively'. Nursing reform and the introduction of trained nurses, often with an independent income and a higher social status than the medical staff, raised different issues however. Doubts were expressed about whether the 'ladies' who wanted to become trained nurses would be suitable; it was hinted that they only had an interest out of morbid curiosity, a desire 'to kill *ennui*' or religious conviction. For the BMJ none of these sentiments was 'likely to result in producing good *staying* workers'. Against a background of opposition to the medical education of women, anxiety also existed

---

[98] Guy's Hospital, memorandum by Lushington, Mar. 1880, LMA, H9/Gy/A224/1–2; Helmstadter, 'Origins of the modern trained nurse', 299–301; BMJ ii (1879), 1045.
[99] Guy's Hospital, minutes of the general court, 29 Sept. 1880, LMA, H9/Gy/A1/3.
[100] Guy's Hospital, 'list of the medical and surgical staff who have not spoken to Burt', June–July 1880, LMA, H9/Gy/A230/1.
[101] Moore, *Zeal for responsibility*, 1–39, 101–69.

that some 'ladies' were using nursing reform as a way to enter medicine.[102] However, the main issue was one of authority. Under the old system nurses were accountable to the doctor; under a reformed system their control was in doubt. Part of the problem lay in a conflict of professional ideals. Any scheme of nursing reform involved a change in the hospital's administration and for a matron to be successful a conflicting power base had to be established. The matrons' and nurses' claim to autonomy was intolerable for the status-conscious medical profession who 'feared that these educated women would undermine their authority'.[103] At the height of the dispute at Guy's, the *BMJ* wrote that the doctors were championing a principle in resisting the self-styled lady-superintendents, who had an 'exaggerated view of their own importance', and were tainted with 'conceit, insubordination, and self-will'.[104] The dispute was more than a parochial disagreement over the nature of reform.

Opposition came rapidly in a series of letters to Lushington. Samuel Osborne Habershon, the senior physician, orchestrated the attack. A former student at Guy's, he was respected by his colleagues and familiar to the governors. Resentful of the High Church party's attempts to establish nursing sisterhoods, Habershon saw the issue as part of a wider crusade and fuelled the conservative feelings of his colleagues. Under his guidance the medical staff overlooked their earlier campaigns for reform and initially claimed that the nurses had been 'tyrannised' by Burt's overbearing manner. An apparent concern for patient welfare (including the colour of the counterpanes) and a manipulation of the nurses' grievances concealed other interests. The medical staff 'utterly opposed' the matron's attempts to establish what they saw as a 'sisterhood to which everything is subservient'. They argued that this opposed 'the great principles which have always been in operation at Guy's'. The governors' authority was recognised, but the doctors felt that they possessed far superior medical knowledge to Lushington or 'a stranger from a country infirmary'. Lushington countered, denying the notion of a sisterhood. He was not unsympathetic to the doctors' interests, but refused to dismiss Burt or alter the new nursing system.[105] Between Lushington and the doctors there was a clash of interests over the legitimate spheres of authority.

Over the following months the medical staff redefined their opposition. There was a gradual shift from a conceptual attack on nursing sisterhoods to an opposition based on the material effects of the reforms, which were shown as jeopardising treatment. At a three-day inquiry in March 1880 the methodical and precise Pavy presented the medical staff's evidence. Particu-

---

102 Dingwall, Rafferty and Webster, *Social history of nursing*, 57–8, cited in Abel-Smith, *History of the nursing profession*, 27.
103 Ibid.
104 BMJ i (1880), 289–90, 400.
105 Medical staff to governors, 1 Dec. 1879, LMA, H9/Gy/A219/7; Lushington to medical staff, 3 Dec. 1879, LMA, H9/Gy/A219/3.

lar attention was given to the new procedures whereby patients were woken at five in the morning or moved so they could be washed. Individual cases were cited where the relocation of trained nurses had left an unskilled probationer in charge of a ward, resulting in inadequate care. Annoyed by Pavy's detailed statement, the governors were unconvinced by evidence that Guy's was now dominated by 'harshness or coercion'. They complained that the doctors 'should not rake up any more bygones which had better be forgotten'.[106]

The death of Louisa Morgan played into the doctors' hands. Pavy had admitted Morgan in June 1880 with signs of tuberculosis and complaining of headaches, nausea and vague pains in her left leg and abdomen. She was considered of 'sensitive organisation' and possibly hysterical. Morgan's condition deteriorated and after she had soiled her bed, she was dragged to the bathroom and placed her in a cold bath for twenty minutes by Louisa Ingle, one of Burt's lady pupils. After adding a little warm water, Ingle left Morgan there for another hour.[107] Pavy in his medical testimony claimed that Morgan had died three days later from a 'tubercular and inflammatory disease of the brain'. He attributed this to the shock of the bath and concluded that Morgan had been grossly ill-treated. Sir William Withey Gull, self-styled intellectual and honorary physician at Guy's and to the prince of Wales, refuted this opinion. He was dismissive of Pavy's physiological and laboratory work and saw himself as superior, a stance that encouraged Gull to be unsympathetic towards Pavy. Although the eminent Gull had never seen the patient or attended the post-mortem, he argued that Morgan had an obvious brain disease that would have progressed rapidly in spite of the bath. Gull's reputation for egocentricity led staff at Guy's to unite behind Pavy.[108] The difference of opinion attracted unwelcome publicity, but Pavy was clear that 'the nursing system in operation' by 'encouraging too much independence' was responsible for Morgan's death. Ingle's explanation that she had treated the patient for hysteria only confirmed the medical staff's fears that the new nurses laid claim to their medical knowledge. Ingle did not make a good impression on the jury who convicted her of manslaughter and sentenced her to three-months imprisonment.[109] *The Times* made the inevitable connection 'that this unfortunate case is not an unnatural result of the controversy about nursing'. For the medical staff and their adherents, the case successfully supported their claim 'to exercise supreme control over the nursing'.[110] In their view, nursing was an extension of treatment and therefore had to be under their

---

[106] Guy's Hospital, minutes of the general court of governors, 3–11 Mar. 1880, LMA, H9/Gy/A225/1–3.

[107] *Lancet* ii (1880), 714.

[108] See Robert Tattersall, 'Frederick Pavy (1829–1911): the last of the physician chemists', *Journal of the Royal College of Physicians of London* xxx (1996), 235–44, for a full discussion of the trial.

[109] Pavy to Lushington, 9 July 1880, LMA, H9/Gy/A223/8.

[110] *Times*, 7 Aug. 1880, 9.

control. Morgan's death implied that when they were not consulted the outcome would be disastrous.

The medical staff feared that the new regulations would destroy the 'traditional relationship between doctors and nurses' and reduce them to a subordinate position.[111] The rotation of probationers and nurses between wards, a practice considered necessary for their training, was seen as a direct threat to the doctors' working practices and ability to allocate nurses as they wanted. They asserted that 'whatever power we had possessed as officers of the Medical Staff with respect to the nursing has been taken from us, if not directly, at all events indirectly, by the matron who has been placed over us, who made rules entirely at variance with our former rules'.[112] Under threat the medical staff's criticisms went further than the daily management of the wards. From the start opposition stemmed from the fact that the reforms had been framed without 'due courtesy' and implemented 'without reference to us'.[113] The medical press seized on this issue. The *Medical Times & Gazette* reflected general medical opinion when it remarked that 'the physicians and surgeons must be consulted about nursing systems, which should certainly be controlled by them rather than by "the torrents of public opinion" '. Even those who supported trained nurses found 'absolute subordination' essential.[114] Once the question of responsibility and authority had been raised the dispute became an arena for a heated discussion on medical representation. The medical press, particularly the *BMJ*, pointed to the wider implications:

> sooner or later, it must be recognised in the City hospitals . . . that the medical officers of the hospital are as much its governors as a layman who administers the funds; that it is essential, for the truly harmonious and effective working of such a hospital, that the medical officers should sit at the Governors' board with the lay Governors; that a mere donation of £30 or £50 does not constitute a unique and particular fitness for governing a medical institution . . . but that living in its wards, the habit of dealing with its patients, with a personal knowledge of what is wanted to make it efficient, are as important factors in the determination of the rules of government as are merely financial qualifications.[115]

Only over finance was *The Lancet* willing to concede that the governors might have a greater claim to knowledge.[116] On these grounds the medical staff at Guy's called for consultation in all matters affecting medical practice, especially nursing. From an awareness that they were basing their opposition

---

111 Cited in Moore, *Zeal for responsibility*, 60.
112 Guy's Hospital, minutes of the general court of the governors, 10 Mar. 1880, LMA, H9/Gy/A225/1.
113 Guy's Hospital, medical staff to Lushington, 1 Dec. 1879, LMA, H9/Gy/A219/1.
114 *Medical Times & Gazette* i (1880), 429; Octavius Sturges, 'Doctors and nurses', *Nineteenth Century* xi (1880), 1093.
115 *BMJ* ii (1880), 593.
116 *Lancet* ii (1880), 583.

on a moral and medical prerogative to intervene and had no legal right under Guy's Act of Incorporation to interfere, they nevertheless sought a greater administrative role. This was expressed as a demand for representation and the medical profession united behind them.

The doctors agreed that 'the nursing of our patients is so closely connected with our treatment of disease that we are not exceeding our duty in being deeply concerned on the subject', but Lushington had other views. In his opinion, 'the medical staff have . . . outstepped the limits of their province in commenting on the minutest details of my administrative proceedings, in impugning the justice of my decisions when dealing with contumacious servants, and in treating with marked disrespect the chief female authority in the Hospital'.[117] Lushington's intractable attitude is not surprising. He had been used to his plans being carried out without dissension, and the medical staff's opposition was the first concerted attack on his authority. It was not only the doctors who felt threatened and even they admitted that the dispute had called Lushington's authority into question.[118]

The governors reacted slowly as they were prepared to allow Lushington, as in the past, to make all the decisions. Only Lord Cardwell felt sufficiently concerned to resign. No opinion was expressed, but the governors placed 'entire confidence' in Lushington. It was hoped that 'the medical staff will find that the future good management of the hospital will thereby be promoted, and that nothing will occur to interfere with the continuation of the cordial understanding between the treasurer and the medical and surgical staff'.[119] It was a forlorn hope as the tradition of informal co-operation had already broken down. Attempts to defuse the situation faltered and in March 1880 the governors appointed a lay subcommittee to investigate.

In April, before the committee reported, the main managing body accepted the medical staff's opinion that a sister should be responsible for each ward, able to administer medicine along their guidelines, and remain in the same ward with no night duties unless 'the interests of the hospital absolutely require'. Burt's regulations were seen as erroneous and centralisation as undesirable and it was admitted that reform required greater collaboration with the medical staff. This was not enough to placate the doctors. With their collective pride offended they continued to insist that Burt be dismissed.[120] The governors refused. The doctors' stubborn attitude in April seemed far less justifiable by June when the subcommittee's report was submitted, a month before it was made public. Reform was identified as a priority and the medical staff's anxiety that changes had been initiated 'without sufficient consultation and preparation' and that Burt had worked under the false assumption that her efforts 'would be acceptable' was acknowledged. However, no 'suff-

[117] Guy's Hospital, printer circular, 5 Feb. 1880, LMA, H9/Gy/A219/18.
[118] Guy's Hospital, medical staff to governors, 13 Aug. 1880, LMA, H9/Gy/A219/25.
[119] Guy's Hospital, minutes of the court of committees, 7 Apr. 1880, LMA, H9/Gy/A3/10.
[120] Ibid.

icient justification for the difficulties which have existed between the medical staff and matron' was found. The subcommittee felt that there had been no fundamental change in the existing rules and that the effect of the reforms had been exaggerated. While the general tone of the report dismissed the dispute, several positive proposals were made. It was admitted that the governors were not always the best body to make informed decisions on medical matters. The solution was to invite the staff to participate formally in the hospital's management to ensure that reorganisation would be satisfactory to both parties. A joint taking-in committee was recommended as a forum for representatives of the medical staff to meet the governors to discuss points of mutual interest, revitalising a body that had become redundant after the doctors had replaced its official control of admissions. Theoretically the committee would allow the governors to become conversant with the internal workings of the hospital and the doctors to come into 'contact with the governors'.[121] Though all the medical staff's other demands had been met, the situation could not be resolved while Burt remained. In protest, Habershon and John Cooper Foster, the senior medical officers and the doctors' representatives, refused to serve on the committee. Both sides were locked in a stalemate.

The publication of the report provided the first real indication outside the medical press of events at Guy's. *The Times* considered the report 'most conciliatory in tone towards the medical staff', but wrongly believed that it was 'likely to restore harmony in the institution'.[122] The dispute, which continued to drag on for another four months, now came under the spotlight of public opinion, making the governors more defensive. With this stalemate a contradictory position developed. The doctors worked with the new nursing system and even collected £2,500 to help the governors in their financial struggles, but there was no growth in co-operation.[123] The medical staff were not in an ideal position. The hospital, for all its apparent problems, held obvious financial and clinical benefits for its staff. Any opposition that went beyond a verbal confrontation would damage individual reputations and practices.

It was the St Saviour's Board of Guardians that finally forced the issue. The board took an interest in the crisis partly because Guy's supplemented its meagre medical services. In an attempt to resolve the dispute, the board issued a memorandum that took the medical staff's line. Their stance is hardly surprising: the only information available to them was from the doctors' statements to the press. The governors were alarmed, feeling that the memorandum contained several accusations that could not go unanswered. They seized the initiative and for the second time used the public forum to express their ideas. The need for reform was defended and it was claimed that

---

121 Guy's Hospital, report of the subcommittee on nursing, 1880, LMA, H9/Gy/A233/1.
122 *Times*, 21 July 1880, 8.
123 *BMJ* i (1880), 784.

the governors had 'endeavoured to comply with the wishes of the medical staff'. The governors argued that their attempts at conciliation had been met with 'renewed acts of opposition either in the form of collective protests or of attacks in public journals, and by the peremptory demand for the dismissal (as the only condition of peace) of an officer whose intentions and acts the staff, in the opinion of the governors, wholly misapprehended'. They closed their statement with a warning that it was they who administered the hospital under an act of parliament and that it might become necessary to act against the staff if the 'struggles for power' continued.[124] The doctors responded clumsily. A protest by Habershon and Cooper Foster on behalf of their colleagues carried an allegation the governors interpreted as an accusation of deliberate mismanagement. Habershon and Cooper Foster were asked to resign when they refused to withdraw their statement. It was a calculated step to frighten the staff into subservience. The real moment of crisis had come. The doctors' resolution and solidarity collapsed as self-interest over-rode professional grievances. The remaining staff withdrew the offending letter and reluctantly agreed to serve on the taking-in committee.

The medical community was disappointed. The *BMJ* noted that the governors had triumphed because the doctors had failed to find unanimity at the crucial moment: 'the governors have ... virtually told the medical staff that the nursing arrangements are no business of theirs; they have not very obscurely intimated that the medical staff must consider themselves as merely occupying a servile position, and that if they object to the matron, they must go, not the matron'.[125] Even *The Times* recognised that the doctors had thrown away their unassailable right to influence 'by injudicious letter-writing'.[126] The dispute, which had lasted for ten months, trailed to an end. The press lost interest, and though Habershon and Cooper Foster were greeted as martyrs, their resignations were not welcomed by their colleagues and had little impact on the internal affairs of the hospital.[127]

Pavy, writing to *The Lancet*, felt that something had been achieved: 'we began with no recognised status in relation to the nursing administration, and we leave off with an official position upon a committee of governors'.[128] *The Lancet* itself was not as optimistic, seeing the taking-in committee as 'a half-hearted and round about way of making a concession'; a compromise that 'cripples while it degrades'.[129] Pavy's view was to prove more accurate. By November 1880 it appeared that 'the committee of governors, in their recent relations with the staff, have shown a disposition to retrace their former position of hostility, and have entered upon a course of deference to the opin-

---

124 Guy's Hospital, minutes of the general court, 29 Sept. 1880, LMA, H9/Gy/A1/3.
125 *BMJ* ii (1880), 593.
126 *Times*, 18 Oct. 1880, 9.
127 Guy's Hospital, minutes of the general court, 25 Nov. 1880, LMA, H9/Gy/A1/3.
128 *Lancet* ii (1880), 714.
129 Ibid. 624, 662.

ions of the physicians and surgeons of the hospital'.[130] Although Lushington later admitted that the committee had a mainly advisory role, it did represent an increased level of medical representation. Within months the taking-in committee had started to adopt a prominent role in the hospital's administration.

When the new nursing arrangements were published in March 1881 all sides claimed victory. The governors secured their nursing reforms and the nurses were placed under the medical staff's authority. Burt no longer proved a problem. She was stripped of her title of lady-superintendent and resigned the following year, not under pressure from her critics but to marry. The BMJ claimed that the main points at issue during the dispute 'are virtually decided in favour of the medical men'.[131] Not all were as enthusiastic: the Medical Times & Gazette noted that authority over the nurses continued to rest with the treasurer, superintendent and matron rather than the taking-in committee.[132] The doctors, left in a better position than when the dispute had started, raised no objections. Informal administrative repercussions followed. During the crisis the medical staff had convened hasty meetings at Habershon's house to formulate their attacks. Between 21 November 1879 and 10 October 1880 there were no less than twenty-nine unofficial meetings. The habit of meeting to discuss matters relevant to the medical staff had been established and it was continued in a more formal manner once the dispute had ended. By November the governors had accepted the medical committee as part of the hospital's administration and it worked in tandem with the taking-in committee. Harmony between the doctors and governors took longer to emerge however. It was only when John Steele was replaced by the young and enthusiastic Edwin Cooper Perry as medical superintendent in 1892 and Lushington was succeeded as treasurer in 1896 by Cosmo Bonsor that co-operation between the two factions took on a more stable form.[133] Neither Cooper Perry nor Cosmo Bonsor had been at Guy's in 1879/80, allowing the dispute to be finally laid to rest.

The events at Guy's were only extraordinary for the public attention they attracted. During 1880 all eyes seemed to turn to the hospital and the issues of medical authority and representation were openly discussed. The dispute, however, was not unique. It symbolised the conflict that evolved between doctors and governors in many hospitals and the way increased formal influence was obtained through stubbornness, apparent defeat and compromise from which the doctors emerged with a stronger administrative position.

130 BMJ ii (1880), 862.
131 Ibid. ii (1881), 438.
132 Medical Times & Gazette i (1881), 403.
133 Cameron, Mr Guy's Hospital, 212, 257, 300–1.

Doctors and hospital management

The Lancet's call that 'medical authority must be supreme in a medical charity' was not practical in the nineteenth century.[134] It foundered on the hospitals' voluntary nature and the governors' important financial role. However, the 'want of union and mutual acquaintance' that the *BMJ* had suggested existed between doctors and governors in the late 1870s had been modified by the 1890s.[135]

The doctor–governor relationship evolved through tension and conflict, and over time. Conflict was required to produce an extension of formal authority, but developments in medical science and a change in the nature of the hospital promoted administrative change. For St Bartholomew's 1868/9 marked a watershed. A retrospective view of its administration shows that from 1868 the doctors' passive position was gradually modified and replaced with a series of medically inspired subcommittees and recommendations.[136] Changes of this type are difficult to explain. Medical journals and hospital reformers did help to establish an environment in which medical representation became a professional goal. Doctors working in the capital's hospitals were undoubtedly influenced by such ideas, but the internal politics of individual hospitals played an important role. An increase in medical authority might also be linked to an altered perception of medical science. Governors, as part of a wealthy London business and social elite, met doctors through the hospital and in private practice, and were influenced by society's altering perceptions of medicine.[137] However, at the centre of these changes was the governors' view of their own medical staff. At St Bartholomew's the extension of the doctors' influence was closely connected with attacks on the hospital's administration in 1868/9. In response, the governors 'requested' the doctors to provide a medical defence of the hospital, giving the medical staff a lever through which they could start to assert their influence.[138]

The London's experiences from the late 1870s clearly show how an alteration in the governors' approach to the hospital required both a formal and informal extension of medical authority. An agreement over the finances of the medical college in 1876 allowed greater formal co-operation, acting as a catalyst in the hospital's administration. The doctors gave up their sole authority over the medical college, but acquired a formal position in the London's administration. From the 1880s onwards the house committee became more closely involved in the hospital's medical administration through its link with the medical college. The governors were now being faced with

134 *Lancet* i (1881), 107.
135 *BMJ* ii (1878), 962.
136 St Bartholomew's, minutes of the medical committee, SBH, MC 1/1.
137 See M. Brightfield, 'Medical profession in early Victorian England', *BHM* xxxv (1961), 238–56.
138 St Bartholomew's, minutes of the board of governors, 22 Dec. 1869, SBH, Ha 1/23.

issues that were beyond their business experience. In response they increasingly referred medical issues to the doctors and invited them to take part in special subcommittees. For example, the doctors were instrumental in proposing plans for the improvement of the hospital's sanitary system in 1890 after outbreaks of typhoid, and were actively consulted over the administration of the out-patients' department in the same year.[139] Sydney Holland's arrival as chairman in 1897 did lead to a more autocratic style of management as he worked to improve the London's financial position. However, he continued to recognise that the medical council played a vital role in the efficient management of the hospital.

Authority, however, was rarely one-sided. Even the most secure doctors at the specialist hospitals still had to negotiate their demands and the governors' decision was always final. However, by the end of the nineteenth century the medical staff of London's hospitals had entered a loose partnership with the governors. Changes in medical science and the public's perception of the medical profession and the value of institutional treatment helped modify the doctors' position in society and within the hospital. Medicalisation and the inclusion of new practices into the hospital environment increasingly forced governors to consult their medical staff. In specialist hospitals this transformation occurred from the hospital's foundation because their specialist nature demanded a greater level of medical involvement, but even at the endowed hospitals changes were taking place. Not all institutions progressed at the same rate and by the end of the Victorian period some doctors were still struggling to get their voices heard. Conflict, tension and an alteration in the nature of the hospital all conspired to increase the level of medical influence. An increase in informal authority was gradual and aroused little opposition, partly because the governors could feel that they dictated the agenda. The direct inclusion of the medical staff in the hospital's management was a different issue and one where conflict seemed inherent. The medical profession and hospital reformers were not arguing for complete medical control. They recognised the hospitals' voluntary nature and sought to uphold it. Separate spheres were established in which the doctors did not attempt to encroach on the governors' financial control. What they wanted was a joint administration in which they could use their professional status and knowledge to help manage the hospital on medical lines. Increasingly governors were being forced to modify their conservative approach. However, if control over the working environment is an indication of professionalisation, then the medical profession in London's hospitals was only at the start of the process by the start of the twentieth century.

Voluntarism remained the key ethic of the hospital and even doctors gave their services without charge. Science and professionalism were insufficient to counter an authority based on charitable contributions and tradition. The

---

139 London Hospital, minutes of the subcommittee (general), 1882–1903, LH, A/9/121–2.

result was a modification of the governors' power, often at their behest, to promote more efficient management. Doctors were left in a better position, with more influence, but they still had to negotiate their recommendations and modify their demands to the financial constraints of the voluntary system and the hospitals' philanthropic basis.

PART III

1897 AND BEYOND

7

State Aid versus Voluntarism

In 1897 the British empire celebrated Queen Victoria's diamond jubilee with all the pomp and pageantry that it could muster. 1897 also represented a significant year for charity. The jubilee was zealously exploited by philanthropists who used it as an excuse to launch new appeals.[1] Hospitals benefited from the patriotic upsurge in benevolence, but the foundation that year of Prince of Wales Hospital Fund as a commemorative fund had a greater impact. The golden jubilee had set the precedent, inaugurating an appeal to support district nursing, while the Sunday and Saturday Funds had established a model of indirect philanthropy that the new fund copied. However, the Prince of Wales Hospital Fund represented a subtle transformation in the nature of hospital philanthropy. It reaffirmed the hospitals' voluntary nature in an attempt to resolve their financial problems and prevent state intervention.

Hopes and fears of state intervention

From the 1880s onwards an increasingly pessimistic assessment of the financial position of the London hospitals came to dominate views on hospital funding. By 1887 latent concerns had been replaced by widespread anxiety. Dr Thomas Gilbart Smith expressed a common opinion in 1882 when he told the SSA that 'the funds now available either for the proper maintenance of nearly all the existing [medical] institutions, or for the extensive relief to districts hitherto unprovided for, are insufficient'.[2] Few governors shared Henry Burdett's optimism when he countered statements in *The Times* in 1894 that charity was 'in extremis'; they believed that their institutions were sinking further into debt. The Sunday Fund added to these fears. In recognition of its own financial inadequacy it admitted that at least £100,000 was needed *per annum* to cover the hospitals' deficit.[3] The fund's assessment of the level of need was widely accepted by hospital philanthropists. Debt was not universal but the image projected by the precarious financial position of Guy's, St Thomas's, King's College Hospital and University College Hospital

---

1 Among these were large national charities such as the NSPCC: Behlmer, *Child abuse*, 143.
2 *SC on Metropolitan Hospitals, First Report*, 15.
3 *Times*, 25 Dec. 1894, 9.

seemed to presage a general crisis. As these hospitals were among London's leading medical institutions, concerned contemporaries wondered what hope there was for smaller hospitals, though ironically these were actually in a better financial position.

An almost universal belief that London's hospitals were facing endemic financial crisis was translated into apprehension that the state might have to intervene. As early as 1881 Burford Rawlings, secretary to the National Hospital for the Paralysed and Epileptic, had predicted the inevitability of state intervention.[4] In the following year these fears had started to enter the vocabulary of hospital appeals. At University College Hospital's annual dinner in 1882, the earl of Kimberley warned that because of the 'unsatisfactory basis' of the finances of most metropolitan hospitals voluntary effort would have to be bolstered by state subsidy.[5] In 1883 the *Charity Record & Philanthropic News* and *The Times* expressed similar concerns, noting that state assistance might be essential to prevent the collapse of the voluntary medical system.[6] Concerns about the possibility of state intervention increased with the hospitals' deepening economic crisis. In 1887 the bishop of London expressed a common feeling among governors that the spectre of public assistance was looming.[7] When several hospitals, including Guy's and University College Hospital, closed wards, the collapse of the voluntary system seemed only a matter of time. Few contemporaries shared Morley's stoicism when he stated that he was prepared to see such a move rather than see hospitals close.[8]

The recurrent fears of state intervention in the London hospitals did not match continental experiences. In many European countries and in America the state played an acceptable and integral role in the provision of public and voluntary healthcare. The two were not often separated. In France a system directed and partially funded by the state had been in existence in Paris since the formation of the hospital council of the Seine *départment* and the *assistance publique* in the 1797. The revolution had confiscated church property and removed the emphasis on private and religious benevolence. With the growth of an idea of participatory citizenship and equality, healthcare was made into a right organised by the state, not a function of charity.[9] The transition met with opposition, but by 1851 communes were obliged to take responsibility for the sick poor. In Paris the *assistance publique* received part of its income from a municipal grant; the rest from the accumulated wealth of

[4] B. Burford Rawlings, 'The honorary element in hospital administration', *Fraser's Magazine* xxiv (1881), 67.
[5] *Lancet* i (1882), 315.
[6] *Charity Record & Philanthropic News* iii (1883), 28; *Times*, 20 Jan. 1883, 9.
[7] *Times*, 13 June 1887, 14.
[8] *Charity Record & Philanthropic News* vi (1886), 37.
[9] Dora B. Weiner, *The citizen-patient in revolutionary and imperial Paris*, London 1993.

charitable bequests.[10] Though the emphasis on healthcare changed between the restoration and the Third Republic, the state retained its influence and in 1893 passed national medical assistance legislation creating a different path to state medical welfare than that offered under the Bismarckian social insurance provisions of the 1880s.[11] In America too the state played an active role, but was more concerned with funding than with direct organisation.[12] Government intervention in Pennsylvania was not unique: by 1910, 141 of the 167 hospitals in the state received a grant. Intervention followed no predetermined strategy and was seen as a natural function of government. The civil war had increased demands for hospital care and mixed private and public initiatives that continued after the war. The result stimulated the growth of voluntary hospitals. Corporate expenditure on hospitals was seen as having material and palliative benefits for business-minded officials, but philanthropists retained their authority and calls in the 1890s for more local control were ignored.[13] In America philanthropy could coexist with state assistance and limited government demands without a challenge to the hospitals' voluntary nature.

In Britain the situation was different. The state, through Sir John Simon's work at the Privy Council and then under the Local Government Board (LGB), was willing to give small grants towards medical research. Intervention was limited: the first auxiliary scientific grant of £2,000 was awarded in 1871, and support was seen as part of the public health initiative.[14] Medical care in an institution partly funded by charity, however, was a different issue. The reasons might be found in the ingrained nature of voluntarism, support for the idea of a limited state and hostility to state action, which was not compensated for by a medical profession geared to market forces and research. Hospital governors, like the mass of the subscribing public, remained hostile to state intervention. They were unaffected by arguments in favour of state action from the 1880s onwards that were fuelled by new revelations about the extent of urban poverty, interest within the Liberal party to use social reform to cement an alliance with the working class and by later concerns about national efficiency.[15] London's voluntary hospitals remained more dogmatic in their antipathy to state intervention than charitable organisations in other

10 Paul Weindling, 'The modernisation of charity in nineteenth-century France and Germany', in Barry and Jones, *Medicine and charity*, 192–3.
11 Evelyn B. Ackerman, *Health care in the Parisian countryside, 1800–1914*, New Brunswick 1990.
12 See Moris J. Vogel, *The invention of the modern hospital, Boston, 1870–1930*, Chicago 1980.
13 Rosemary Stevens, 'Sweet charity: state aid to hospitals in Pennsylvania 1870–1910', BHM lviii (1984), 288–9, 311–13.
14 Theodore L. Stourkes, 'John Simon, Robert Lowe and the origins of state-supported biomedical research in nineteenth-century England', *Journal of the History of Medicine* xlviii (1993), 436–53.
15 See Harris, 'Political thought and the welfare state', 116–41; Stefan Collini, *Public*

areas, which were prepared to work with government agencies. Governors continued to view the state in terms of centralisation; any growth in its power was seen as an attack on the 'spontaneous efforts of individuals or voluntary groups'.[16]

Despite the expansion of the metropolitan poor law's medical services and mounting anxiety over social hygiene, a similar reluctance to intervene in voluntary provision was shared by the state.[17] A faith in minimal government joined with the Gladstonian belief that charity had an important role to play in welfare, helped ensure that no Victorian government was willing to interfere with voluntary healthcare. The public health movement, expanding poor-law medical services and the development of the Metropolitan Asylums Board created an alternative arena of state interest in healthcare for those classes that the London hospitals did not claim to assist. However, the state did have an indirect effect. Changes in the local taxation system added to hospitals' precarious financial position. Charitable institutions had been excluded from imperial taxation, but Gladstone threatened their right to tax exemption in 1863 and in 1866 a court decision in Liverpool made them liable for local rate assessment. The decision had national implications, forcing hospitals to contribute towards the poor rate and sponsored a periodic and unsuccessful reform movement to reverse the decision.[18] It was not until 1875, once the City of London had effectively established St Thomas's rate liability, that the London hospitals were included. In response governors enthusiastically joined the rate exemption campaign.[19] Predictably this new taxation incensed vested interests and did nothing to enhance governors' opinions of the state.

Antipathy to state intervention in the London hospitals was not total and debate existed in a muted form. It was part of a wider discussion on the role of the state and new attitudes to welfare. According to Thane, 'the problem that was increasingly evident by the 1890s was that for all the high-minded principles underlying the Victorian consensus on the minimal state, the liberal economy, decentralisation, probity in public life and the responsible involvement of the citizenry, serious social problems visibly remained'.[20] A renewed awareness of poverty showed that charity was not enough and philanthropists found themselves increasingly prepared to encourage legislation

---

moralists: political thought and intellectual life in Britain, 1850–1930, Oxford 1991; Paul Weiler, The new liberalism, New York 1982; Bernard Semmel, Imperialism and social reform, London 1960.

[16] Stefan Collini, Liberalism and sociology: L. T. Hobhouse and political argument in England, 1880–1914, Cambridge 1979, 23.

[17] See M. A. Crowther, The workhouse system, 1834-1929: the history of an English social institution, London 1981; Gwendolyne Ayers, England's first state hospitals and the Metropolitan Asylums Board, 1867–1930, London 1971; Greta Jones, Social hygiene in twentieth-century Britain, London 1986.

[18] Owen, English philanthropy, 341–3.

[19] Charity, Dec. 1889, 169.

[20] Thane, 'Government and society', 48.

where individualistic efforts had failed. At an intellectual level, liberal theorists proposed a changing conception of the state as an agent of communal responsibility.[21] These arguments joined with practical developments. Outside healthcare, the state was beginning to take a more active role in social policy and by the 1890s these concerns had started to become issues of 'first-rate national importance'.[22] By 1914 the approach to social policy had profoundly changed and government felt forced to resort to an interventionist role, partly because politicians had come to believe that voters were motivated by social welfare issues. Under these conditions the boundaries between the state and charitable provision began to be re-negotiated.[23] Progressive hospital reformers were part of this development and from the 1880s onwards they began to question the voluntary system and see a role for the state in healthcare beyond the poor law. Two strands emerged in the debate, one linked to finance, the second rooted in the need to promote co-ordination between healthcare sectors to solve the problems of institutional overcrowding in north London. Those who advocated state support because hospitals were a public utility like gas and water were on the margins of the debate and few contemporaries connected London's hospitals to municipal socialism.[24] It was state intervention, not local control, that was feared and discussed. The impetus came mainly from concerns that hospitals faced mounting debt and this was linked to an awareness that reforms could no longer be avoided.

Rate-supported schemes were suggested in 1858 and in 1883, but Burdett was one of the first hospital reformers to discuss the boundaries between the state and voluntary hospitals.[25] Burdett was already recognised as an expert on hospitals having previously helped the BMA compile evidence on hospital abuse. Aware of the problems of running a London hospital, he argued in his influential *Hospitals and the state* that hospitals were in urgent need of reform. Two years later, in an article in the *Nineteenth Century*, he again called for parliamentary action to encourage reorganisation. After outlining the manifest problems facing London's hospitals, from a lack of organisation to overcrowding and nursing difficulties, Burdett suggested that a controlling authority should be formed and a royal commission appointed. Whether Burdett, himself a hospital governor and committed to the voluntary system, fully believed these ideas or was trying to shock civil society, hostile to state intervention, into action is uncertain. Rivett certainly believed that Burdett was trying to 'shake the complacency of his audience'. Burdett ultimately

---

21 Collini, *Liberalism and sociology*, 23; Harris, 'Political thought and the welfare state', 116–41.

22 Cited in idem, 'Transition to high politics in English social policy, 1880–1914', in M. Bentley and J. Stevenson (eds), *High and low politics in modern Britain*, Oxford 1983, 61.

23 See Finlayson, *Citizen, state and welfare*.

24 BMJ ii (1892), 964; Harry Roberts, *Public control of hospitals*, London 1895, 3.

25 *Medical Times & Gazette* xxxvii (1858), 104.

avoided the need for state intervention by calling on the SSA, in which he played a leading part, to take an active role in hospital reform.[26]

Burdett was not alone in his views however. Gilbart Smith raised the issue of state control at the 1882 SSA conference and in the following year the association discussed in detail Frederick Mouat's proposals for an integrated health service. Mouat had trained as a doctor at Edinburgh and University College Hospital before entering public service in India where he had played an energetic role in stimulating and remodelling medical and higher education. On his return to Britain in 1871 he had joined the staff on the LGB. At the board, Mouat flair for organisation led him to become interested in the need to organise hospital services in London through his work with Henry Saxon Snell on hospital design, and he had already published a number of articles on the issue in *The Lancet* in 1881.[27] Given his background in public service, he suggested a state-financed system in which existing poor-law infirmaries would be gradually converted into general hospitals. London was to be organised into five districts with separate boards to regulate management and care. Mouat aimed to distance medical care from poor relief and argued that his scheme would solve the problem of poor distribution of hospital services, increase accountability and promote a unified system of medical education.[28] Although Mouat's ideas generated considerable debate they were not considered acceptable. They did, however, serve to keep the issue in front of the SSA, the medical press and the benevolent public, encouraging others to look into the question of the financial future of London's hospitals. A number of rate-support schemes continued to be put forward and after two years of further discussion a conference of hospital governors was called, out of which the Hospitals Association was formed.[29] It was anticipated that the new association would be a voluntary alternative to state action, but it did little to end the debate over state intervention.

Few schemes were discussed as extensively as the one put forward by Robert Reid Rentoul, a general practitioner in Liverpool interested in obstetrics. Having won the Sturge Prize with an essay on the 'Financial condition of London hospitals', he considered himself an expert on London's hospitals. An awkward and passionate man, Rentoul was a popularist who delighted in finding radical solutions to controversial subjects, although he tired quickly of individual problems. A staunch defender of the interests of less affluent general practitioners, Rentoul launched a vitriolic attack in 1889 on the out-patient system, which he claimed was the subject of flagrant abuse by the middle classes. He argued that medical relief within the non-endowed hospi-

[26] Burdett, *Hospitals and the state*, and 'Our hospitals', *Nineteenth Century* xiii (1883), 359–84; Rivett, *London hospital system*.
[27] *BMJ* i (1897), 628; *Lancet* i (1881), 73, 409.
[28] Mouat and Snell, *Hospital construction*.
[29] Michael Millman, 'The influence of the Social Science Association on hospital planning in Victorian England', *Medical History* xviii (1974), 128–32.

tals was inadequate and public recognition of this had led to a fall in income. Rentoul believed that a 'public medical service' would solve all the hospitals' problems. He also felt it would aid general practitioners by eliminating counter prescribing by chemists and reduce the influence of medical clubs on fee setting.[30] The medical journals attacked Rentoul's ideas and a lively debate was stimulated on the possibility of a state co-ordinated or organised scheme. In response the BMA appointed a special committee in 1890 to investigate. The doctors consulted by the BMA expressed a need for reform, but Rentoul's ideas aroused fears that a government body would reduce fees and a clear majority rejected the scheme as impractical and undesirable.[31] In such a climate, Rentoul's arguments were discredited. However, his views had helped generate debate and encouraged others to come to similar conclusions, though he himself quickly abandoned his interest in hospital reform and became embroiled in debates over the licensing of midwives, abortion, social hygiene and sterilisation of the mentally ill.[32]

Mounting pressure from the COS, the Hospitals Association and the press for reform forced a situation where the state had to take an active interest in the voluntary system, if only to defend it.[33] Where reformers and the government would not contemplate state intervention, both gradually accepted the need for a parliamentary inquiry. As early as March 1879, discussions were initiated by Fowell Buxton, chairman of the London, for a select committee, but no coherent plan emerged. According to the BMJ fear of state control or 'something of this sort' had retarded 'the movement in favour of a public inquiry'. The journal itself, and many hospital reformers, supported a royal commission in the hope that it would 'educate the public into recognising the public importance of voluntary hospitals' and stimulate charity.[34] Sir William Harcourt, the diplomatic Liberal chancellor, had acknowledged the need for an inquiry following the nursing dispute at Guy's in 1879/80, but public interest was not stimulated until 1888 when the COS took up the issue and formed a special committee to promote hospital reform as part of its campaign to organise charity. Aware of its unfavourable image of 'cringe or starve', the COS was careful to explain that it did not wish to discredit the voluntary system, only to promote 'some improvement in their organisation that will make them [the hospitals] even more useful than they are now'.[35]

---

30 BMJ ii (1880), 1067.
31 Brand, Doctors and the state, 154.
32 See Jean Donnison, Midwives and medical men: a history of the struggle for the control of childbirth, London 1977, 129–31, 138–9; Robert Reid Rentoul, The dignity of women's health and the nemesis of its neglect, London 1890; Proposed sterilisation of certain mental and physical degenerates, Newcastle 1903; and Race culture; or race suicide, London 1906.
33 Hospitals were not the only philanthropic objects that underwent investigation in the 1890s: the NSPCC in 1895–6 and the RNLI in 1897 were exposed to searching inquiries and then vindicated: Behlmer, Child abuse, 145–9.
34 BMJ ii (1881), 87.
35 SC on Metropolitan Hospitals, First Report, 6.

With the support of leading hospital governors and doctors, the COS circulated a petition which Lord Sandhurst, chairman of the Middlesex and active member of the COS special committee, presented to the House of Lords in July 1889. The BMA welcomed the initiative; for its part the Hospitals Association was antagonistic but realistic enough to claim some credit for creating a climate of opinion that favoured reform. Other supporters of reform clearly had axes to grind and used the campaign to promote their own ends.[36] With governors sensitive to a royal commission, Lord Cranbrook, the minister responsible, decided upon a select committee.

The House of Lords' Select Committee on Metropolitan Hospitals met under the chairmanship of Sandhurst from 1890 to 1892. The long duration of the inquiry was testimony to the complexity of the issues involved. The press responded with extensive coverage of the committee's proceedings, and time was wasted discussing the intricacies of nursing at the London and the sanitary arrangements at St Bartholomew's. From the beginning the committee recognised that state interference was incompatible with the principle of voluntarism and completely vindicated the existing system in its final report.[37] *The Times* felt that the committee had been appointed with this purpose in mind: 'to furnish the Government with good reasons for leaving the hospitals alone'.[38] Ultimately it made weak recommendations, but proposed a modicum of informal centralisation. The COS was disappointed, believing that the final report was 'as good as could be expected from a body of amateurs'.[39] Others were more enthusiastic because the Lords' unqualified support of voluntarism seemed to place the emphasis firmly on reform within a voluntary context and to remove any threat of state intervention.

The dismissal of Rentoul's 'public medical service' and the select committee's final report did not, however, end debate. The Lords had supported the voluntary system, encouraged nursing reform at the London and sanitary improvements at St Bartholomew's, and relieved public pressure for action, but it had done nothing to solve the problems facing London's hospitals. Progressive reformers therefore continued to see a role for the state. In 1892 Mathers and Sydney Buxton introduced a private member's bill to allow local authorities to support voluntary hospitals and have full subscribers' rights.[40] Buxton was the Liberal MP for Poplar and although under-secretary for the colonies he was practically committed to welfare reform and extending provision in the East End of London. The bill partly recognised that poor-law guardians and municipal authorities already subscribed to specialist hospitals

---

[36] FWA, minutes of the medical advisory subcommittee, July 1889, LMA, A/FWA/C/A26/9.
[37] SC on Metropolitan Hospitals, Second Report.
[38] BMJ i (1893), 30.
[39] Charity Organisation Review, Jan. 1893, 28.
[40] Hansard, 4th ser. i. 106.

and sent patients to general hospitals for treatment they could not provide.[41] The bill received no discussion. When questioned over the possibility of a grant to the hospitals in Belfast, the minister responsible indicated the general feeling of the House towards state assistance. He noted that 'I am not aware of any proposal to make grants from public money to the hospitals in Belfast or in other cities in the United Kingdom, nor even if such a proposal were made do I think it would meet the approval of the House.'[42] Mathers and Buxton were discouraged and let the bill drop, but interest in state intervention resurfaced in 1896. Knowsley Sibley, in *State aided v. voluntary hospitals*, called for a state medical service and pointed to a current of opinion favouring reorganisation. Similar schemes were proposed and though many of these focused on using the rates, few were prepared to go as far as Colonel Gordon Wilson in suggesting a 1*d*. levy on income tax to replace benevolence.[43]

The press debated the merits of these schemes in a critical light, but even the more sympathetic felt that hospitals could not be surrendered to 'economy and political expediency'.[44] John Eric Erichsen, consulting surgeon at University College Hospital, was just one among many actively involved in hospital management who believed that state support would 'dry up' charity and multiply the very problems it sought to solve.[45] Hospital reformers warned that any form of subsidy would inevitably lead to a demand for representation and ultimately to state dominance, manipulating public prejudice against intervention. The public was more critical. Many claimed that state support was morally objectionable and went against an ethic of voluntarism that was an integral part of the social fabric. In their defence of voluntarism they appeared to forget the philanthropic chaos the COS had highlighted. The *Hospital* shared this opinion, but warned governors that they should take note of the developments in education.[46]

Governors and hospital reformers certainly feared the possibility of state intervention and constantly used it in the 1890s as a shibboleth to invoke public support. Two movements emerged from these concerns as voluntary alternatives to state funding and organisation. The foundation of the Prince of Wales Hospital Fund in 1897 and the Central Hospitals' Council for London in the following year saw the embodiment of reformers' hopes that a voluntary means could be found that would permanently remove the need for state intervention. The foundation of these two bodies served to check the

---

41 *Times*, 19 Mar. 1892, 5.

42 *Hansard*, 4th ser. i. 448.

43 *Lancet* i (1896), 723; *Charity Record & Philanthropic News* xvii (1897), 335; *Lancet* i (1896), 723.

44 *Hospital*, 12 Dec. 1896, 175; 3 Oct. 1896, 15.

45 *Charity Record & Philanthropic News* xv (1895), 90.

46 *Hospital*, 26 Nov. 1892, 130.

debate over the role of the state until the issue re-emerged during the 1905–9 Royal Commission on the Poor Law.

Royal support: the Prince of Wales Hospital Fund for London

The Prince of Wales Hospital Fund (later known as the King's Fund) built on the fashionable awareness that London's hospitals faced a financial crisis that would ultimately lead to state intervention unless an alternative remedy were found. The recent successes of the Sunday Fund in 1895 and the launch of an endowment appeal by Guy's in 1896 only seemed to confirm the strength of charity. Given the income structure of hospitals that faith was ultimately misplaced. The Prince of Wales Hospital Fund stood at the intersection of opposition to state funding initiatives and the perceived need to place the capital's hospitals on a firm financial footing with a guaranteed source of income.[47]

The fund's aim to prevent state intervention was clear from the start. Introducing the appeal, the prince of Wales stated that

> public opinion has shown itself on more than one occasion, and I think wisely, in favour of the voluntary system for support for our hospitals, combined with an adequate system of representation of the body of subscribers in their control and management. It is obvious, however, that if these institutions are to be saved from the state or parochial aid, their financial condition must be secured.[48]

The Sunday Fund had attempted to resolve this dilemma, but its interventionist aims had been submerged beneath the practicalities of administering general maintenance grants. The Prince of Wales Hospital Fund built on the Sunday Fund's experiences and attracted many of its supporters. It adopted the contemporary analysis that an additional assured income of £100,000 was needed *per annum* to prop up the voluntary system and ignored suggestions that rationalisation might solve the hospitals' problems. No attempt, however, was made to account for rising expenditure or institutional expansion which would only multiply the existing problems the fund sought to solve. The Sunday Fund had shown that there was a limit to the amount that could be raised annually so the Prince of Wales Hospital Fund adopted the controversial policy of endowment, a policy that reflected the prince's opposition to annual appeals. By December 1897 the optimism placed in endowment had receded as the fund's organisers realised that the endowed income

---

[47] For a recent history of the fund see Prochaska, *Philanthropy and the hospitals of London*, a meticulous account of the fund's confused genesis, highlighting the crucial role played by Burdett and the prince's enthusiasm for medical charity.
[48] Prince of Wales Hospital Fund, annual report 1897, LMA, A/KE/300/1.

could initially only raise £5,000 and the anticipated annual income of £100,000 was not reached until 1909.[49]

According to Frank Prochaska, 'in a society fascinated by the royal family, and with an increasing demand for hospital provision, the fund had every hope of success'.[50] Contemporaries viewed the £227,551 12s. 5d. collected in 1897 as an undoubted success and for one enthusiast it had ended the 'days of doubt'.[51] However, many voiced disappointment that more had not been accomplished. The BMJ, The Times and the COS had predicted in 1897 that the fund would have problems after the jubilee and this was borne out by the dramatic fall in revenue after 1897, as 'enthusiasm, even when most glaring, is not always convertible into a satisfactory equivalent in cash'.[52] Dissatisfaction increased between 1898 and the coronation in 1902 because collections remained modest in comparison to 1897. Disappointment and the fall in collections after 1897 conceal the fund's impact. The jubilee collection was the largest single amount raised in any one year for the London hospitals, and in the following years the fund provided a welcome source of income. It also symbolised a new departure in fundraising by exploiting the traditional modes of direct philanthropy and adding its own innovative tactics.

Previous benevolent funds had attempted to extend charity beyond the traditional subscribing public and the Prince of Wales Hospital Fund tailored its appeal to this purpose, 'to both great and small, private individuals and capitalist organisations'.[53] Burdett, as one of the fund's main organisers, recognised that 'money must now be collected not from the few, but from the many, and every one must be interested in the process' to prevent the voluntary system from collapsing.[54] Influential with the prince of Wales, it was his conception of the fund that dominated. The aim was to democratise benevolence and ensure that every sector of society contributed. The fund argued that this would not damage other institutions because these new subscribers had no established tradition of giving, while it would encourage self-help among those who had previously only benefited. Success was not complete. The mass of contributions continued to come from the middle classes, from 'munificent gifts' and from the new plutocracy of businessmen. Only £51 was raised from contributions under 5s. in 1897 and it was felt as early as June that the working and lower-middle classes were not being encouraged to contribute.[55] The fund redoubled its efforts, though with little apparent success, and founded the League of Mercy in 1898 to appeal directly to these groups.[56] The fund's inability to compete with local networks of working-class charity,

---

49 Prochaska, *Philanthropy and the hospitals*, 34-9.
50 Ibid. 23.
51 *Hospital*, 20 Feb. 1897, 341.
52 BMJ i (1897), 413.
53 *Daily Chronicle*, 6 Feb. 1897, 4.
54 *Hospital*, 13 June 1896, 181.
55 BMJ i (1898), 1341; *Times*, 10 Oct. 1898, 9.
56 Like the NSPCC's League of Pity, the League of Mercy intended to bring local traditions

Table 23: Prince of Wales Hospital Fund: income, 1897–8

| Income | 1897 | | 1898 | |
source	amount	%	amount	%
Donations	£98,605	43.4	£8,864	22.6
Investments	£1,469	0.6	£5,334	13.6
Legacies	–	0.0	£10	*
Mayoress Fund	£5,373	2.4	–	0.0
Newspaper collections	£42,681	18.7	£181	0.5
Programme sales	£2,041	0.9	–	0.0
Retained as capital	£21,161	9.3	£564	1.4
Stamps	£34,776	15.3	–	0.0
Subscriptions	£21,443	9.4	£23,318	59.4
Trustees	–	0.0	£1,000	2.5
TOTAL	£227,551	100.0	£39,271	100.0

* Figure for this item represents 0.03% of collection
Source: Annual reports 1897–8, LMA, A/KE/300/1–2

built on community and familial ties, or rival established provident dispensaries and benefit societies, came from the fact that they offered practical returns where the fund gave none.

If the fund had difficulty tapping working-class benevolence, it did exploit every charitable imperative and played on guilty consciences, social aspirations, compassion for the sick, and 'love and loyalty to the throne'.[57] No effort, however, was made to capitalise on the imperial federation movement and its concern with 'national efficiency' and latent opposition to state welfare.[58] Little was left to chance and personal contacts were taken advantage of, becoming a hallmark of the fund's tactics. Collections were not taken on a single day as it was envisaged that the fund would receive money all year round. As such it was more of a charitable society comparable to the COS than a benevolent fund. The mechanisms of direct philanthropy were used to the full, forming the most traditional aspect of its activities (see table 23). Donations were welcomed, but it was subscriptions that were solicited to

of community service to the hospitals' benefit within a hierarchical organisational structure which stressed the reciprocal duties between the hospital and the recipient of medical aid. The league initially faced enormous difficulties and both Loch and Sydney Holland actively resisted it, but the prince rallied to the idea and after a slow start the movement snowballed, increasing the fund's prestige and income.

[57] Prochaska, *Philanthropy and the hospitals*, 22.
[58] The Prince of Wales Hospital Fund did not appear to be influenced by these ideas as it

ensure a reliable income. Such was the confidence expressed in the fund, that the trustees of the London parochial charities, a body formed to rationalise out-moded posthumous benevolence, contributed £1,000 *per annum* from 1898 to distribute to convalescent homes.[59] Public subscription lists were analysed and appeals made to those most likely to give, while obituaries were scoured for relatives with money left to undefined charitable purpose.[60] All contributions received a thank-you note; those who gave over £5,000 received personal letters from the prince, invitations to royal events or gifts of game from Sandringham. Several large West End hospitals suffered as a result. At St George's, according to Sir George Turner, many of the traditional supporters switched to the Prince of Wales Hospital Fund. One subscriber explained to him: 'you don't mind, dear George, I hope, if I leave off subscribing to St George's, and give my subscription to the King's fund'. Turner felt that this was a common attitude among the aristocratic supporters of St George's.[61]

Effort was not only directed at individuals: 28,200 companies were approached in 1897. Banking support was canvassed by Lord Rothschild and eighty direct appeals were issued, though the result was initially disappointing.[62] City livery companies retreated behind the claim that they already helped individual hospitals, but as the fund matured they increased their contributions with twenty-one companies giving £240,000 between 1897 and 1940.[63] It is unlikely that many would have been as generous without the knowledge that the prince desired it and the recognition or prestige that was gained from subscribing.

Although subscriptions and donations provided the bulk of the fund's support, they were supplemented by revenue that marked a new departure in fundraising. Investments, which were supposed to furnish the main body of income, initially provided a small percentage. This proportion increased over time, rising in the first two years from 0.6 per cent to 13.6 per cent. It was not, however, until after 1909 that investments attained the position that the

---

failed to adopt the liturgy of imperial federation or national efficiency. Certainly the fund did aim to promote efficiency and opposed state welfare, but the prominent supporters of these ideas did not form a substantial element in the subscription list. Although Alfred Harmsworth, Lord Strafford and Lord Rothschild were all represented on the fund's management, only Lord Rothschild had an influential role. The presence of such names should not negate the view that other charitable motives were more important and such was the nature of the fund's appeal that the supporters of imperial federation would probably have contributed independently of their imperial ideology: see R. Smith, 'British nationalism, imperialism and the City of London, 1880–1900', unpubl. PhD diss. London 1985.
59 Prince of Wales Hospital Fund, annual report 1898, LMA, A/KE/300/2.
60 Prince of Wales Hospital Fund, minutes of the executive council, LMA, A/KE/27/1.
61 Turner, *Unorthodox reminiscences*, 76.
62 Prince of Wales Hospital Fund, minutes of the executive council, 27 May 1897, LMA, A/KE/27/1.
63 Prochaska, *Philanthropy and the hospitals*, 28.

founders had intended.[64] The fund extended the role of endowments from an institutional source of capital to a metropolitan source of revenue as it was hoped that this would provide a permanent solution to debt and offset the need for public assistance. In 1897, 75 per cent of the collection was invested. Thereafter a varying proportion of the collection was invested annually until the target income was reached. The fund modified the idea of posthumous benevolence, adopting the hospitals' conception of endowment as a permanent source of funding by using endowed revenue to finance an organisation that would be administered to address the problems of the present rather than the troubles of the past. It was a far-reaching and innovative approach, though one ultimately flawed as it failed to anticipate that expenditure was not static.

The other components of income for the first year were no less innovative. The jubilee was exploited to the full: jubilee procession programmes were sold and the Lady Mayoress Jubilee Appeal was redirected to hospitals and administered by the fund. Hospital stamps were designed to recruit small subscribers and were advocated by Burdett who took most of the credit for them.[65] In the first collection they raised £34,776 5s., accounting for a large proportion of that year's grants. The COS thoroughly disapproved of this means of raising money and claimed that charity should be a sacrifice without reward, but the fund was aware that subscribers expected something for their money.[66] Unfortunately the stamps' initial popularity was not enough to ensure that they remained a permanent feature. Dedicated philatelists and stamp dealers refused to buy them, and with no commemorative function after the jubilee or any postal value many subscribers quickly lost interest.[67] As a result they were abandoned. A diverse source of income was not enough to ensure that successive collections preserved the 1897 level.

Hospital governors complained that the entire 1897 collection had not been directed to resolve their accumulated debts. Sydney Holland, the reforming chairman of the London, voiced the concern shared by smaller institutions that the distribution was unfair. A shameless publicist, he was determined to maximise the London's income and wanted additional funds to carry out long overdue rebuilding. With a shrewd and ruthless sense of financial management he felt the Prince of Wales Hospital Fund had mishandled the distribution and not sufficiently recognised certain hospital's needs. When the Mary Wardell Convalescent Home in Stanmore, Middlesex, received an unusually large grant in recognition of the princess of Wales's support for the institution, these criticisms were supported.[68] Distribution

[64] Prince of Wales Hospital Fund, annual reports 1897–8, LMA, A/KE/300/1–2.
[65] *Standard*, 4 Feb. 1898, 3.
[66] *Charity Organisation Review* iii (1898), 63.
[67] Prince of Wales Hospital Fund, press cuttings, LMA, A/ KE/750/10; stamps sold in aid of fund, 1897–8, LMA, A/KE/751/3.
[68] Prochaska, *Philanthropy and the hospitals*, 34.

was not always perfect, but generally grants were 'dis-imbursed', as *The Lancet* acknowledged in 1899, with discernment and fairness.[69] Most welcomed the fund, especially as it could be a generous body: the Hospital for Sick Children was awarded £50,000 in 1902 to build a new out-patients' department. Grants mostly remained small however.[70] For example, in 1898 the Royal Hospital for Diseases of the Chest received £100, though the larger hospitals could receive grants of over £5,000.[71] The idea was 'to do the greatest good to the greatest number of the sick, not the greatest good to the greatest number of hospitals'.[72] This conceals the impact of the fund's grants which on average represented 5 per cent of individual hospitals' income. Institutional experiences differed: for the Hospital for Sick Children the 1899 grant represented 3.4 per cent of the total income; for Guy's this was 7.7 per cent raising the proportion of the hospital's revenue from charity to 37.2 per cent.[73] Critics claimed that the fund could not increase the aggregate resources available to hospitals, only redirect the income obtainable within the benevolent economy.[74] This was not entirely true. Both the Sunday and Saturday Funds were indeed damaged by the new movement, despite attempts to limit rivalry and promises from the Prince of Wales Hospital Fund that it would not trespass on the other funds' territory.[75] Hospitals, however, benefited from the competition and the fund opened 'new fields of practical benevolence'.[76] In 1897 the income of ninety-three hospitals showed an increase, and in 1898 ordinary income was £35,000 higher than in 1897.[77] The existence of the Prince of Wales Hospital Fund must account for part of this rise. The effect was to provide a fresh source of charitable income at a time when philanthropists were afraid that the state might have to intervene.

The Prince of Wales Hospital Fund not only raised income but also embodied a new opportunity to influence hospitals through financial incentives and as such it received advice from all quarters about how its income should be distributed. Many governors sympathised with Dr Thomas Glover Lyon's view that the fund should distribute the entire collection rather than 'hoard' the income, but this opinion did not make much headway.[78] The secretary of the Westminster Ophthalmic Hospital, Beatrice Campbell, sug-

---

69 *Lancet* i (1899), 42.
70 Prince of Wales Hospital Fund, report on the Hospital for Sick Children, LMA, A/KE/250/1.
71 RCH, annual report 1898, LMA; Guy's Hospital, annual report 1898, LMA.
72 Prochaska, *Philanthropy and the hospitals*, 52.
73 Hospital for Sick Children, miscellaneous financial records, GOSH, 3/4/7; Guy's Hospital, annual report 1898, LMA.
74 *Charity Organisation Review* iii (1898), 63: the COS remained a stern critic, disliking the fund for the attention it had taken away from its own schemes for a central board.
75 Prince of Wales Hospital Fund, minutes of the executive council, 15 Mar. 1897, LMA, A/KE/27/1.
76 *Lancet* i (1897), 1656.
77 *Times*, 21 Dec. 1898, 8.
78 Ibid. 23 Dec. 1897, 4.

gested that the coal, corn and finance committee of the Corporation of London should be used to distribute grants.[79] Such an approach through local government was clearly unacceptable when the fund aimed to uphold charity. The COS urged that the mistakes of the Sunday Fund should not be repeated and the BMA picked up the hidden meaning by proposing that the collection should be distributed publicly through a body similar to the COS's proposed central board (see below).[80] From within the fund, Lord Lister, pioneer of antiseptics and the first medical peer, propounded this view, explaining that the proposed board was 'a body which represents all that is best in the Medical Profession in London, combined with the widest experience in Hospital management'.[81] The prince, however, wanted no outside influence and pushed for a separate distribution committee. This was not initially possible. The fund was too preoccupied with the basic organisation to adopt any firm policy on distribution. At first it utilised the information collected by the Sunday Fund as it was 'conscious that they were not qualified to undertake that thorough investigation into the merits of individual hospitals which is needed'.[82] A distribution committee was finally established in December 1898 and subsequently met for one month annually to allocate grants. As a non-elected body it reflected the autocratic nature of the movement, breaking with the established cultural norm for a voluntary society and even with the hybrid benevolent funds as no effort was made to duplicate the voluntary associations' 'subscriber democracy'. All members of the fund's administration were personally selected by the prince to ensure a breadth of opinion and to defuse any potential disputes. Lord Lister, however, strongly influenced the distribution committee's foundation. Though he was unable to persuade the prince to agree to any co-operation with the proposed central board, he did involve Sir Trevor Lawrence, treasurer of St Bartholomew's and an important force behind the central board, in the committee's activities. This was supplemented by a visiting committee primarily selected by Lister. It sent two 'dispassionate' representatives, one medical, one lay, to investigate each application for a grant. This was the first committee of its kind, but strangely, given the fund's reforming intentions, it refused to publicise the information collected as it did not want unduly to embarrass the hospital concerned.[83]

The Prince of Wales Hospital Fund employed the Sunday Fund's procedures as reformers continued to believe that improvement could only be effectively secured through a voluntary model of centralisation supported by financial incentives. Lord Rothschild expressed concern that the fund would be criticised as a body that wanted to influence hospital management by only

---

[79] Beatrice Campbell to Prince of Wales Hospital Fund, 1897, LMA, A/KE/568/7.
[80] Rivett, *London hospital system*, 148.
[81] Lister to Prince of Wales Hospital Fund, 16 Mar. 1898, LMA, A/KE/751/2.
[82] *BMJ* i (1898), 37–8.
[83] Ibid. ii (1898), 196.

distributing money 'to the hospitals which they thought were best managed'.[84] This was precisely how the fund was conceived and hospital reformers gave their support to the movement on these grounds. It departed from the Sunday Fund by not using grants to reflect an individual hospital's utility, but reinvigorated the principle of using them to stimulate reform guided by a humanitarian, patient-centred ethic.[85] In effect it became a mass subscriber through its grants and therefore assumed the right to influence management for the benefit of the patients and not from individual institutional interests. The promise of an annual grant remained a powerful reforming incentive, though no formal pressure was initially applied.

Grants were at first set at a maximum of £5,000 in recognition of the fund's limited resources. Begging letters were received from all directions, but the movement was dedicated to the hospitals' cause and initially devoted special attention to the seventeen hospitals with over 100 beds within seven miles of Charing Cross, believing that these institutions held the greatest benefit for the nation.[86] Each grant had a specific intention and it was felt that any hospitals that co-operated should receive a similar grant for the following year. A clear idea of what was expected was always given. The London Lock Hospital, for example, was awarded £500 on condition that the drainage was improved and overcrowding reduced; the West London Hospital received the same amount to reduce overcrowding. Other grants had a direct medical purpose: the East London Hospital for Children received £250 towards a new operating theatre.[87] However, it was generally assumed that because bureaucracy was modest any improvement in administration that the grants would promote could be equated with an advancement in healthcare. The Sunday Fund had never been so precise, merely using its grants to promote efficiency.

Grants did have a positive effect. In 1898 the governors of the London were asked if they had used the previous year's grant of £5,000 to improve the hospital's wards. The fund had made its annual subscription of £5,000 conditional on rebuilding and Holland replied anxiously that a building committee had been appointed to spend £100,000 on improvements, and asked for patience. The inquiry had had the desired effect. Under the circumstances the fund agreed to award a further £5,000 and by 1901 a new isolation block and pathological department had been opened.[88] Influence is perhaps more clearly displayed in the fund's initial policy to use grants to reopen wards, which was equated directly with medical progress. Within the first four years

84 *Standard*, 4 Feb. 1898.
85 Prochaska, *Philanthropy and the hospitals*, 53.
86 Prince of Wales Hospital Fund, minutes of the executive committee, 9 Nov. 1898, LMA, A/KE/27/1.
87 *Times*, 31 Dec. 1898, 6.
88 Prince of Wales Hospital Fund, minutes of the distribution committee, 15 Dec. 1897, LMA, A/KE/20/1.

433 beds were reopened, the equivalent of two large hospitals.[89] University College Hospital immediately agreed to this policy; Guy's proved obstinate. Although Guy's had been awarded £6,600 of a £7,912 grant to reopen beds, the governors insisted that the money would be better used to build a nursing home. They argued that paying patients would have to be removed if they reopened all the beds and that this would ultimately prove more expensive. In the end a compromise was reached: forty-three of the 154 closed beds were reopened, ironically reducing hospital provision for the middle classes.[90]

The Prince of Wales Hospital Fund rapidly assumed the influential position that Adrian Hope, secretary of the Hospital for Sick Children, had envisaged at the inaugural lecture of the Hospital Officers' Association in 1902.[91] Its influence was almost guaranteed because of the financial pressure it wielded. This was not unique given the Sunday Fund's activities, but it marked a new departure in hospital philanthropy. The view that contributions could be used to influence hospital administration was reinvigorated by the fund, which took over the role of the active citizen by replacing the citizen with a funding institution. The link between funding and reform was explicitly made and the fund set about using its influence in what it considered a positive manner. Charitable influence was revitalised, even if the benevolent economy lacked the resources to solve the problems of hospital finance.

A bid for co-ordination: development of a central hospital board

The second strand of the debate on state intervention focused on the need for co-ordination. Some form of central organisation had long been a tenet of hospital reformers' ideas as a possible solution to the problems of competition, duplication of services and overcrowding in London's central and northern districts. In an atmosphere openly hostile to state intervention arguments for organisation were conducted within the language of voluntarism. The debate focused on calls for a voluntary central board as a counter to state organisation and mirrored debates within the London County Council over the need to centralise services.[92]

As early as 1796 Sir William Blizzard, surgeon to the London and founder of the medical school, had suggested a central board, as had the *Pall Mall Gazette* in 1868, but it was not until the 1880s that these views resurfaced into the public domain.[93] In 1883 Burdett, dissatisfied with the Sunday Fund's achievements, proposed a voluntary central body. Five years later a

---

[89] Abel-Smith, *The hospitals*, 183.

[90] Guy's Hospital, sundry court papers, LMA, H9/Gy/A1/4/6.

[91] *Hospital*, 22 Nov. 1902, 133–5.

[92] Rivett, *London hospital system*, 144.

[93] *Charity Record & Philanthropic Messenger*, 31 Mar. 1868, 103.

similar scheme was suggested to the BMA.[94] These views fitted within more practical moves to establish voluntary co-ordination through the COS's efforts and Graham Wallas's ultimately unsuccessful attempts to co-ordinate those charitable organisations in London providing meals for needy school-children.[95] However, it was the suggestion made by the Select Committee on Metropolitan Hospitals that an informal central board should be established to help solve the problems facing London's hospitals that acted as a major stimulus to debate. Sandhurst, as chair of the committee, was aware that support for a voluntary central board would help promote charity and prevent state action, and suggested it on these grounds.[96] The select committee found these views more acceptable than a state-oriented approach, but was not confident enough to give them a full endorsement. Because of the vague nature of its proposals, uncertainty prevailed and there was no immediate effort to carry out its suggestions. Without any firm agenda the matter was left hanging and parochial concerns and the sheer number of interests involved slowed the development of a positive solution.

The select committee helped to establish a consensus that favoured a definite central board. For Burdett and *The Lancet* this could be achieved by revitalising the Sunday Fund. In 1892 a conference called in the wake of the select committee to discuss the issue ascribed an important role to the Sunday Fund.[97] However, partly because Douglas Galton, general secretary of the British Association and an authority on hospital construction, successfully resisted all moves towards centralisation, the conference only recommended a further investigation.[98] Predictably the COS took over. In calling for a voluntary and representative central body, the COS shared the opinions voiced by Sandhurst and believed that it would counter moves to municipalisation. For the COS a central board was the 'universal panacea' for the hospitals' problems. Burdett realistically regarded the COS's proposed arrangements, which had 169 representatives and included general practitioners, as impractical.[99] He disagreed with the COS's ill-informed meddling and overt emphasis on character, arguing that the society lacked the necessary experience of hospital management to be effective. He believed its intervention would prevent any concerted improvement, frustrating the aims of reformers like himself. Burdett's assessment proved accurate: the COS's recommendations were cumbersome and were dismissed by governors who had never been extensively canvassed for their opinion.[100]

The COS did not form the first central board, but its involvement in the

94 Loch, 'Confusion in medical charities', 308; Burdett, 'Our hospitals', 381–2.
95 A. M. McBriar, *An Edwardian mixed doubles: the Bosanquets versus the Webbs: a study of British social policy*, Oxford 1987, 91.
96 *Charity Record & Philanthropic News* xii (1892), 251.
97 *BMJ* i (1893), 312, 184.
98 Ibid. ii (1892), 314–15.
99 *Times*, 11 Nov. 1897, 6
100 See FWA, minutes of the medical advisory subcommittee, LMA, A/FWA/C/A/26/9–10;

debate and the antagonism it generated was influential in its foundation. The twelve teaching hospitals met independently and established their own Central Hospitals' Council for London in 1898, effectively excluding the COS.[101] At a time when changes were being introduced into the structure of university education in London, concerns over hospital reform and the COS's interests may have been less significant than would at first appear.[102] Certainly the council was a central board that hoped to discuss the provision of medical care in the metropolis, but it may also have been an attempt by the teaching hospitals to strengthen their hand in the negotiations over the reorganised London University. Without any real power and lacking the authority and financial incentives of the Sunday Fund or the Prince of Wales Hospital Fund, the council proved ineffective. The *Charity Record & Philanthropic News* warned that a central board would drive away many of those active in hospital management, but governors took little interest in its work, and the council seldom assumed the lead, preferring to procrastinate until the hospitals had virtually decided policy of their own accord.[103] However, never before had a body existed in which the capital's hospitals, albeit of a limited number and character, co-operated with the general aim of organising a representative body. The council reinforced the notion of voluntary centralisation in a practical representative context rather than through funding or state intervention. In the twentieth century the model it pioneered was adopted by other bodies such as the British Hospital Association and the London Voluntary Hospitals Committee that succeeded it.

Neither the Prince of Wales Hospital Fund nor the Central Hospitals' Council were ideal solutions to the problems facing London's hospitals at the end of the nineteenth century. The two movements were founded in a climate in which state intervention had become an object of anxiety; as a result they were attempts to counter the need for public assistance within a voluntary framework. Ultimately both proved unsuccessful. The Prince of Wales Hospital Fund was an effective funding body and became the champion of the voluntary system, but it addressed a situation of escalating financial demands which charity was unable to meet. The fault did not rest with the fund, but with the changing nature of the hospital and the demands of medical care. In the late 1890s voluntarism had reasserted itself in the face of state intervention. The result was only to postpone the eventual outcome as healthcare created problems and demands that charity could not successfully meet.

minutes of the general committee for the promotion of a central board, LMA, A/FWA/C/A/44/1.
[101] *BMJ* ii (1897), 1608.
[102] Negley Harte, *The University of London, 1836–1986*, London 1986, 146–58.
[103] Rivett, *London hospital system*, 152.

8

Conclusion:
1898 and Beyond

1898 was a more stable year for London's hospitals in comparison to the uncertainties of the early 1890s. Governors and concerned contemporaries had worried about hospitals' level of debt, but now this seemed more of an institutional problem than a metropolitan one. Debates over the abuse of the capital's out-patient departments continued to rumble in the medical press, revealing general practitioners' persistent antagonism to the hospital, but fewer calls were now being made for state intervention. Advances in medicine had increased the medical profession's status and helped alter the public's perception of the hospital. Admissions remained high and many patients who had previously shunned hospital care now appeared willing to wait up to six hours for treatment.[1] Although charitable contributions were still unpredictable, the foundation of the Prince of Wales Hospital Fund for London had created a new mood of optimism. This concealed half a century of accumulated structural problems. Hospitals had been forced to evolve with medical science and changing attitudes to poverty and welfare so that by the 1890s they had moved further away from their philanthropic origins to become the top level of the medical care hierarchy, though delays remained between external changes and the adoption of new practices. The sick poor continued to be the prime objects of attention, but now the hospitals' aim was to heal the sick as best they could; moral reform and religious observation were marginalised in its objectives. In admissions a distinction continued to be made between 'deserving' and 'undeserving', especially in the debate over hospital abuse, but many now admitted that there had been a shift towards a more medical perspective as the governors' moral and superficial medical assessments had been replaced by a system guided by the doctors. Changes in medicine altered the hospital's theoretical basis and slowly introduced new techniques into it, depersonalising treatment.

In such a climate a paradox existed. The medical profession had acquired an increased social status, though not the prosperity it aspired to. Within the hospital, however, the profession's scientific rhetoric, improving social status, and surgical ability only made the medical staff junior partners in the administration rather than placing them in the dominant position that the hospitals' increasing medicalisation would suggest. In specialist hospitals doctors played a more prominent role than their counterparts in other medical insti-

---

1 *Charity Record & Philanthropic News* xviii (1898), 380.

211

tutions, but even here their authority was still restricted. Nowhere was the transition a smooth one. The hospitals' function might have altered, but as institutions they continued to be dominated by the voluntary ethic.

The structural transformation of welfare provision, encouraged by the increasing scale of economic organisation, the inadequacies of local government finance, demographic change, the impact of collectivist arguments and an altered attitude to poverty, suggested 'a mixed economy of welfare'. Between 1906 and 1949 welfare provision moved from the responsibility of the 'active citizen' to the 'active state'. The process was far from a linear one. Voluntarism remained an important component with the state willing to delegate provision in certain areas, but the balance was increasingly to favour the state.[2]

In 1898 many of these changes still seemed unthinkable. Charity retained the upper hand in welfare. Even where social welfare programmes were to be initiated by the state it was believed that they should be administered by elected local authorities in association with voluntary organisations. By 1914 increased taxation and extended state services had not dramatically affected the level of voluntary contributions. Civil society was practically committed to voluntarism, despite mounting concern that charity was becoming unable to solve social problems and the influence of the emerging collectivist school of thought which favoured an extension of the state's role. A new 'politics of conscience' had partly replaced the religious basis of voluntarism, but no single impulse guided charity; it continued to appeal to a multitude of factors from guilt to gratitude. In comparison to the view that state aid through the poor law was impersonal – a view encouraged by means testing – many continued to praise philanthropy for its conviction, enthusiasm, freedom from restraint and individualism, overlooking the unco-ordinated nature of benevolence and the duplication of services. Hospitals were the 'flagships' of this benevolent system and internalised its ethics. At the end of the nineteenth century their continued reliance on voluntary principles reflected charity's social importance. Changes, however, were already being seen. The rhetoric of philanthropy was becoming less socially significant to the middle classes or useful as an arena for mediating class relations than it had been during the mid Victorian period. To a certain extent London's hospitals were immune from this. In the twentieth century they were the last major institutional bastions of voluntarism, outside provincial attempts to secure greater co-operation between the voluntary and statutory welfare sectors.[3]

The permanence of the voluntary ethic in hospital management was not

[2] Prochaska, *The voluntary impulse*; Finlayson, 'A moving frontier', 183–206; N. Johnson, *Reconstructing the welfare state*, Brighton 1990.
[3] Daunton, 'Payment and participation', 189; M. Moore, 'Social work and social welfare: the organisation of philanthropic resources in Britain, 1900–14', *Journal of British Studies* xvi (1977), 85–104; M. Cahill and T. Jowett, 'The new philanthropy: the emergence of the Bradford City Guild of Help', *Journal of Social Policy* ix (1980), 359–82.

matched in hospital finance where other sources of income had always been necessary. Contemporaries wanted to believe that hospitals were supported by voluntary contributions and in doing so they ignored its other sources of funding. Governors shared this preoccupation, inventing new strategies to encourage support from London's highly competitive benevolent economy. However, in 1873 the *BMJ* had already concluded that on average London's hospitals only received approximately 30 per cent of their income from charity.[4] By the 1890s it was becoming increasingly evident that they could no longer rely on the 'sweepstake' of philanthropy if they wanted to survive. As one contemporary wrote in 1894, 'a glance at the advertising columns of any of the leading newspapers reveals only too clearly that the existing [charitable] sources of hospital income are fatally deficient'.[5] Governors and reformers exaggerated the hospitals' economic problems, but it was inescapable that charity's relative financial contribution was falling. Over time, as the pressures on the hospital and the benevolent economy increased, financial diversification became the key characteristic of hospital finance. The finances of the Royal West Sussex Hospital, Chichester, the Bristol Infirmary and the Norfolk and Norwich Hospital, reveals that this process was not just limited to the metropolitan hospitals, though in London diversification was more marked.[6] It was a product of the institutional provision of healthcare that developed beyond the point where traditional sources of funding (be they the poor rate or philanthropy) could meet spiralling expenditure. An anonymous hospital secretary explained to the *Charity Record & Philanthropic News* in 1894 that governors spent too much time worrying about the future, but 'somehow or other the hospitals were maintained in spite of the anxieties of the committees'.[7] It is perhaps because governors did not rely on any one source of income, but haphazardly developed a diverse financial framework that they managed to survive institutional expansion and the transition away from their philanthropic base. In the twentieth century these changes were to become more pronounced.

Twentieth-century hospital finance

The optimism of 1898 quickly waned. The Prince of Wales Hospital Fund did not save the London hospitals as contemporaries had hoped, and its continued popularity threatened the other benevolent funds' level of support.

4   *BMJ* ii (1873), 611.
5   *Hospital*, 28 Apr. 1894, 83.
6   Royal West Sussex Hospital, annual reports 1850–98, West Sussex County Record Office, Chichester; Bristol Infirmary, annual reports 1850–98, Bristol Record Office; Norfolk and Norwich Hospital, annual reports 1850–98, Norwich Record Office, City Library.
7   *Charity Record & Philanthropic News* xiv (1894), 87; iv (1884), 189.

The fund was able to stimulate charity temporarily to provide a short-term solution to the London hospitals' apparent financial crisis, but no realistic attempt was made to address the fundamental problems that the Select Committee on Metropolitan Hospitals had outlined in 1892. Voluntary contributions through the Prince of Wales Hospital Fund were a substitute for reform, leaving a system of medical overcrowding and competition as charitable institutions scrambled for funds.

A change in how social problems were viewed saw a gradual modification of the accepted solutions to the dilemmas facing London's voluntary hospitals. Between 1880 and 1914 the consensus that the 1834 Poor Law had taken social policy out of politics collapsed. A new feeling came to take its place. 'Social issues', noted José Harris, 'were no longer marginal to the major concerns of high politics' and 'among those whose main interest was in social questions, social policy was increasingly viewed as central to the effectiveness, the stability, and even the legitimacy of the state'.[8] Late nineteenth-century debates on the relationship of the London hospitals to the state were revived by the Liberal government's welfare reforms and the 1905–9 Royal Commission on the Poor Law. The poor-law medical service, freed from its pauper stigma by the separation of the infirmary from the workhouse, increasingly provided the main source of medical care for the sick poor. 'The small end of the wedge in breaking down status barriers between paupers and the wider community' had already been introduced into the poor law with the inclusion of non-pauper patients through the Metropolitan Asylum Board (MAB) before the Local Government Board's decision in the 1900s to allow a system of 'statutory disregards', which permitted people to claim relief without forfeiting small private savings.[9] Both marked a change in attitudes towards relief. However, the poor law lacked the sophisticated medical services and educational function associated with the voluntary hospitals. This left a gap in provision and raised important questions over the nature of healthcare. A number of poor-law medical officers giving evidence to the Royal Commission called for the establishment of a national health service, developing the earlier muted sympathy for co-ordination of Sidney Webb and Henry Burdett.[10] The BMA was scandalised and again declared its opposition to state intervention. Neither the majority nor minority report of the commission approved of government intervention, but both recognised the need for reorganisation.[11] The 1911 National Insurance Act provided a political substitute for any revision of the existing arrangements. Few at the time seemed seriously prepared to counter any other solution than a voluntary one in hospital provision. London's hospitals maintained their independence

8 Harris, 'Transition to high politics', 62–3.
9 Ibid. 72
10 Sidney Webb, 'Reform of the poor law', *Contemporary Review* lviii (1890), 95–120; Burdett, 'Our hospitals', 359–84.
11 Brand, *Doctors and the state*, 201–5.

until the 1940s but co-operation and the desirability of a state-run service increasingly became a matter of political discussion. The growing complexity of poor-law provision, an overlap of services for the sick and the education of the population in municipal socialism though the MAB, made many aware by the 1910s that the system was in need of a radical overhaul.

An increasing awareness that the state might have to intervene in the voluntary hospitals was intensified by their financial condition. The growth of the 'active state' was part ideological, part economic and part social, but within the London hospital sector it was practical financial issues that served to alter governors' attitudes towards the state. A growing system of payment from local government for the treatment of sexually transmitted diseases and tuberculosis, and for provision of infant and child welfare clinics and medical care for schoolchildren in the 1910s all involved hospitals accepting some money from the state.[12] If this was not a new departure, and the amounts paid were not significant, the First World War created a short-term reliance on government funding that by 1919 left London's hospitals facing an acute financial crisis. Under these conditions fears resurfaced about the possibility of state intervention. The Medical Consultative Council set the tone in 1920, realising that any government assistance would be 'the beginning of the end, and not many years would pass before the hospitals would be "provided" for out of public funds'.[13] It could not escape, however, the need for state aid and recommended that financial assistance should be made the reward for greater co-ordination. The new Board of Health was uninterested and with the government determined to cut spending and to avoid positive action, the Voluntary Hospital Council was established under Lord Onslow to distribute a £500,000 grant.[14] Of the first year's grants 80 per cent went to London only to be quickly discontinued once it was felt that the 'financial position of the hospitals was more favourable' than anticipated. Inter-war governments were all too aware of the economic and ideological value of the voluntary sector and wanted to underpin it to prevent the need for a centralised bureaucratic welfare system.[15] Further exchequer grants were refused in 1925, though some indirect aid continued to be given. Covenanted gifts, for example, were exempted from tax under the 1922 Finance Act and the 1930 Road Traffic Act required insurance companies to pay for long-term treatment. Working-class contributory schemes proved more effective at reducing hospital debt but only at a price. Institutions that benefited were placed on a quasi-insurance basis.[16]

Ideologically grants and contribution schemes challenged the hospitals'

---

12 Cherry, 'Before the National Health Service', 315–16.
13 Robert W. Chalmers, *Hospitals and the state: a popular study of the principles and practice of charity*, London 1928, 119.
14 J. E. Pater, *The making of the National Health Service*, London 1981, 12.
15 Daunton, 'Payment and participation', 168–72, 182.
16 Abel-Smith, *The hospitals*, 325; Cherry, 'Beyond national health insurance', 466.

voluntary status, but in many respects they built on existing arrangements. To meet the problems of wartime healthcare, local authorities between 1914 and 1918 had negotiated contractual agreements with the hospitals on a financial basis, adapting their existing financial relationship with poor-law unions. After the war the relationship was strengthened and hospitals became increasingly reliant on the income these agreements generated. In Manchester, government contributions provided 7 per cent of hospital income; in Norfolk and Suffolk this was between 4 and 9 per cent in the inter-war period. By the 1930s both the London County Council and the London hospitals had accepted that grants were a necessity.[17]

The London hospitals' financial position had introduced short-term government grants and long-term financial dependence on state funding into the voluntary system where in the 1890s it had been resisted. An unwilling precedent had been set and the development of the hospital further away from its charitable origins made state funding increasingly more attractive in practical, if not ideological terms. It gradually became clear that voluntarism was ill-suited to effective medical administration and that charity was unable to meet the hospitals' financial needs without limiting provision and leading to the widespread closure of beds. The same phenomenon had been apparent much earlier in other welfare sectors. Under these conditions few avenues seemed open other than state funding and control, though debates over the nature of such a health service and the strength of the voluntary ethic in hospitals and within the medical profession slowed the adoption of any scheme. In 1947 the same state intervention, even taking over the hospitals' accumulated debts, helped ease the acceptance of the NHS where governors had previously objected to the 1944 White Paper.

In the twentieth century the hospitals' finances became a central feature in the state's gradual assumption of the full economic burden of healthcare. In the nineteenth century financial concerns underlay the debate over hospital reform. A new charitable 'zeal' was suggested because no other alternative to voluntarism could be realistically considered. Money from direct philanthropy, however, was already insufficient to meet the London hospitals' needs and where the administration remained dominated by voluntarism, charity had long been diluted in the hospitals' finances. The two were not incompatible. Governors continued to seek charitable funding, but as the hospital developed the unacceptable possibility of state intervention increasingly became the only realistic option.

---

17 Pickstone, *Medicine and industrial society*, 252; Cherry, 'Beyond national insurance', 465.

APPENDIX

Financial Sources and Methodology

Problems of evidence

This study has, in part, been based on the information contained in the financial records (mainly cash books, receipt books and ledgers), annual reports and public financial statements of the seven hospitals studied.[1] Contemporaries complained that hospital accounts were idiosyncratic, complicated and confusing. They believed that this presented problems that prevented satisfactory institutional comparisons. For administrators, as Robert Pinker has shown, this could be beneficial, allowing them to conceal any debt or irregularity.[2] Lax procedures were publicised, often with an incredulous tone. In 1890 the *Hospital* reported that St John's Hospital for Diseases of the Skin kept its accounts 'upon loose sheets of paper' that had become muddled. In the records 'amounts appeared twice' and items could not 'be traced and totals cannot be made to agree'.[3] Many believed that these problems were widespread. Concern manifested itself in a campaign led by Henry Burdett and the Metropolitan Hospital Sunday Fund (founded in 1873) for a uniform system of accounts, a move partly inspired by a desire to prevent embezzlement and to allow a comparison of institutions so that their relative utility and efficiency could be assessed as a guide to contributions. The Metropolitan Hospital Saturday Fund (founded in 1874) also applied pressure for uniform accounts, borrowing the Sunday Fund's schema. Their efforts were not entirely successful and not all hospitals were willing to follow their suggestions. For example, in 1886 Burdett could still complain that University College Hospital's accounting was 'not intelligible'.[4]

For the historian this would present numerous problems, especially as time and storage have ensured that many financial records are no longer available or appear out of context. However, hospital accounts are not as confusing as contemporaries wanted to make out. The foundation of the Sunday Fund and Saturday Fund forced a measure of standardisation and all hospitals that wanted to receive a grant from the funds had to adopt their classifications. Most accounts, however, were already arranged in a double-entry format. By balancing the hospital's internal financial records with financial decisions

---

1   See bibliography for each hospital and financial records used.
2   Pinker, *English hospital statistics*, 142–3.
3   *Hospital*, 1 Feb. 1890, 286.
4   UCH, abstract of UCH committees, UCL, UNOF/2/3 (2).

made in committee meetings, the balance sheets bound in annual reports, and contemporary evidence in journals and periodicals, it is possible to create an accurate picture.

Classification

Hospitals and contemporaries used a standard terminology in their classification of income. In 1869 Burdett and William Laundry drew up a uniform system of accounts that was adopted by the Sunday Fund and Saturday Fund and revised by the Prince of Wales Hospital Fund in 1906.[5] The funds presented the ideal model for accounts and when they framed their classification they used the terminology hospitals used. Most terms are self-explanatory and follow standard dictionary definitions. In this study, these classifications have been used to analyse hospital finance.

Hospitals divided their income and expenditure into two categories: 'ordinary', which included income and expenditure that were seen as annual and 'reliable', and 'extraordinary', income and expenditure that were infrequent or unpredictable. In this last category such items as legacies or the cost of building were covered. For income, the term 'extraordinary' allowed hospital governors to present income in terms that would not create the image that they were a well-funded institution, an impression that would limit their public appeal. For expenditure it concealed extravagance and presented the image that the hospital was normally run on economical lines. This vocabulary was used to ensure that the right impression was created.

Philanthropic income was separated into donations (one-off gifts), subscriptions (annual payment of a set sum), legacies (amounts left by will, including those for endowed beds which were usually listed separately as extraordinary income), income from various benevolent funds recorded under their names (i.e. Sunday Fund, Saturday Fund, Prince of Wales Hospital Fund etc.), collections (collection boxes, street collection, church collections) and entertainments (plays, concerts etc.). Each annual report contained a list of contributors that recorded the amount given as a donation or subscription. Where an individual gave both these were listed separately. Charity bazaars, annual dinners, balls and public appeals, if not listed separately, were included in the accounts as a donation, though the figure they raised was always recorded in the minutes. Not all hospitals used the separate terms for entertainments and collections. These could be listed as separate events or more commonly placed with donations.

Non-charitable income was less complex and related more closely to the source of income. This wide category included dividends (interest on investments), rent (from land or houses – the two were not separated), sale of

---

[5] See Henry Burdett, *Uniform system of accounts for hospitals and institutions*, London 1893.

Table 24: Classification of income

Category	Sources of income included
Direct philanthropy	Donations, subscriptions, legacies, entertainments, collections, any money given as a voluntary gift.
Indirect philanthropy	Sunday Fund, Saturday Fund, Prince of Wales Hospital Fund, individual hospital collection schemes
Property	Rent, dividends, deposits, sale of stock/property, sale of waste material, insurance.
Function	Patient payments, nursing, fees, medical services (i.e. patient baths), public authorities (i.e. poor-law)
Loans	
Balance	Income from previous year
Sundries	Small amounts not classified

investments/property, sale of waste material, loans, deposits (money held on deposit, not the income from the interest it generated which was included under dividends), nursing (probationers' payment for their training and additional money from the hire of nurses was distinguished), payment from patients (separated into money from in-patients and out-patients), payment from public authorities (i.e. poor law, Metropolitan Asylum Board) though this was often listed as patient payments, money from additional services (includes use of hospital baths etc.), college or medical fees, insurance (premiums or a claim made) and trust funds for scholarships or prizes. Contemporary classification can be further subdivided, as shown in table 24. These classifications are illustrated and explained in more detail in chapter 3.

Method of calculation

Three reference periods have been selected to illustrate change and development over the period: 1850–5, 1870–5 and 1890–5. For each period a five-year average has been calculated to produce an overall figure. By using such an average, annual fluctuations in income are smoothed to present a more accurate representation of the relative financial contribution of each source of income to the overall structure of funding.

Bibliography

Unpublished primary sources

London, Bethlem Royal Hospital
Minutes of the court of governors, 1835

London, Hospital for Sick Children, Peter Pan Gallery and Archive, Great Ormond Street (GOSH)

1/2/1–21	Minutes of the committee of management, 1850–1900
1/5/1–12	Minutes of the medical committee, 1852–99
1/5/52	Medical committee papers, 1894–5
1/6/1	Minutes of the board of governors, 1869–94
1/7/1	Minutes of the joint committee, 1894–1908
1/8/1–2	Minutes of the finance committee, 1858–60
1/11/1	Subcommittee minutes, 1884–5
3/1/1	General ledger, 1887–92
3/1/20	Balance sheets, 1890–1902
3/4/7	Miscellaneous financial records
5/1/3	Staff rules
5/2/2	List of patrons and officers
6/1/1	Register of life governors, 1852–90
6/1/2	List of life donors
6/1/4	Register of donors, 1890–7
6/1/8	Register of legacies, 1855–85
6/1/25–37	Register of special cots, 1868–1918
6/2/1	Royalty correspondence file
6/6/1	Miscellaneous donors file
8/151–4	Press cuttings
8/162	Patients' correspondence
8/168	Complaints and scandals
9/1/1	Admissions register, 1852–5
9/1/2	Medical reports, 1855–7
9/1/6	Admissions book, 1859–64
9/1/7	Medical reports, 1859–62
9/1/20	Register of in-patients, 1891–2
9/1/22	Register of applicants for admission, 1881–92
14/18	Specimen of appeals, 1852–93

London, London Metropolitan Archive (LMA), Northampton Road, Clerkenwell
Charitable Organisation Society (A/FWA)

C/A11/1	Council minutes, 1894–8

221

C/A26/1–10	Minutes of the medical advisory subcommittee, 1871–98
C/A42/1	Minutes of the special committee on the reform of the metropolitan medical charities, 1888–93
C/A42/2	Petition to the House of Lords, 1889
C/A44/1	Minutes of the general committee for the promotion of a central board, 1897–1900
C/D52/1	Hospital for Sick Children, 1875–1934
C/D61/1	Metropolitan Hospital Saturday Fund, 1875–1939

General Lying-In Hospital (H1/GLI)

| A2/5 | Weekly board minutes |
| A29/1–21 | Minutes of the committee of inquiry, 1880 |

Guy's Hospital (H9/Gy)

A1/2/1	Minutes of the general court, 1815–60
A1/3–4/1	Minutes of the general court, 1861–98
A1/4	Sundry court papers, 1881–98
A3/8–11	Minutes of the court of committees, 1850–99
A3/11/1–3	Committee papers, 1883–99
A5/1/1	Clerks' minute book, 1854–1903
A5/1/2–4	Memoranda, 1854–1903
A17/1	Minutes of the committee re accommodation for patients, 1849–55
A18/1/1	Minutes of the committee of finance and estates, 1855–61
A19/1	Minutes of the taking-in committee, 1880–96
A20/1–2	Minutes of the medical committee, 1881–1906
A21/1–2	Minutes of the estate committee, 1887–1903
A23/1	Minutes of the staff and school committee, 1896–1906
A24/1	Minutes of the finance committee, 1896–1934
A25/1	Minutes of the house committee, 1896–8
A40/1	Agenda books of the general court and court of committees, 1830–93
A41/1–2	Agenda papers, 21 Oct. 1896
A48/5	Will and Act of Incorporation, 1725
A53/1	'Regulations for the management of Guy's Hospital', 1874
A54/1–4	Act to amend Act of Incorporation, 1897–8
A67/1–8	Weekly reports of superintendence, 1857–1903
A68/1	Medical officers' book, 1880–2
A69/2	House physicians' journal, 1893–9
A72/1	Report on Guy's Hospital and its property, 1868
A73/1	Supplementary report by committee of physicians and surgeons, 21 Mar. 1869
A73/2	Memorandum on the payment of staff, 1882–1913
A74/1	Report of medical committee on payment by out-patients, 30 May 1883
A74/2	Report of subcommittee on financial position of hospital, 19 June 1883
A75/1	Report of committees of management, 28 Oct. 1896
A93/1–5	Treasurer's reports, 1887–92

A94/2	Annual reports, 1898–1902
A96/1–14	Printed lists of presidents and governors, 1865–78
A97/1	List of governors, 1893
A99/1–12	Members of court of committees, 1863–74
A101/1	List of medical men made governors, 1725–1884
A104/1–17	Letter book of treasurer, 1857–97
A107/1–2	Letter book of clerk, 1875–1901
A112–122	Letter boxes
A118/1–24	Correspondence with Charity Commission, 1882–7
A164/1/1–2	Memorandum book of John Steele, 1855–77
A172/1–3	Correspondence with Charity Commission re scheme for receiving paying patients, Mar. 1884
A219/1–28	Correspondence regarding nursing dispute, 1879–80
A219/19	Printer circular, 5 Feb. 1880
A220/1–9	Gull to Lushington, 1879–80
A221/1–2	Habershon to Lushington, 1879–80
A222/1–3	Petition from thirteen sisters, 5–10 Dec. 1879
A223/1–14	Correspondence on nursing dispute, 1879–80
A224/1–2	Memorandum by Lushington, Mar. 1880
A224/3	Statement by Lushington, 12 July 1880
A225/1–3	Minutes of the general court of governors, 3–11 Mar. 1880
A227/1	Medical staff to governors, 12 Apr. 1880
A229/1–13	Correspondence regarding demonstration of students, 16–24 June 1880
A229/1–13	Nursing dispute miscellaneous cuttings, 1879–80
A230/2	List of changes made in nursing staff, June–July 1880
A230/3	List of medical and surgical staff who had not spoken to Burt, June–July 1880
A233/1	Report of the subcommittee on nursing, 1880
A235/1–3	Correspondence of medical staff to treasurer and governors relating to report on taking-in committee, 4 Aug.–25 Oct. 1880
A235/1–3	General court of governors, 3–11 Mar. 1880
A262/1	Patient statistics, 1868
A263/1	Volume of statistics, 1863–75
A270/1–2	Salters Company to Lushington on endowment of 5 beds, 5–10 Aug. 1894
A281/1/1–7	Register of officers, 1829–1918
B2/1–5	Register of admission and discharge: medical cases, 1854–92
B3/1–12	Register of admission and discharge: surgical cases, 1854–92
D1/8–12	Ledger, 1842–1905
D5/13–19	Financial journal, 1850–99
D11/8–13	Cash book, 1848–90
D19–20	Abstracts of accounts, 1852/3–96
D45/1	Appeals cash book, 1886–98
Y74/1	Special appeal, 1886
Y121/1–2	St Thomas's, annual statements, 1895–6

Prince of Wales Hospital Fund (KE)

A/KE/2/1	Minutes of the general council, 1897–1901
A/KE/20/1	Minutes of the distribution committee, 1897–1917
A/KE/27/1	Minutes of the executive council, 1897–1903
A/KE/250/1	Report on the Hospital for Sick Children
A/KE/259/1	Report on University College Hospital
A/KE/300/1–2	Annual reports, 1897–8
A/KE/568	Correspondence, 1898–9
A/KE/750	Press cuttings, 1897–1903
A/KE/751/2	Lister to prince of Wales, 16 Mar. 1898
A/KE/751/3	Stamps sold in aid of fund, 1897–8

Royal Hospital for Diseases of the Chest (H33/RCH)

A1/1–3	Governors' minute book, 1848–67
A1/4–8	Council minute book, 1868–1902
A2/1–2	Minutes of the court of governors, 1867–1921
A3/1–2	Minutes of the medical council, 1867–1907
A4/1–5	Minutes of the house committee, 1867–99
A5/1–2	Minutes of the finance committee, 1878–1901
D1/1	Register of subscribers and donors, 1890–2
Y1/1	Visitors book, 1886–1921

Whitechapel Union (St.B.G)

G/Wh/21	Board of Guardians' minutes, 1857

London, Public Record Office

CHAR3/12	Taxation of charities
CHAR3/22	City livery companies
CHAR3/38	Charity Commissioners
CHAR3/57	Select Committee on the Charity Commission

London, Royal London Hospital Archive and Museum, St Augustine with St Philip's Church, Newark Street

A/1/17	Copy charter, bye-laws and standing orders, 1888
A/1/22	Copy charter and London Hospital Act, 1884
A/1/24	Agreement between the governors and the medical and surgical officers for establishment of college board, 4 June 1879
A/2/10–15	Minutes of the court of governors, 1846–98
A/4/11–16	Reports of the house committee, 1849–1907
A/5/26–47	Minutes of the house committee, 1847–1900
A/9/2–3	Minutes of the accounts committee, 1846–1912
A/9/41	Minutes of the estates subcommittee, 1885–1903
A/9/51	Minutes of the finance committee, 1897–1914
A/9/113	Minutes of the subcommittee on payment of patients, 1878
A/9/121–2	Minutes of the subcommittee (general), 1882–1903
A/10/8	Minutes of public meeting in aid of the London, 13 Apr. 1883
A/16/5–6	House visitors' book, 1849–1924

A/17/7	Physicians and surgeons' report book, 1836–67
A/17/15	Report by William Nixon *re* relative costs of the hospital compared with the Metropolitan Free Hospital, 18 Feb. 1873
A/17/17	Report by William Nixon on analysis of expenditure, 15 Mar. 1880
A/17/49	Report by house committee on allegations against nursing department, Dec. 1890
A/19/2–3	Register of life governors, 1859–1907
A/25/1	Draft correspondence of Sydney Holland, 1898–1900
A/26/3–9	Press cuttings, 1875–99
A/26/31	Scrapbook, 1870–98
D/3/21	Schedules of leases, 1866–97
D/4/1–9	Endowments, trusts and investments, 1824–87
D/22–3	Register of leases, 1888–1935
D/24	Register of assignment of leases, 1862–1929
F/1/9–14	Treasurer's ledgers, 1847–1901
F/9/3–4	Legacy book, 1844–98
F/9/8	'E' revisionary legacy book, 1871–1918
F/9/31	Register of endowed beds and cots, 1880–1924
F/10/6	Estate ledger, 1890–6
M/1/11–26	Physicians and surgeons' inpatients, 1883–98
M/3/74	Register of surgical operations, 1852–62
Mc/A/1/1–3	Minutes of the medical council, 1846–80
LM/1	Minutes of college council, 1880–1901

London, St Bartholomew's Hospital Archives (SBH), West Smithfield
German Hospital

GHA 2/1–10	Minutes of the hospital committee, 1843–1907
GHA 4/1	Gülich to duke of Cambridge, 22 Mar. 1894
GHA 5/1–2	Minutes of the annual general court, 1846–1923
GHA 6/1	Notice of general court meeting, *c.* 1890
GHA 6/2	Official shorthand report of proceedings of general court, 1894
GHA 8/1–12	Minutes of board of household management, 1849–1903
GHA 9/2	Memorandum book of the board of household management, 1849–59
GHA 14/1–2	Minutes of the bazaar committee, 1847–69
GHA 14/3	Income from bazaars and list of ladies to have stalls, 1858–69
GHA 18/1–2	Opening of German Hospital, 15 Oct. 1845
GHA 18/3	'A word in season to the governors and friends of the German Hospital', 1894
GHA 19/1–2	Letter book, 1846–74
GHA 19/21–34	Letters concerning royal patronage, 1862–1936
GHA 19/35–58	Letters concerning attendance and stewarding of anniversary festival dinners, 1883–1912
GHA 20/1	Draft petition to Lord Mayor and City of London for financial support for new building, *c.* 1863
GHA 21/1	List of committee members, 1845–1918

GHA 21/2	Copy of answers given to the hospitals committee of the House of Lords, 1891
GHA 23/1/1	Visitors' book, 1845–1929
GHA 23/2	Interim visitors' reports, 1859–71
GHB 2/1–2	Cash books, 1845–56
GHB 4/1	Income analysis ledgers, 1891–1908
GHB 10/21	Papers concerning a bed endowment, 1901
GHB 11/1	Investment ledgers, 1870–1934
GHB 14/1	Circular letter requesting ladies to contribute donations to new building, c. 1862
GHM 1/1	Minutes of the medical committee, 1845–94
X 5/26	Memoirs of William Henry Cross, 1866–1905

St Bartholomew's Hospital

FD 7/5/2	Charity Commission to governors, 10 Feb. 1877
Ha 1/21–7	Minutes of the board of governors, 1854–1903
Hb 5/3	Register of legacies, 1764–1917
Hb 19	Trusts register, 1843–1972
Hb 23/3–4	General account books, 1863–1901
Hc 9/4–6	View and survey books, 1843–1906
Hc 15/1–3	Register of leases, 1835–1923
MC 1/1–2	Minutes of the medical committees, 1843–1903
MC 3/1	Staff regulations
MR 3/1–6	Admission register (female), 1870–1903
MR 9/58–86	Statistical tables of medical and surgical registrars, 1861–1900

London, University College Hospital Archive, D. M. S. Watson Library, University College (UCH)

A/1/1	Minutes of the medical committee, 1834–1900
A/1/2/1–7	Minutes of the general committee, 1844–96
A/1/3/2–4	Minutes of the house and finance committee, 1880–99
A/1/4/1	Samaritan fund, 1880–91
A/1/5/1–2	Subcommittee minutes, 1884–1905
A/2/1/1–319	Legacy papers
MR/3A/1–8	Medical and surgical registrars' reports, 1872–1901
UNOF/2/3	Abstract of UCH committees, 1849–1900

London, Wellcome Institute, Contemporary Medical Archive Centre

| GC/181/B.4 | Bowlby to Sir Trevor Lawrence |

Annual reports

Bristol Infirmary, annual reports, 1850–1900 (Bristol Record Office)
Charitable Organisation Society, annual reports, 1872–1900 (LMA)
German Hospital, annual reports, 1850–1900 (SBH)
Hospital for Sick Children, annual reports, 1850–1900 (GOSH)
London Hospital, annual reports, 1850–70, 1872–1900 (Royal London Hospital Archive)

Norfolk and Norwich Hospital, annual reports, 1850–98 (Norwich Record Office, City Library, Norwich)

Royal Hospital for Diseases of the Chest, annual reports, 1850–1900 (LMA)

Royal West Sussex Hospital, annual reports, 1826–1900 (West Sussex County Record Office, Chichester)

St Bartholomew's Hospital, report, 1889 (SBH)

Society of St Vincent De Paul, annual reports, 1885–95

University College Hospital, annual reports, 1850–1900 (UCH)

Published primary sources

Official documents and publications (in date order)

Select Committee on Medical Education, PP 1834 xiii

Thirty-Second report of the Charity Commission, PP 1840 xxxii

Select Committee on Metropolitan Local Government etc., PP 1867 xii

Report on Candidates for the Medical Department, PP 1878–9 xliv

Royal Commission on the Medical Acts, PP 1882 xxix

Hansard, 3rd ser. cccxxx–cccxc, 1880–90

Hansard, 4th ser. i, 1892

Select Committee of the House of Lords on Metropolitan Hospitals etc., First Report, PP 1890 xvi; Second Report, PP 1890/1 xiii; Third Report, PP 1892 xiii

Returns of Official Expenses in Connection with the Election of Governors, PP 1894 lxxxv

Royal Commission on Agricultural Depression, PP 1897 xv

Newspapers and periodicals

British Medical Journal

Charity

Charity Organisation Reporter

Charity Organisation Review

Charity Record & Philanthropic Messenger

Charity Record & Philanthropic News (after 1890 continued as *Charity Record, Philanthropic News, Hospital Times & Official Advertiser*)

City Press

Contemporary Review

Cornhill Magazine

Daily Mail

Daily Telegraphy

Economic Journal

Economic Review

Examiner

Fortnightly Review

Fraser's Magazine of Town and Country

Graphic

Hospital

Hospital Gazette & Students' Journal
Hospital Saturday Fund Journal
Illustrated Times
Journal of the Royal Statistical Society
The Lancet
Medical Examiner
Nineteenth Century
Nursing Record
Medical Times & Gazette
Morning Leader
Morning Post
Pall Mall Gazette
Philanthropist
Political Science Quarterly
Punch
Quarterly Review
Star
The Times
Truth
Westminster Review and Foreign Quarterly

Contemporary books and articles

Acland, H. W., *Medicine in modern times*, London 1869

Acland, Reginald B. P. (ed.), *Hospital Saturday and medical charities*, London 1898

Addams, J. and others, *Philanthropy and social progress*, New York 1893

Anon., 'A visit to the Hospital for Sick Children', *Fraser's Magazine of Town and Country* xlix (1854), 62–7

Anon., *Almsgiving destroying charity, and, the reverse, charity nourishing almsgiving*, Bath 1862

Anon., *Charity: a tract for the times*, London 1874

Anon. [Robert Louis Stevenson], 'A charity bazaar', *Cornhill Magazine* iv (1861), 338–9

Anon., *Christian charity*, London 1859

Anon., *Confessions of an old almsgiver, or three cheers for the Charity Organisation Society etc.*, London 1871

Anon., 'Confusion in medical charities', *Nineteenth Century* xxxii (1892), 298–310

Anon., 'The modern hospital', *Quarterly Review* clxxvii (1893), 464–94

Anon., 'Philanthropy of the age and its relation to social evils', *Westminster Review and Foreign Quarterly* xxxv (1869), 437–57

Antrobus, Edmund, *Christian charity, its characteristics and channels*, London 1852

Arnot, William, *Christian philanthropy*, London 1856

Ashwell, William, *Essay on charity or, bits and scraps selected from various eminent authors*, London 1852

Aveling, Thomas W. B., *Christian philanthropy*, London 1874

Bacon, Francis, *Goodness, and goodness of heart*, London 1625

Barnet, Henrietta, 'Women as philanthropists', in T. Stanton (ed.), *The woman question in Europe*, London 1884

Barrett, Jonathan, *Observations on endowments for charitable purposes*, London 1852

Bartley, George C. T., *The work of charity in promoting provident habits*, London 1879

Bickersteth, R., *The labourer's friend*, London 1855

Blaikie, William G., *Leaders in modern philanthropy*, London 1884

Bogot, Daniel, *Faith, hope and charity*, London 1878

Booth, Charles, *Life and labour of the people of London*, i, London 1889

Bosanquet, Charles B., *London: some account of its growth, charitable agencies and wants*, London 1868

———— 'Principle and chief dangers of the administration of charity', in Miss J. Adams and others, *Philanthropy and social progress*, New York 1893

Buckle, Fleetwood, *Vital and economical statistics of hospitals and infirmaries etc of England and Wales for the year 1863*, London 1865

Buckler, Henry R., *The perfection of man by charity*, London 1889

Burdett, Henry C., *Hospital Sunday and Hospital Saturday: their origin, progress and development together with suggestions for making both funds more useful to hospitals*, London 1884

———— *Hospitals and asylums of the world*, iii, London 1893

———— *Hospitals and charitable annual: 1895*, London 1895

———— *Hospitals and charitable annual: 1901*, London 1901

———— *Hospitals and the state with an account of the nursing at London hospitals and statistical tables showing the actual and comparative cost of management*, London 1881

———— 'Our hospitals', *Nineteenth Century* xiii (1883), 359–84

———— *Pay hospitals and pay wards throughout the world: facts in support of a re-arrangement of the English system of medical relief*, London 1879

———— *Uniform system of accounts for hospitals and institutions*, London 1893

Burford Rawlings, B., *The Church, the laity and the hospitals*, London 1886

———— 'The honorary element in hospital administration', *Fraser's Magazine* xxiv (1881), 57–67

Carter, R. Brundell, 'The London medical schools', *Contemporary Review* xxxiv (1878/9), 582–93

Chudleigh, M., *Charity: its essence and operation*, London 1882

Clifford-Smith, J. L. (ed.), *Hospital management*, London 1883

Constable, H., 'Measure of Christian liberality', in *Gold and the gospel*, London 1853

Davis, Henry, *Our hospitals: their difficulties and remedy*, London 1894

Davis, William, *Hints to philanthropist, or a collective view of practical means for improving the condition of the poor and labouring classes of society and of a careless administration of funds left for charitable purposes*, Bath 1821

Dawes, Richard, *The evils of indiscriminate charity and of careless administration of funds left of charitable purposes*, London 1856

Day, George T., *Christian philanthropy*, London 1852

Engels, Frederick, *The condition of the working class in England in 1844*, New York 1844

Fairman, Edward, *Philanthropy in 1886: a word of warning to the truly benevolent*, London 1886

Farrar, Frederick W., *Social and present-day questions*, London 1891

Foote, Henry W., *Bountiful return of charity*, Boston 1869

Ford, Gabriel E., *Religion and philanthropy*, London 1894

Foster, Balthazar W., *Political powerlessness of the medical profession: its causes and remedies*, London 1883

Galton, Douglas, *Healthy hospitals: observations on some points connected with hospital construction etc.*, Oxford 1893

Gilbart, James W., *Moral and religious duties of public companies*, London 1856

Greenwood, James, *Seven curses of London*, London 1869

Gull, William W., *Clinical observation in relation to medicine in modern times etc.*, London 1869

Guy, William A., *Rescued from beggars; or how to support our hospitals*, London 1853

Hake, A. E., *Suffering London*, London 1892

Hawksley, Thomas, *Charities of London and some errors in their administration*, London 1869

Higginson, T. W., 'The word philanthropy', in Committee of the Free Religious Association (ed.), *Freedom and fellowship in religion*, Boston 1875

Hobhouse, Arthur, *A lecture on the characteristics of charitable foundations in England etc.*, London 1868

———— *The dead hand*, London 1880

Holyoake, George J., *Patriotism by charity*, Leicester 1885

Horsford, John, *Philanthropy: the genius of Christianity*, London 1862

Howe, W. F. (ed.), *Twenty-forth annual edition of the classified directory to the metropolitan charities for 1899*, London 1899

Huntington, J., 'Philanthropy: its success and failure', in Miss J. Adams and others, *Philanthropy and social progress*, Boston 1893

James, John A., *Christian philanthropy*, London 1859

'A Lady', *On charity*, London 1861

Lambert, Brook, 'Charity: its aims and means', *Contemporary Review* xxiii (1873/4), 460–5

Lane, Edward W., *Thesis: notes on medical subjects, comprising remarks on the constitution and management of British hospitals*, Edinburgh 1853

Loch, Charles S., 'Charity: noxious and beneficent', *Westminster Review and Foreign Quarterly* iii (1853), 62–88

———— *Charity organisation*, London 1890

———— *Charity and social life: a study of religious and social thought in relation to charitable methods and institutions*, London 1910

———— *Cross purposes in medical reform*, London 1884

———— *Some necessary reforms in charitable work etc.*, London 1882

Low, Sampson, *The charities of London, comprehending the benevolent, educational and religious institutions: their origins, progress, and present-position*, London 1850

Mackay, Thomas, *The state and charity*, London 1898

Mackenzie, Morrell, 'The use and abuse of hospitals', *Contemporary Review* lviii (1890), 501–19

Maguire, Robert, *Christian charity*, London 1863

Mill, John Stewart, *Autobiography*, New York n.d.

Miram, [?], *What is charity?*, Dublin 1850

Mouat, Frederick and Henry Saxon Snell, *Hospital construction and management*, London 1883

Nelson Hardy, H., *The London hospitals and the jubilee*, Bristol 1887

Nightingale, Florence, *Notes on hospitals*, London 1863

Oppert, Franz, *Hospitals, infirmaries and dispensaries: their construction, interior arrangements and management, etc.*, London 1867

Ormsby, Lambert, *The social, scientific and political influence of the medical profession in 1886*, Dublin 1886

Paton, Chalmers I., *Freemasonry: the three Masonic graces, faith, hope and charity*, London 1878

Peck, Benjamin D., *Reflex influence of benevolence*, London 1852

Peck, Francis, *The uncharitableness of inadequate relief*, London 1879

Phelps, Lancelot R., *Poor law and charity*, Oxford 1887

Pope, George V., *Faith, hope and charity*, London 1870

Pretyman, John R., *Voluntary v. legal relief*, London 1879

Rathbone, William, *Social duties considered with reference to the organisation of efforts in works of benevolence and public utility*, London 1867

Reid Rentoul, Robert, *The dignity of women's health and the nemesis of its neglect*, London 1890

———— *Proposed sterialisation of certain mental and physical degenerates*, Newcastle 1903

———— *Race culture; or race suicide*, London 1906

———— *Reform of our voluntary medical charities*, London 1891

Ritchie, David G., *The principles of state intervention*, London 1891

Roberts, Harry, *Public control of hospitals*, London 1895

Scalpel, A., *Dying scientifically*, London 1888

———— *St Bernard's: the romance of a medical student*, London 1888

S. E., 'The poor and the hospital', *Fraser's Magazine* xiii (1876), 715–27

Sherlock, Thomas, *The measure of Christian charity and their rewards*, Daventry 1851

Sibly, Walker K., *State aided v. voluntary hospitals: an exposition of the abuse of English hospitals*, London 1896

Steele, John, 'Agricultural depression and its effects on a leading London hospital', *Royal Statistical Journal* (1892), 1–14

———— *Summary of information relative to the working of the outpatient departments in thirteen London hospitals*, London 1878

Stevenson, Robert Louis, *Charity bazaar: an allegorical dialogue*, London 1868

Sturge, Octavius, 'Doctors and nurses', *Nineteenth Century* xi (1880), 1089–96

Timewell, James, *The state carriage*, London 1895

Warner, Amos G., *Evolution of charities and charitable institutions*, London 1893

Watson, A. W. (ed.), *Sermons for Sundays, festivals, and fasts and other liturgical occasions*, 2nd ser. iii, London 1847

Webb, Sydney, 'Reform of the poor law', *Contemporary Review* lviii (1890), 95–120

West, Charles, *On hospital organisation, with special reference to the organisation of hospitals for children*, London 1877

Withington, Charles F., *Relation of hospitals to medical education*, Boston 1886

Wright, Joseph H., *Charity organisation*, London 1883

Secondary sources

Abel-Smith, Brian, *A history of the nursing profession*, London 1960
—— *The hospitals, 1800–1948: a study in social administration in England and Wales*, London 1964
Ackerman, Evelyn B., *Health care in the Parisian countryside, 1800–1914*, New Brunswick 1990
Andrew, Donna T., *Philanthropy and police: London charity in the eighteenth century*, Princeton 1989
Ayers, Gwendolyne, *England's first state hospitals and the Metropolitan Asylums Board, 1867–1930*, London 1971
Baly, Monica E., *Nursing and social change*, London 1982
Banks, J. A., *Prosperity and parenthood: a study of family planning among the Victorian middle classes*, Aldershot 1954
Barker, Theo and Michael Robbins, *A history of London transport*, London 1963
Barry, Jonathan, and Colin Jones (eds), *Medicine and charity before the welfare state*, London 1994
Behlmer, George K., *Child abuse and moral reform in England, 1870–1908*, Stanford, Ca. 1982
Belcher, Victor, *The City Parochial Foundation, 1891–1991: a trust for the poor of London*, Aldershot 1991
Berry, Amanda, 'Community sponsorship and the hospital patient in late eighteenth-century England', in Peregrine Horden and Richard Smith (eds), *Locus of care: communities, institutions, and the provision of welfare since antiquity*, London 1998, 126–50
Bishop, P. and others, *The seven ages of the Brompton*, Guildford 1991
Black, Eugene C., *The social politics of Anglo-Jewry, 1880–1980*, Oxford 1988
Borsay, Ann, 'Cash and conscience: financing the General Hospital at Bath, c. 1738–50', *SHM* iv (1991), 207–29
—— ' "Persons of honour and reputation": the voluntary hospital in the age of corruption', *Medical History* xxxv (1991), 281–94
Bradley, Ian, *The call to seriousness: the evangelical impact on the Victorians*, London 1976
Brand, Jeanne L., *Doctors and the state: the British medical profession and government action in public health, 1870–1912*, Baltimore 1965
Bremer, Robert H., *Giving: charity and philanthropy in history*, New Brunswick 1996
Briggs, Asa, and Anne Macartney, *Toynbee Hall: the first hundred years*, London 1984
Brightfield, M., 'The medical profession in early Victorian England', *BHM* xxxv (1961), 238–56
Brockbank, William, *Portrait of a hospital, 1752–1948*, London 1952
Brown, Ford K., *Father to the Victorians: the age of Wilberforce*, Cambridge 1961
Bullough, V. and M. Vogt, 'Women, menstruation and nineteenth-century medicine', *BHM* viii (1973), 66–82
Bynum, W. F., 'Medical philanthropy after 1850', in Bynum and Porter, *Companion encyclopedia*, ii. 1480–94
—— *Science and the practice of medicine in the nineteenth century*, Cambridge 1996

———— and Roy Porter (eds), *Common encyclopedia of the history of medicine*, ii, London 1997

Cahill, M. and T. Jowett, 'The new philanthropy: the emergence of the Bradford City Guild of Help', *Journal of Social Policy* ix (1980), 359–82

Cameron, H. C., *Mr Guy's Hospital, 1726–1948*, London 1954

Cannadine, David N., *Lords and landlords: the aristocracy and the towns 1774–1967*, Leicester 1980

———— *Patricians, power and politics in nineteenth-century towns*, Leicester 1982

Carlin, Martha, 'Medieval English hospitals', in Granshaw and Porter, *The hospital in history*, 21–39

Carr Saunders, Alexander M. and Paul A. Wilson, *The professions*, Oxford 1933

Cavallo, Sandra, 'Motivations of benefactors: an overview of approaches to the study of charity', in Barry and Jones, *Medicine and charity*, 46–62

Chalmers, Robert W., *Hospitals and the state: a popular study of the principles and practice of charity*, London 1928

Cherry, Steven, 'Accountability, entitlement and control issues and voluntary hospital funding, c. 1860–1939', *SHM* ix (1996), 215–33

———— 'Before the National Health Service: financing the voluntary hospitals', *EcHR* c (1997), 305–26

———— 'Beyond national health insurance: the voluntary hospitals and the hospital contributory schemes', *SHM* v (1992), 455–82

———— 'The role of a provincial hospital: the Norfolk and Norwich Hospital, 1771–1880', *Population Studies* xxvi (1972), 291–306

Clark-Kennedy, A. E., *The London: a study in the voluntary hospital system*, ii, London 1963

———— *London pride: the story of a voluntary hospital*, London 1979

Collini, Stefan, 'Idealism and "Cambridge idealism" ', *Historical Journal* xviii (1975), 171–7

———— *Liberalism and sociology: L. T. Hobhouse and political argument in England, 1880–1914*, Cambridge 1979

———— *Public moralists: political thought and intellectual life in Britain, 1850–1930*, Oxford 1991

Cooter, Roger (ed.), *Studies in the history of alternative medicine*, Basingstoke 1988

Cox, Jeffrey, *English churches in a secular society: Lambeth, 1870–1930*, Oxford 1982

Crowther, M. A., *The workhouse system, 1834–1929: the history of an English social institution*, London 1981

Croxson, Bronwyn, 'Public and private faces of eighteenth-century London dispensary charity', *Medical History* xli (1997), 127–49

Cunningham, Andrew and Roger French (eds), *The medical enlightenment of the eighteenth century*, Cambridge 1990

Currie, Robert, *Methodism divided: a study in the sociology of ecumenicalism*, London 1968

———— Alan D. Gilbert and Lee Horsley, *Churches and churchgoers*, London 1977

Dandeker, C., *Surveillance, power and modernity: bureaucracy and discipline from 1700 to the present day*, Cambridge 1990

Daunton, Martin, *Coal metropolis: Cardiff, 1870–1914*, Leicester 1977

———— 'Payment and participation: welfare and state formation in Britain 1900–51', *Past and Present* cl (1996), 169–216

———— (ed.), *Charity, self-interest and welfare in the English past*, London 1996

Davidoff, Leonore and Catherine Hall, *Family fortunes: men and women of the English middle class, 1780–1850*, London 1987

Davies, John, 'Aristocratic town-makers and the coal metropolis', in Cannadine, *Patricians, power and politics in nineteenth-century towns*, 17–67

Davies, T. G., *Deeds not words: a history of the Swansea General and Eye Hospital, 1817–1948*, Cardiff 1988

Davis, John, *Reforming London: the London government problem, 1855–1900*, Oxford 1988

Dennis, Richard, *English industrial cities of the nineteenth century: a social geography*, Cambridge 1984

Digby, Anne, *Making a medical living: doctors and patients in the English market of medicine, 1720–1911*, Cambridge 1994

Dingwall, Robert, Anne Marie Rafferty and Charles Webster, *An introduction to the social history of nursing*, London 1988

———— and Philip Lewis (eds), *The sociology of the professions: lawyers, doctors and others*, London 1983

Donajgrodzki, A. P. (ed.), *Social control in nineteenth-century Britain*, London 1977

Donnison, Jean, *Midwives and medical men: a history of the struggle for the control of childbirth*, London 1977

Dyos, H. J. and D. A. Reeder, 'Slums and suburbs', in H. J. Dyos and M. Wolff (eds), *The Victorian city*, i, London 1973, 359–86

———— *Victorian suburbs: a study of the growth of Camberwell*, Leicester 1967

Earle, Peter, *The making of the English middle class: business, society and family life in London, 1660–1730*, London 1989

Evans, Neil, ' "The first charity in Wales": Cardiff Infirmary and South Wales society, 1837–1914', *Welsh History Review* ix (1978/9), 319–46

———— 'Urbanisation, elite attitudes and philanthropy: Cardiff, 1850–1914', *International Review of Social History* xxvii (1982), 290–323

Eyler, John M., *Victorian social medicine: the ideas and methods of William Farr*, Baltimore 1979

Feinstein, Charles H., *Statistical tables of national income, expenditure and output in the United Kingdom, 1855–1965*, Cambridge 1976

Figlio, K., 'Chlorasis and chronic disease in nineteenth-century Britain: the social construction of somatic illness in a capitalist society', *Social History* iii (1978), 167–97

Finlayson, Geoffrey, *Citizen, state, and social welfare in Britain, 1830–1990*, Oxford 1994

———— 'A moving frontier: voluntarism and the state in British social welfare, 1911–49', *Twentieth Century British History* i (1990), 183–206

Fissell, Mary E., *Patients, power and the poor in eighteenth-century Bristol*, Cambridge 1991

Fitzherbert, L., *Charity and the National Health Service*, London 1989

Foster, John, *Class structure and the industrial revolution: early industrial capitalism in three English towns*, London 1974

Foucault, Michel, *The birth of the clinic: an archaeology of medical perceptions*, trans. A. M. Sheridan, London 1972

———— *Discipline and punishment: the birth of the prison*, London 1979

Freidson, Eliot, *Professional dominance: the social structure of medical care*, New York 1970

―――― *Professional powers: a study of the institutionalisation of formal knowledge*, London 1986

French, Richard D., *Antivivisection and medical science in Victorian society*, Princeton 1975

Garrard, John, *Leadership and power in Victorian industrial towns, 1830–80*, Manchester 1983

Garside, Patricia, 'London and the home counties', in Thompson, *Cambridge social history of Britain*, i. 471–539

Gauldie, Enid, *Cruel habitations: a history of working-class housing*, London 1974

Gelfand, Toby, 'Decline of the ordinary practitioner and the rise of the modern medical profession', in S. Staum and D. E. Larson (eds), *Doctors, patients and society: power and authority in medical care*, Ontario 1981

Gilbert, Alan D., *Religion and society in industrial England: Church, Chapel and social change, 1740–1914*, London 1976

Gore, J. F., *Sydney Holland: Lord Knutsford, a memoir*, London 1936

Gorsky, Martin, *Patterns of philanthropy: charity and society in nineteenth-century Bristol*, Woodbridge 1999

Gourvish, T., 'The rise of the professions', in T. Gourvish and A. O'Day (eds), *Later Victorian Britain*, Basingstoke 1988, 12–35

Granshaw, Lindsay, ' "Fame and fortune by means of bricks and mortar": the medical profession and specialist hospitals in Britain, 1800–1948', in Granshaw and Porter, *The hospital in history*, 199–220

―――― 'The hospital', in Bynum and Porter, *Companion encyclopedia*, ii. 1180–203.

―――― 'Introduction', in Granshaw and Porter, *The hospital in history*, 1–17.

―――― 'Knowledge of bodies or bodies of knowledge?: surgeons, anatomists and rectal surgery, 1830–1985', in Lawrence, *Medical theory, surgical practice*, 232–62

―――― 'The rise of the modern hospital in Britain', in Andrew Wear (ed.), *Medicine in society: historical essays*, Cambridge 1994, 197–218

―――― *St Mark's Hospital, London: a social history of a specialist hospital*, London 1985

―――― ' "Upon this principle I have based a practice": the development of antisepsis in Britain', in Pickstone, *Medical innovation*, 17–46

―――― and Roy Porter (eds), *The hospital in history*, London 1989

Gray, Bernard Kirkman, *A history of English philanthropy: from the dissolution of the monasteries to the taking of the first census*, London 1905

―――― *Philanthropy and the state, or social politics*, London 1908

Haley, Bruce, *The healthy body and the Victorian culture*, Cambridge, Mass. 1978

Hamilton, David, 'The nineteenth-century surgical revolution: antisepsis or better nutrition?', *BHM* lvi (1982), 30–40

Hamilton, [?], *The economical management of an efficient voluntary hospital*, London 1906

Hamlin, Christopher, 'State medicine in Great Britain', in Dorothy Porter (ed.), *The history of public health and the modern state*, Amsterdam 1994, 132–64

Hannah, Leslie, *The rise of the corporate economy*, London 1983

Hardy, Anne, *Epidemic streets: infectious disease and the rise of preventive medicine, 1856–1900*, Oxford 1993

—— 'Tracheotomy versus intubation: surgical intervention in diphtheria in Europe and the United States, 1825–1930', *BHM* lxvi (1992), 536–59

—— 'Urban famine or urban crisis?: typhus in the Victorian city', *Medical History* xxxii (1988), 401–25

Harris, José, 'Political thought and the welfare state, 1870–1940: an intellectual framework for British social policy', *Past and Present* cxxxiv/v (1992), 116–41

—— 'Transition to high politics in English social policy, 1880–1914', in M. Bentley and J. Stevenson (eds), *High and low politics in modern Britain*, Oxford 1983, 58–79

Harrison, Barbara, 'Women and health', in June Purvis (ed.), *Women's history: Britain, 1850–1945*, London 1995, 157–92

Harrison, Brian, *Peaceable kingdom: stability and change in modern Britain*, Oxford 1982

—— 'Philanthropy and the Victorians', *Victorian Studies* ix (1966), 353–74

—— 'Religion and recreation in nineteenth-century England', *Past and Present* xxxviii (1967), 98–125

Hart, H., 'Some notes on the sponsoring of patients for hospital treatment under the voluntary system', *Medical History* xxiv (1980), 447–60

Harte, Negley, *The University of London, 1836–1986*, London 1986

Heasman, Kathleen, *Evangelicals in action: an appraisal of their social work in the Victorian era*, London 1962

Hector, W., *The life of Mrs Bedford Fenwick*, London 1973

Helmstadter, Carole, 'Robert Bentley Todd, Saint John's House, and the origins of the modern trained nurse', *BHM* lxvii (1993), 282–319

Hennock, E. P., 'Poverty and social theory in England: the experience of the eighteen-eighties', *Social History* i (1976), 67–92

Hodgkinson, Ruth G., *The origins of the National Health Service: the medical services of the new poor law, 1834–71*, London 1967

Holcombe, L., *Victorian ladies at work*, Newton Abbot 1973

Hollis, Patricia, *Ladies elect: women in English local government, 1865–1914*, Oxford 1987

Holloway, S. W. F., 'All Saints Sisterhood at University College Hospital, 1862–99', *Medical History* iii (1959), 146–56

—— 'Medical education in England, 1830–1858: a sociological analysis', *History* xlix (1969), 299–324

Holt, R., *Sport and the British: a modern history*, Oxford 1989

Howie, W. B., 'Complaints and complaints procedures in the eighteenth- and early nineteenth-century provincial hospitals in England', *Medical History* xxv (1981), 345–62

Jackson, J. (ed.), *Professions and professionalism*, Cambridge 1970

Jewsbury, Eric C. O., *The Royal Northern Hospital, 1856–1956*, London 1956

Johnson, N., *Reconstructing the welfare state*, Brighton 1990

Johnson, Paul, *Saving and spending: the working-class economy in Britain, 1870–1939*, Oxford 1985

Johnson, T. J., *Professions and power*, London 1972

Jones, Colin, and Roy Porter (eds), *Reassessing Foucault: power, medicine and the body*, London 1994

———— 'Some recent trends in the history of charity', in Daunton, *Charity, self-interest and welfare*, 51–63

Jones, Greta, *Social hygiene in twentieth-century Britain*, London 1986

Jordan, A., *Who cared?: charity in Victorian and Edwardian Belfast*, Belfast 1994

Jordan, Wilbur K., *Philanthropy in England, 1460–1660: a study of the changing pattern of English social aspirations*, London 1959

Kent, J., 'The role of religion in the cultural structure of the late Victorian city', *Transactions of the Royal Historical Society* xxiii (1973), 158–73

Kidd, Alan, J., 'Outcast Manchester: voluntary charity, poor relief and the casual poor, 1860–1905', in Alan J. Kidd and K. W. Roberts (eds), *City, class and culture: studies of social policy and cultural production in Victorian Manchester*, Manchester 1985, 48–73

———— 'Philanthropy and the "social history paradigm"', *Social History* xxi (1996), 180–92

Kilpatrick, R., ' "Living in the light": dispensaries, philanthropy and medical reform in late eighteenth-century London', in Cunningham and French, *Medical enlightenment*, 254–80.

King's Fund, *Enquiry into the management of out-patients departments*, London 1912

Kosky, Jules, *Mutual friends: Charles Dickens and Great Ormond Street Children's Hospital*, London 1989

Kuhn, Thomas, *The structure of scientific revolution*, Chicago 1970

Larkin, Gerald, *Occupational monopoly and modern medicine*, London 1983

Larson, M. S, *The rise of professionalism*, London 1978

Lawrence, Christopher, 'Incommunicable knowledge: science, technology and the clinical art in Britain, 1850–1914', *Journal of Contemporary History* xx (1985), 502–20

———— (ed.), *Medical theory, surgical practice*, London 1992

Lawrence, Susan, *Charitable knowledge: hospital pupils and practitioners in eighteenth-century London*, Cambridge 1996

Le Grand, Julian, David Winter and Francis Woolley, 'The National Health Service: safe in whose hands?', in John Hills (ed.), *The state of welfare: the welfare state in Britain since 1974*, Oxford 1990, 88–134

Lewis, Jane, *The voluntary sector, the state and social work in Britain*, Aldershot 1995

Loudon, Irvine, *Medical care and the general practitioner, 1750–1850*, Oxford 1986

McBriar, A. M., *An Edwardian mixed doubles: the Bosanquets versus the Webbs: a study of British social policy*, Oxford 1987

McKellar, C., *The German Hospital, Hackney: a social and architectural history*, London 1991

McLeod, Hugh, *Class and religion in the late Victorian city*, London 1974

MacLeod, Roy, 'Introduction', in Roy MacLeod (ed.), *Government and expertise: specialists, administrators and professionals, 1860–1919*, Oxford 1988, 1–24

Maggs, Christopher, *A century of change: story of the Royal National Pension Fund for Nurses*, London 1987

———— *The origins of general nursing*, London 1983

Marks, Lara, 'Medical care for pauper mothers and their infants: poor law provision and local demand in East London, 1870–1920', *EcHR* xliii (1993), 518–42

Marland, Hilary, 'Lay and medical conceptions of charity during the nineteenth century', in Barry and Jones, *Medicine and charity*, 149–71

——— *Medicine and society in Wakefield and Huddersfield, 1780–1879*, Cambridge 1987

Martin, Mary Clare, 'Women and philanthropy in Walthamstow and Leyton', *London Journal* xix (1994), 119–50

Martin, R. H., *Evangelicals united: ecumenical stirrings in pre-Victorian Britain, 1795–1830*, London 1983

Meacham, S., 'The evangelical inheritance', *Journal of British Studies* iii (1963/4), 88–104

Medvei, Victor C. and John L. Thornton, *The royal hospital of Saint Bartholomew's, 1123–1973*, London 1974

Meller, Helen E., *Leisure and the changing city, 1879–1914*, London 1976

Merrington, W. R., *University College Hospital and its medical school*, London 1976

Millman, Michael, 'The influence of the Social Sciences Association on hospital planning in Victorian England', *Medical History* xviii (1974), 122–37

Milne, Alan J., *The social philosophy of English idealism*, London 1962

Minney, R. J., *The two pillars of Charing Cross: the story of a famous hospital*, London 1967

Mooney, Graham, Bill Luckin and Andrea Tanner, 'Patient pathways: solving the problems of institutional mortality in London during the late nineteenth century', *SHM* xii (1999), 227–71

Moore, Judith, *A zeal for responsibility: the struggle for professional nursing in Victorian England, 1868–83*, London 1988

Moore, M., 'Social work and social welfare: the organisation of philanthropic resource in Britain, 1900–14', *Journal of British Studies* xvi (1977), 85–104

Morris, E. W., *A history of the London*, London 1926

Morris, Robert J., *Class, sect and party: the making of the British middle class, Leeds, 1820–50*, Manchester 1990

——— 'Clubs, societies and associations', in Thompson, *Cambridge social history of Britain*, iii. 395–443

Mowat, Charles L., *The Charity Organisation Society, 1869–1913*, London 1961

Nead, Lynda, *Myths of sexuality: representations of women in Victorian Britain*, Oxford 1988

Nicholls, Philip A., *Homeopathy and the medical profession*, London 1988

Olsen, Donald J., *The growth of Victorian London*, London 1976

Owen, David E., *English philanthropy, 1660–1960*, Cambridge, Mass. 1964

Panayi, Panikos, *The enemy in our midst: Germans in Britain during the First World War*, New York 1991

Parkin, Frank, *Marxism and class theory: a bourgeois critic*, London 1979

Parry, Noel and José Parry, *The rise of the medical profession: a study of collective social mobility*, London 1976

Pater, J. E., *The making of the National Health Service*, London 1981

Paton, Monica, 'Corporate East End landlords: the example of the London Hospital and the Mercer's Company', *London Journal* xviii (1993), 113–28

Pennington, T. H., 'Listerism, its decline and its persistence: the introduction of aseptic surgical techniques in three British teaching hospitals, 1890–9', *Medical History* xxxix (1995), 35–60

Pennybacker, Susan D., *A vision for London, 1889–1914: labour, everyday life and the LCC experiment*, London 1995

Perkin, Harold, *The rise of professional society: England since 1880*, Princeton 1989

Peterson, M. Jeanne, *The medical profession in mid Victorian London*, Berkeley 1978

Pickstone, John V., *Medicine and industrial society: a history of hospital development in Manchester and its region, 1752–1946*, Manchester 1985

—————— (ed.), *Medical innovation in historical perspective*, New York 1992

Pinker, Robert, *English hospital statistics, 1861–1938*, London 1966

Porter, Roy, 'The gift relationship: philanthropy and provincial hospitals in eighteenth-century England', in Granshaw and Porter, *The hospital in history*, 49–78

—————— *London: a social history*, London 1994

Prochaska, Frank K., 'Charity bazaars in nineteenth-century England', *Journal of British Studies* xvi (1976/7), 62–84

—————— 'Philanthropy', in Thompson, *Cambridge social history of Britain*, iii. 357–94

—————— *Philanthropy and the hospitals of London: the King's Fund, 1897–1990*, Oxford 1992

—————— *Royal bounty: the making of a welfare monarchy*, New Haven 1995

—————— *The voluntary impulse: philanthropy in modern Britain*, London 1988

—————— *Woman and philanthropy in nineteenth-century England*, Oxford 1980

Rafferty, Anne Marie, *The politics of nursing knowledge*, London 1996

Rawcliffe, Carole, 'Hospitals of later medieval London', *Medical History* xxviii (1984), 1–21

Reiser, Stanley J., *Medicine and the reign of technology*, Cambridge 1990

Richter, Melvin, *The politics of conscience: T. H. Green and his age*, London 1964

Risse, Guenter B., *Hospital life in enlightenment Scotland: care and teaching at the Royal Infirmary of Edinburgh*, Cambridge 1986

Rivett, Geoffrey, *The development of the London hospital system, 1832–1982*, London 1986

Roberts, David, *Paternalism in early Victorian England*, London 1979

Roberts, Richard, 'Leasehold estates and municipal enterprise: landowner, local government and the development of Bournemouth', in Cannadine, *Patricians, power and politics*, 175–218

Rooff, Madeleine, *A hundred years of family welfare: a study of the Family Welfare Association (formerly the Charity Organisation Society), 1869–1969*, London 1972

Rosenberg, Charles E., *Care of strangers*, New York 1987

Ross, Ellen, 'Survival networks: women's neighbourhood sharing in London before World War One', *History Workshop* xv (1983), 4–27

Rubin, Miri, 'Development and change in English hospitals, 1100–1500', in Granshaw and Porter, *The hospital in history*, 41–59

Rueschemeyer, D., 'Professional autonomy and the social control of expertise', in Dingwall and Lewis, *Sociology of the professions*, 38–58

Russell, Colin A., *Science and social change, 1770–1900*, London 1983

St Bartholomew's Hospital Medical School Session 1877–79, London 1898/9

Saul, S. B., 'House building in England, 1890–1914', *EcHR* xiii (1962), 119–36

Schmiechen, James, *Sweated industries and sweated labour: the London clothing trade, 1860–1914*, London 1984

Semmel, Bernard, *Imperialism and social reform*, London 1960

Shortt, S. E. D., 'Physicians, science and status: issues in the professionalisation of Anglo-American medicine in the nineteenth century', *Medical History* xxvii (1983), 51–68

Shryock, Richard H., *The development of modern medicine*, London 1948

Simey, Margaret B., *Charitable effort in Liverpool in the nineteenth century*, Liverpool 1951

Slack, Paul, 'Social policy and the constraints of government, 1547–58', in Jennifer Loach and Robert Tittler (eds), *The mid-Tudor polity, c. 1540–60*, London 1980, 94–115

Smalley, G., *The life of Sir Sydney H. Waterlow*, London 1909

Smith, F. B., *Florence Nightingale: reputation and power*, London 1982

———— *The people's health, 1830–1910*, London 1990

Spring, D., *The English landed estate in the nineteenth century: its administration*, Baltimore 1963

Squire Sprigge, Samuel, *Medicine and the public*, London 1905

Stedman Jones, Gareth, *Outcast London: a study of the relationship between classes in Victorian society*, London 1984

Stevens, Rosemary, *Medical practice in modern England: the impact of specialisation and state medicine*, New Haven 1966

———— 'Sweet charity: state aid to hospitals in Pennsylvania, 1870–1910', *BHM* lviii (1984), 474–95

Stourkes, Theodore L., 'John Simon, Robert Lowe, and the origins of state-supported biomedical research in nineteenth-century England', *Journal of the History of Medicine* xlviii (1993), 436–53

Summers, Ann, 'The mysterious demise of Sarah Gamp: the domiciliary nurse and her detractors, c. 1830–60', *Victorian Studies* xxxii (1988/9), 365–86

Tattersall, Robert, 'Frederick Pavy (1829–1911): the last of the physician chemists', *Journal of the Royal College of Physicians of London* xxx (1996), 235–44

Taylor, Jeremy R. B., *Hospital and asylum architecture in England, 1840–1914: buildings for health care*, London 1991

Thane, Pat, 'Government and society in England and Wales 1750–1914', in Thompson, *Cambridge social history of Britain*, iii. 1–62

Thompson, F. M. L., 'The English great estate in the nineteenth century', *Contributions and communications to the first international conference of economic history*, Paris 1960

———— *English landed society in the nineteenth century*, London 1963

———— *Hampstead: building a borough, 1650–1970*, London 1978

———— 'Social control in Victorian England', *EcHR* xxxiv (1981), 189–208

———— (ed.) *The Cambridge social history of Britain, 1750–1950*, I: *Regions and communities*; III: *Social agencies and institutions*, Cambridge 1990

Titmus, Richard, *The gift relationship*, London 1950

Tomlinson, Bernard, *Report of the inquiry into London's health service, medical education and research*, London 1992

Tompson, Richard, *The Charity Commission and the age of reform*, London 1979

Trainor, Richard H., *Black Country elites: the exercise of authority in an industrialised area, 1830–1900*, Oxford 1993

———— 'Peers on an industrial frontier: the earls of Dartmouth and of Dudley in the Black Country, c. 1810–1914', in Cannadine, *Patricians, power and politics*, 69–132

Trueman, B. E. S., 'The purchase and management of Guy's Hospital's estates, 1726–1806', in C. Chalkin and J. R. Wordie (eds), *Town and countryside: the English landowners in the national economy*, London 1989, 52–82

Turner, George, *Unorthodox reminiscences*, London 1931

Vicinus, Martha, *Independent women: work and community for single women*, London 1985

Vincent, Andrew and Raymond Plant, *Philosophy, politics and citizenship: the life and thought of the British idealists*, London 1984

Vogel, Morris J., *The invention of the modern hospital, Boston, 1870–1930*, Chicago 1980

────── and Charles E. Rosenberg, *The therapeutic revolution: essays in the social history of American medicine*, Philadelphia 1979

Wade Martins, S., *A great estate at work: the Holkham estate and its inhabitants in the nineteenth century*, Cambridge 1980

Waddington, Ivan, *The medical profession in the industrial revolution*, Dublin 1984

Waddington, Keir, ' "Bastard benevolence": centralisation, voluntarism and the Sunday Fund, 1873–1898', *London Journal* ix (1995), 151–67

────── ' "Grasping gratitude": hospitals and charity in late Victorian London', in Daunton, *Charity, self-interest and welfare*, 181–202

────── 'The nursing dispute at Guy's Hospital, 1879–80', *SHM* viii (1995), 211–30

────── ' "Unsuitable cases": the debate over out-patient admissions, the medical profession and late Victorian London hospitals', *Medical History* xlii (1998), 26–46

Walkowitz, Judith R., *City of dreadful delight: narratives of sexual danger in late Victorian London*, London 1992

Waller, P. J., *Town, city and nation: England, 1850–1914*, Oxford 1991

Warner, John H., 'Therapeutic explanation and the Edinburgh bloodletting controversy: two perspectives on the medical meaning of science in the mid nineteenth century', *Medical History* xxiv (1980), 241–58

────── *The therapeutic perspective*, Cambridge 1986

Watkins, C. K., *Social control*, London 1975

Weatherall, Mark, 'Making medicine scientific', *SHM* ix (1996), 175–94

Webster, Charles. 'The crisis of the hospital during the industrial revolution', in E. G. Forbes (ed.), *Human implications of scientific advance*, Edinburgh 1978, 214–33

Weiler, Paul, *The new liberalism*, New York 1982

Weinbren, David, 'Against all cruelty: the Humanitarian League, 1891–1919', *History Workshop* xxxviii (1994), 86–105

Weindling, Paul, 'The modernisation of charity in nineteenth-century France and Germany', in Barry and Jones, *Medicine and charity*, 190–206

Weiner, Dora B., *The citizen-patient in revolutionary and imperial Paris*, London 1993

Whitehand, J., 'Building cycles and the spatial pattern of urban growth', *Institute of Geographers (Transactions)* lvi (1972), 39–55

Williams, Guy R., *The age of miracles: medicine and society in the nineteenth century*, London 1981

Williams, Ian, *The alms trade: charities, past, present and future*, London 1989

Wilson, Adrian, 'Politics of medical improvement in early Hanoverian London', in Cunningham and French, *Medical enlightenment*, 4–39

Winter, A., 'Mesmerism and the introduction of inhalation anaesthesia', SHM iv (1991), 1–27

Witz, Anne, *Professions and patriarchy*, London 1992

Wohl, Anthony S., *Endangered lives: public health in Victorian Britain*, London 1983

———— *The eternal slum: housing and social policy in Victorian England*, London 1977

Woodroofe, Kathleen, *From charity to social work in England and the United States*, London 1962

Woodward, John, *To do the sick no harm: a study of the British voluntary hospital system to 1875*, London 1974

Worboys, Michael, 'The sanatorium treatment for consumptives in Britain', in Pickstone, *Medical innovations*, 47–71

Yeo, Stephen, *Religion and voluntary organisation in crisis*, London 1979

Youngson, A., *The scientific revolution in Victorian medicine*, London 1979

Unpublished theses

Barnes, N., 'The Docker's Hospital', unpubl. BSc. diss. London 1993

Berry, Amanda, 'Charity, patronage and medical men: philanthropy and provincial hospitals', unpubl. DPhil. diss. Oxford 1995

Craig, S., 'A survey and study of hospital records and record keeping in London (England) and Ontario (Canada), c. 1850 to c. 1950', unpubl. PhD diss. London 1988

Gorsky, Martin, 'Philanthropy in Bristol, 1800–50', unpubl. PhD diss. Bristol 1995

Granshaw, Lindsay, 'St Thomas's Hospital, London, 1850–1900', unpubl. PhD diss. Bryn Mawr 1981

Humphreys, R., 'Poor law and charity: the Charity Organisation Society in the provinces, 1870–1890', unpubl. PhD diss. London 1991

Morris, Robert J., 'Organisation and aims of the principal secular voluntary organisations of the Leeds middle class, 1830–51', unpubl. DPhil. diss. Oxford 1970

Shapley, P., 'Voluntary charities in nineteenth-century Manchester: organisational structure, social status and leadership', unpubl. PhD diss. Manchester Metropolitan University 1994

Smith, R., 'British nationalism, imperialism and the City of London, 1880–1900', unpubl. PhD diss. London 1985

Index

accounts: and H. Burdett, 217–18; and
Metropolitan Hospital Sunday Fund,
145, 217; uniform, 145, 217–18
acts of parliament: Apothecaries Act
(1815), 10; Finance Act (1922), 215;
Labouring Classes Dwellings House
Act (1866), 54; Medical Act (1858),
162; Medical Amendment Act (1886),
162; Mortmain Act (1736), 39, 40;
National Insurance Act (1911), 74,
214; Road Traffic Act (1930), 215
agricultural depression, 10, 44, 75, 80, 99,
110; and Guy's Hospital, 10, 44, 97,
125–6; impact on hospital income, 10,
75, 80, 123, 125–7; and St Thomas's
Hospital, 10, 75, 80, 125, 126
All Saints nursing sisterhood, 108, 145–6,
198
antivivisection, 127–8, 166; impact on
hospital funding, 127–8; and London
Hospital, 128
appeals, 116, 121, 122, 156, 191, 200; for
Guy's Hospital, 44, 64, 122, 125–6,
177, 200; for Hospital for Sick
Children, 28; for London Hospital,
44–5, 101–2, 108, 122, 156; by Norfolk
and Norwich Hospital, 101; by Royal
Hospital for Diseases of the Chest, 28,
44, 59; use of sympathy in, 28–9;
weariness over, 14, 45
aristocracy: influence of, 149, 151, 206
Aunt Judy Magazine: endowment of beds
by, 40–1
Austin, J., 151, 156, 175–6; attack on
doctors, 175–6

Baly, E., 28
Barber Wright, T., 51
Barclay, C., 27
Barclay, R., 27
Bath Infirmary, 62
bazaars, 14, 47–9, 148; attitudes to, 47–8,
49; at German Hospital, 48, 113; image
of, 49; income from, 49, 113; at
London Hospital, 49; at University
College Hospital, 48–9
Bedford Fenwick, E., 129

beds, 109, 121, 123, 126, 160, 171; closure
of, 45; endowed, 40–1; at Hospital for
Sick Children, 40–1; opposition to
endowed at German Hospital, 41;
paying, 91, 92–5; reopening of, 207–8.
See also Aunt Judy Magazine, H. Burdett
Belfast, 147, 149, 199
Bence Jones, H., 11
benevolence, *see* charity
benevolent economy, 3, 6, 15, 17, 24, 61,
73, 91, 96, 99, 118, 121–4, 147, 205,
208
Bentley, J., 38
bequests, *see* legacies
Bethlem Hospital: fraud at, 156
Birmingham General Hospital, 51, 117
Black Country, 23
Blizzard, W., 208
Board of Health, 215
Bonsor, C., 185
Booth, C., 6, 120
Booth, General, W., 122
Bowlby, A., 169
Bristol: influence of doctors in, 160
Bristol Infirmary, 160, 213
British Association, 209
British and Foreign Bible Society, 50, 53
British Foreign School Society, 59
British Hospital Association, 210
British Medical Association (BMA): and
hospital reform, 127, 206; and medical
influence, 166, 169; and patients, 91,
195; on role of the state, 197, 198
British Medical Journal (BMJ): on
benevolent funds, 73; and Guy's
Hospital, 179, 181, 184, 185; on
hospital funding, 41, 79, 100, 120, 122,
124, 125; on hospital management,
156, 197; and medical influence, 54,
166, 170, 177, 179, 181, 184, 185, 186
British Nurses Association, 129
Brock Lambert, Revd, A., 27
Brodie, B., 159
Brompton Hospital, 79, 113, 151
Burdett, H., 43–4, 62, 110–11, 112, 117,
157, 191; attitudes to state
intervention, 195–6; on a central

243

Printed and bound by CPI Group (UK) Ltd, Croydon, CR0 4YY

09/06/2025

14685776-0003